ANAESTHESIA AND ANALGESIA
IN
DENTISTRY

ANAESTHESIA AND ANALGESIA
IN DENTISTRY

by

RONALD A. GREEN

M.A.(Cantab.), M.B., B.Chir., F.F.A.R.C.S.(Eng.), D.A.
Consulting Anaesthetist, The Royal Free Hospital and St. George's Hospital, London

and

MICHAEL P. COPLANS

M.B., B.S.(Lond.), F.F.A.R.C.S.(Eng.), D.A.
Consulting Anaesthetist, St. George's Hospital and the Royal Dental Hospital

With 166 illustrations.

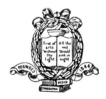

LONDON

H. K. LEWIS & Co. LTD.

1973

First published 1973

©

H. K. LEWIS & Co. Ltd.
1973

I.S.B.N. 0 7186 0394 X

PRINTED AND BOUND IN GREAT BRITAIN
BY HAZELL WATSON AND VINEY LTD, AYLESBURY, BUCKS

PREFACE

It has been our aim in this book to offer both practical and theoretical guidance to all those engaged in the practice of pain relief in dentistry. It has been necessary, therefore, to cater for a wide spectrum of readership, from dental undergraduate to consultant anaesthetist, and many would consider our aim to have been over-ambitious. We hope, however, that selective reading will provide something of value for all, and that consequently, the book will fulfil the need for a complete work of instruction in this important subject. Whilst we have attempted to present a wide range of techniques which should satisfy all the needs of the modern dental anaesthetist, we do not claim that this range is necessarily comprehensive; for only those methods of which we have personal experience are described in detail.

In our coverage of most theoretical concepts, we have assumed that the reader possesses a basic knowledge of physiology and clinical medicine but, in those areas which are of particular relevance to dental anaesthesia, we have discussed the subject matter comprehensively. We have not included references in the text, but at the end of each chapter we have compiled a list of recommended reading which is designed to include the maximum number of important references. The chapter on local anaesthesia, however, adopts the customary full reference technique, in addition to a list of recommended reading.

Although the subject matter discussed in the text is orientated towards dental anaesthesia, it can, nevertheless, be equally applied to other anaesthetic situations, particularly those involving the outpatient. It is therefore, hoped that the book will be of value as a practical manual to all students of anaesthesia.

We are grateful to Mr K. Ray and Dr P. Moore for their contributed chapters on Local Anaesthesia and Maxillo-facial Anaesthesia respectively. We are also grateful to Professor Howe and the dental and nursing staff of the Royal Dental Hospital unit, St George's Hospital, Tooting, for their co-operation; to Mrs Mary Green for typing the manuscripts; to Miss Jo Underhill and the Photographic Department, St George's Hospital, for the bulk of the clinical photographic work; and to Miss Anne Gooch for 'modelling' many of the photographs; to Miss Jenny Middleton for providing all the illustrations; and finally to Claudius Ash, British Oxygen Company, Medical and Industrial Equipment Ltd., McKesson, Virilium Company, Cyprane Ltd., and the Longworth Scientific Instrument Company for their help in providing illustrations of equipment.

January 1973
R.A.G.
M.P.C.

CONTENTS

ANAESTHESIA AND ANALGESIA IN DENTISTRY

CHAPTER ONE

PREOPERATIVE CONSIDERATIONS

The initial assessment of any planned dental treatment involves the practitioner in a decision as to the intended nature of pain relief. He has to decide between local and general anaesthesia, and discuss with his patient the implications of that choice. Thus, preoperative assessment, as carried out by the dental practitioner, demands that he shall acquire sufficient information to enable him to make the following decisions:

A. To make a choice between local and general anaesthesia.
B. To decide where the operation should be performed.
C. To form an opinion as to the probable nature of the general anaesthetic.
D. To prepare the patient adequately, and issue all relevant instructions to him, whatever anaesthetic method is chosen.

These decisions are normally made at a preoperative visit, but under emergency circumstances, the preoperative assessment may have to be made immediately prior to treatment.

A. LOCAL OR GENERAL ANAESTHESIA

Overall Considerations

In all out-patient procedures requiring the provision of pain relief, there should be a bias towards the use of local rather than general anaesthesia for the following reasons:

1. The patient's normal eating and drinking routine need not be disturbed.
2. Adult patients do not necessarily require to be accompanied.
3. Patients are usually able to return to work immediately following completion of treatment.

These advantages, inherent in local anaesthesia, are of course minimized should the operative procedure *per se* demand that the patient be accompanied or forbid his return to work. In addition to these advantages of local anaesthesia for out-patient treatment, there are certain factors of specific relevance to dentistry.

1. The local anaesthetic techniques in common dental use carry a high success rate, involve the use of very small quantities of local anaesthetic solution, and are generally acceptable to a high proportion of patients.

A.A.D.—1*

2. The use of general anaesthesia in dentistry is characterized by difficulties inherent in the necessity for anaesthetist and operator to share the patient's upper airway.
3. The majority of dental procedures do not involve the patient in post-treatment loss of work, and it is thus desirable that the anaesthetic technique should not do so either.
4. In terms of professional man-power, economy and overall organization, local anaesthesia is superior to general under most routine circumstances.
5. The information relating to comparative morbidity is scanty, but the mortality rate associated with general anaesthesia, although small, is significantly higher than that associated with the use of 'local'.

It will be seen from the foregoing, that the authors believe that most of the inherent advantages in dentistry lie with local anaesthesia and that general anaesthesia should be preferred only in the presence of a valid indication. In very broad terms, the indications for general anaesthesia are as follows:

1. Acute inflammatory lesions requiring surgical intervention, where local anaesthesia is both likely to prove ineffective and to increase the risk of the spread of infection.
2. Multiple quadrant work which would entail excessive discomfort to the patient, and where the use of general anaesthesia enables the practitioner to complete his work at one sitting, without accepting the disadvantage of bilateral inferior dental block, or other multiple injections. This is of particular importance when dental treatment has to be covered by chemotherapy, as in heart disease, since it avoids exposure to repeated episodes of bacteraemia and the risk of the development of penicillin-resistance.
3. A history of adverse reactions to local anaesthesia such as:

  (i) Failure to achieve adequate anaesthesia.
 (ii) Allergy or sensitivity to the 'local' or adrenaline.
(iii) Repeated fainting following intraoral injections.
(iv) Distressing postinjection symptoms, including dry socket.

4. Inability of the patient to tolerate dental treatment whilst conscious. This may be associated with mental disorder, neurological illness characterized by involuntary motor activity, or emotional instability.
5. Haemophilia (see page 296).

Specific Considerations

Certain additional specific features have a direct bearing upon the choice of anaesthetic method, and indeed upon the overall management of the case in all its aspects. It is convenient to consider these specific features under three separate headings, namely disease, drugs and pregnancy.

1. **Disease**
(a) **Cardiovascular Disease.**—The presence of cardiovascular disease will be suggested by a history of the patient having suffered from one of the following complaints.

(i) Congenital heart disease which may have been corrected by operative treatment.
(ii) Valvular disease, which is usually the result of rheumatic fever, Sydenham's chorea (St Vitus's Dance), or occasionally scarlet fever.
(iii) Coronary infarction, normally characterized by cardiac pain and collapse; or attacks of anginal pain indicating some degree of coronary insufficiency.
(iv) Other disorders of the circulatory system, such as high blood pressure.

The patient may either present with symptoms of cardiac decompensation, or the cardiovascular illness may be purely a matter of historical record, the patient being symptom-free. This latter situation is sometimes an indication for the use of general anaesthesia, which will enable multiquadrant extractions to be performed at one sitting. Antibiotic cover prior to dental treatment is essential (page 274). Cardiac illness in which there is a degree of impairment of function will also influence the choice of anaesthetic technique. Broad assessment of the situation may be made with an elementary but sound knowledge of the signs and symptoms associated with cardiac dysfunction. Dyspnoea is probably the most reliable guide; if present at rest or on mild exertion it indicates a serious degree of decompensation, as does also orthopnoea (shortness of breath on lying flat). Anginal pain is indicative of coronary insufficiency. Congestion of neck veins, oedema of the ankles, palpable liver and abnormalities in pulse rate or rhythm are amongst the readily discernible clinical signs of serious disease. Whenever the dental practitioner suspects that cardiac dysfunction exists, he should delay active dental treatment until a fuller assessment has been made, and the appropriate treatment instituted.

When the patient's cardiac condition is unlikely to benefit further from treatment and dental extraction is considered necessary, the choice between local and general anaesthesia has to be made. It is a difficult choice, requiring considerable experience. Under no circumstances should general anaesthesia be selected in the absence of an experienced, medically qualified anaesthetist. Given, however, that the services of such an anaesthetist are available, general anaesthesia has much to recommend it. The avoidance of fear and tension is extremely important in the management of cardiac patients, and general anaesthesia with smooth intravenous induction is frequently the best way of achieving this aim. Moreover, the use of local anaesthesia carries with it the problems associated with exogenous adrenaline administration (page 306). Careful intravenous induction with 1% methohexitone (Brietal, Brevital) and maintenance with inhalation agents incorporating a high oxygen content often constitutes the safest method for the cardiac case. The pulse must be continuously palpated during the induction and meticulous attention given to the patency of the airway. Such cases are liable to develop cardiac dysrhythmias in response to dental stimulation under light general anaesthesia, and therefore it may be judged advisable to infiltrate the operation site with adrenaline-free 'local', when general anaesthesia is maintained at a light level. Patients suffering from aortic valvular incompetence present a special hazard during the induction of general anaesthesia, since even the most careful intravenous administration may lower the already reduced diastolic blood pressure sufficiently to imperil the coronary circulation. A history of recent coronary infarction or 'stroke' in any patient is a powerful reason for delaying treatment, if such delay is possible; the administration of a general anaesthetic to such a patient carries with it the obligation for all concerned to consider very carefully any possible clinical and legal sequelae.

Initial experience with the use of intravenous diazepam (Valium) and 'local' in the nervous dental patient suggests that this technique may be of considerable value in the cardiac case, thus avoiding some of the hazards of general anaesthesia and minimizing the harmful effects of anxiety so often associated with unsupplemented 'local'.

The detailed management of dental patients suffering from cardiovascular disease is dealt with on page 274.

(b) **Respiratory Disease.**—In many respiratory disorders, excess secretions are a prominent feature of the illness, and in these cases general anaesthesia is often stormy and characterized by bouts of coughing, laryngeal stridor and bronchospasm. Intubation may prove the only way of gaining satisfactory control over the airway, and local anaesthesia should thus be preferred whenever possible. The conditions commonly associated with these difficulties are:—coryza, sinusitis, 'smoker's cough', bronchiectasis, bronchitis and emphysema. Asthmatics usually tolerate general anaesthesia well, but the anaesthetist must be capable of dealing with a severe attack of bronchospasm should it occur. Where long-standing or old respiratory disease has resulted in impairment of respiratory function without excess secretions, general anaesthesia is not contraindicated. It must, however, be remembered that the patient may require artificial respiratory assistance as a result of drug depression of the respiratory centre, or simply as a consequence of inability to use the accessory muscles of respiration whilst unconscious.

Ludwig's Angina (pages 143, 185, 282).—This condition is characterized by the spread of inflammatory oedema beyond the confines of the jaw, affecting the tissues of the neck, pharynx or larynx. It results in impairment of swallowing and/or breathing accompanied by trismus, and *on no account should an intravenous anaesthetic be given*. If a general anaesthetic is absolutely essential—as it occasionally is—this should always be administered in hospital by an experienced medical anaesthetist, in the presence of a surgeon capable of performing rapid tracheostomy. Indeed, preanaesthetic tracheostomy under local anaesthesia may be indicated in severe cases.

For detailed anaesthetic management of serious respiratory disease see page 280.

(c) **Metabolic Disorders**
Diabetes.—Diabetics may attend for dental treatment either as emergency or as planned cases.

(i) *Emergency Cases*

Acute inflammatory lesions—to which diabetics are particularly susceptible—often throw the diabetes temporarily out of control. Should urine testing or any other sign or symptom suggest that this has occurred, the patient should be admitted to hospital, where the diabetic state can be closely controlled before, during and after surgical treatment, irrespective of whether local or general anaesthesia is administered.

(ii) *Planned Cases*

Whenever possible local anaesthesia should be used in a controlled diabetic, since this method of treatment does not involve any alteration in eating habits, and therefore does not interfere with the diabetic stability. General anaesthesia on other grounds may prove desirable and the detailed management is described on page 287.

Thyroid Disease.—Uncontrolled thyrotoxicosis is rarely encountered nowadays, but it should be remembered that hyperthyroidism may result in hypersensitivity to catecholamines. Thus, local anaesthetic solution containing adrenaline or nor-adrenaline is best avoided. For this reason general anaesthesia may be preferred, but assessment of the cardiovascular state is of paramount importance. Any evidence suggestive of auricular fibrillation or other major circulatory disturbance will demand further investigation prior to general anaesthesia. Should the clinical history, the physical examination, or the x-ray evidence suggest tracheal compression or any other form of airway obstruction, general anaesthesia is strictly contraindicated unless supervised by an experienced physician anaesthetist in hospital. If local anaesthesia appears to be more appropriate, prilocaine with felypressin is the agent of choice (page 312).

(d) **Gastro-Intestinal Disorders.**—The increased risk of vomiting or regurgitation of stomach contents must always be borne in mind in cases of pyloric stenosis, hiatus hernia, pharyngeal pouch and oesophageal obstruction. Local anaesthesia should be selected whenever possible. If general anaesthesia proves necessary, it must be remembered that the risk of regurgitation (pharyngeal pouch, hiatus hernia) is considerably increased in the supine posture, which should be avoided (page 179). Undiagnosed hiatus hernia must be suspected when there is a history of heartburn or regurgitation on lying flat, and is more common in obese subjects.

(e) **Epilepsy.**—Whilst epilepsy is the most common cause of 'fits', it should be stressed that patients will sometimes describe 'black-outs' as 'fits'. 'Black-outs' may not only be due to the *Petit Mal* of epilepsy but also to congenital heart disease associated with Stokes-Adams attacks, and in particular the cardiomyopathies, which carry a serious anaesthetic risk. Epilepsy, however, does not constitute a contraindication to general anaesthesia, but a quiet induction and meticulous avoidance of hypoxia are essential. The barbiturates are used in the control of epilepsy, and intravenous thiopentone (Pentothal) holds a time honoured place in the treatment of *status epilepticus*, and can thus be considered the induction agent of choice. Methohexitone, with its motor excitatory tendencies, should be avoided. If rapid recovery from anaesthesia is especially desirable, propanidid (Epontol) or Althesin should be used.

When local anaesthesia is chosen, it may with benefit be accompanied by diazepam Valium), given either orally or intravenously.

The patient may be receiving routine treatment with one or more of the following drugs: phenobarbitone or methylphenobarbitone, phenytoin sodium (Epanutin), primidone (Mysoline), diazepam; even this list is not comprehensive. In general, established treatment should not be disturbed. It must be remembered that epileptic patients on large doses of phenytoin depend upon active hydroxylation by the liver to avoid toxic effects. Thus, any anaesthetic such as trichlorethylene or halothane, particularly when associated with hypoxaemia, may disturb liver function and result in phenytoin poisoning, with consequent delay in recovery, pyrexia and coma.

The management of epileptic fits is described on page 290.

(f) Blood Disorders

(i) *Anaemia.*—In simple hypochromic iron-deficiency anaemia, general anaesthesia is not contraindicated, but whenever possible the anaemia should be corrected prior to dental treatment. Anaemic patients generally require lower doses of all anaesthetic agents than do normal patients, and in view of the reduced oxygen-carrying capacity of the blood, the anaesthetic technique should incorporate liberal oxygenation. The same principles apply to patients with hyperchromic pernicious anaemia.

(ii) *Thalassaemia.*—This condition is a genetically determined blood dyscrasia in which there is a suppression of normal haemoglobin A, resulting in severe hypochromic anaemia. For reasons discussed on page 283, general anaesthesia should be avoided.

(iii) *Sickle-cell Disease.*—Sickle-cell disease is a chronic, familial haemolytic anaemia which is usually found in the negro race. For reasons discussed on page 283, general anaesthesia should be avoided whenever possible.

(iv) *Haemophilia.*—Owing to the special hazard of excessive bleeding from any injection site, local anaesthesia is contraindicated. Full management of these cases is discussed on page 285.

(v) *Polycythaemia Rubra Vera.*—Patients suffering from polycythaemia have a raised haemoglobin, increased viscosity of the blood and high blood pressure, and therefore, general anaesthesia is best avoided, but not strictly contraindicated (page 287).

(g) Renal and Hepatic Dysfunction (page 288).—For broad guidance, it may be prudent to avoid general anaesthesia on the grounds of interference with drug detoxification and elimination; the possible hepatotoxic actions of certain anaesthetic agents (e.g. halothane) must also be borne in mind (page 107). In expert hands, general anaesthesia is permissible.

(h) Porphyria.—Porphyria is a congenital metabolic defect characterized by the passage of red or brown urine, and an absolute and often fatal intolerance to barbiturates together with some degree of sensitivity to many other drugs. The disease may be either European or South African in origin. Propanidid and Althesin are tolerated normally, but general anaesthesia should be avoided if possible, and only undertaken in hospital (pages 26 and 287).

(i) Skeletal and Neurological Disease.—When gross deformity, spasm or involuntary movement seriously impede access to the operation site, a general anaesthetic may be essential.

(j) **Travel Sickness.**—Patients who suffer from travel sickness almost invariably experience some degree of nausea or vomiting during recovery from general anaesthesia. This may be controlled by administering their usual 'cure' $1\frac{1}{2}$ hours prior to the administration of an anaesthetic (page 39). Local anaesthesia is preferable whenever possible.

2. Drugs

Many drugs used in medical practice affect the course of both general and local anaesthesia, and influence the choice of anaesthetic technique selected. It is vital that the anaesthetist should be fully informed of *all* drugs that the patient is taking, and aware of the significance of these drugs in relation to the proposed anaesthetic. The problem of drug interaction is likely to worsen so long as the output of new drugs continues to outstrip the pharmacological and clinical knowledge of the anaesthetist. It is hard enough for the full-time specialist anaesthetist to keep up to date in this complex field, in spite of his ready access to the opinions of colleagues in other spheres of medicine and his own widely-based training; it would therefore seem wise for the dental practitioner, in his position of relative isolation, to restrict his anaesthetic practice to those cases not in receipt of drug therapy, unless he is certain that the drug concerned is devoid of potentially dangerous interactions or side effects.

The following is a brief account of those drugs which are most likely to demand the dental anaesthetist's special attention.

Antidepressant Drugs

(a) **Mono Amine Oxidase Inhibitors** (M.A.O.I. Drugs) Table I.—These drugs are used in the treatment of exogenous or reactive depression, and patients receiving treatment, although often uncommunicative, will usually admit to having been forbidden to eat cheese and other tyramine-containing foods. Treatment with M.A.O.I.s carries significant consequences where anaesthesia and analgesia for dental practice are concerned, as a number of drugs which may be used show dangerous interactions.

TABLE I.—*Monoamine Oxidase Inhibitors*

Approved or Chemical Name	Trade Name
Mebanazine	Actomol (I.C.I.)
Etryptamine	Monase (Upjohn)
Iproniazid	Marsilid (Roche)
Isocarboxazid	Marplan (Roche)
Nialamide	Niamid (Pfizer)
Pargyline	Eutonyl (Abbott)
Pivazin, Pivazide	Tersavid (Roche)
Phenelzine	Nardil (Warner)
Pheniprazine	Catron, Cavodil (Benger)
Phenoxypropazine	Drazin (Smith & Nephew)
Tranylcypromine	Parnate (S.K.F.)
Tranylcypromine + Trifluoperazine (Stelazine)	Parsteline (S.K.F.)

Drugs which are absolutely contraindicated

 (i) Pressor amines such as amphetamine and mephenteramine.
 (ii) Nasal decongestants, such as ephedrine and phenylephrine. These are sometimes recommended for use prior to nasal intubation.
(iii) Ephedrine by injection which may be used for the treatment of bronchospasm and asthma.

   In the presence of M.A.O.I.s these drugs may produce dangerous hypertension. It should be noted that the amphetamines and ephedrine are themselves M.A.O.I.s, hence their vasopressor activity; however, their action in this respect is very weak and in therapeutic doses leaves intact sufficient enzyme activity to obviate the necessity for special precaution when used in combination with other drugs and foodstuffs.

Drugs contraindicated except in special circumstances

 (i) Pethidine, especially when used intravenously as in the Jorgensen technique, is contra-indicated. Respiratory depression, hypotension and coma may occur. This is due to inhibition of the liver enzyme which metabolizes pethidine. Under special circumstances intramuscular pethidine may be justified in reduced dosage.
(ii) Morphine, codeine and other narcotic analgesics have been claimed to cause interaction, but the evidence is less convincing.

Drugs where special care is required

   As a general principle, any drug normally metabolized in the liver might be potentiated by M.A.O.I.s. These will include the long acting barbiturates, tranquillizers (diazepam) and the phenothiazines. These drugs should therefore be used in reduced dosage. When used intravenously in a single induction dose, the barbiturates should be used with caution but are unlikely to be potentiated.

   Whenever possible, treatment for patients on M.A.O.I.s should be delayed until the drug has been withheld for at least 3 weeks. If this is not possible, local anaesthesia should be preferred. There is no contraindication to the inclusion of adrenaline and noradrenaline in the local anaesthetic solution, since these substances are destroyed in the body, not by monoamine oxidase but by catechol-o-methyl transferase.

   If general anaesthesia proves essential, inhalational methods are preferred by many anaesthetists, but both methohexitone and propanidid have been used successfully on many occasions.

Treatment of Interactions.—A hypertensive reaction must be reversed by an alpha-adrenergic blocking agent. Phentolamine Mesylate (Rogitine) 5 mg intravenously is the drug of choice. The ganglionic blocking agents are ineffective. Other interactions must be treated symptomatically.

(b) **Tricyclic Antidepressants.**—This group of drugs, of which imipramine (Tofranil) and amitriptyline (Triptizol) are the most popular, are used in the treatment of endogenous depression. They produce increased sensitivity to noradrenaline and adrenaline, but not to felypressin (Octapressin). There is no contraindication to general anaesthesia.

Corticosteroids

Prolonged steroid therapy may result in suprarenal suppression giving rise to inability to tolerate 'stress'. Operative procedures, whether undertaken under general or local anaesthesia, provide such a stress stimulus, and when performed upon patients not receiving, but who have received steroid therapy within the past 2 months, should be covered by an appropriate course of steroid treatment. Table II shows the commonly used steroid preparations with their equivalent doses. General anaesthesia in the dental out-patient is best avoided.

TABLE II.—*Steroid Preparations*

Steroid	*Comparable Dosage*
Cortisone	100 mg
Hydrocortisone	80 mg
Prednisolone	20 mg
Prednisone	20 mg
Betamethasone (Betnelan)	3 mg

The preparation suitable for direct intravenous injection in emergency is hydrocortisone hemi-succinate (Efcortesol).

It is advantageous for the anaesthetist to know those medical conditions for which steroid therapy is most likely to be administered, so that in his history taking he will be alerted to this possibility. The majority of patients being so treated will carry a special card. Below is a list of the most important of these diseases.

1. **Adrenal Insufficiency**

   (a) Addison's disease
   (b) Hypopituitarism

2. **Skin Conditions**

   (a) Exfoliative dermatitis
   (b) Pemphigus
   (c) Lupus erythematosus
   (d) Eczema

3. **Blood Disorders**

   (a) Acute lymphatic leukaemia
   (b) Haemolytic anaemias
   (c) Thrombocytopoenic purpura
   (d) Agranulocytosis

4. **Sensitivity and Allergic Diseases**

   (a) Asthma
   (b) Severe nasal allergy (hay-fever) and other acute sensitivity reactions

5. **Collagen Diseases and Degenerative Diseases**

    (a) Rheumatic fever
    (b) Rheumatoid arthritis
    (c) Polyarteritis nodosa
    (d) Scleroderma
    (e) Polymyositis
    (f) Ankylosing spondylitis
    (g) Ulcerative colitis
    (h) Regional ileitis (Crohn's disease)

6. **Miscellaneous**

    (a) Aphthous ulcers of mouth
    (b) Acute polyneuritis
    (c) Certain types of acute cardiac failure

For a full discussion of the significance of steroid therapy in anaesthesia see page 290.

Hypotensive Agents

Many hypertensive patients are in receipt of drugs which lower the blood pressure. Mild hypertension may be adequately controlled by simple sedatives, but in severe cases the blood pressure may have to be controlled by specific hypotensive drugs. Patients in receipt of these drugs are prone to suffer sudden changes in blood pressure in relation to both general anaesthesia and posture. Dental procedures should be carried out under local anaesthesia with the patient in a comfortable reclining position with legs raised. Should general anaesthesia prove necessary, all drugs known to be capable of producing hypotension (e.g. intravenous barbiturates, halothane) must be administered cautiously. The subject is fully discussed on page 292.

Table III lists the main drugs used in the routine treatment of hypertension.

Anticoagulants

Patients on anticoagulant therapy generally require hospitalization from both the medical and surgical point of view. There is no particular contraindication to general anaesthesia, but the use of local anaesthesia, as in haemophilia, constitutes a special risk owing to the dangers associated with excessive haemorrhage into soft tissues (page 296).

Alkalis

Patients being treated with large doses of alkalis (e.g. for duodenal ulcer) may develop temporary alkalosis following a bout of hyperventilation. Transient tetany may sometimes be exhibited.

TABLE III.—*Hypotensive Agents*

Group	Approved Name	Trade Name
Anti-adrenergic agents	Guanethidine	Ismelin
	Bethanidine	Esbatal
	Guanoxan	Envacar
	Debrisoquine	Declinax
Methyldopa	Methyldopa	Aldomet
Rauwolfia	Reserpine	Serpasil
Ganglion-blocking agents	Hexamethonium	Vegolysen
	Pempidine	Perolysen
	Mecamylamine	Inversine
Alpha-adrenergic blocking agents	Phenoxybenzamine	Dibenyline
	Phentolamine	Rogitine
Beta-adrenergic blocking agents	Propranolol	Inderal
	Practolol	Eraldin
Thiazides	Hydrochlorothiazide	Hydrosaluric
		Direma
		Esidrex
	Chloroithiazide	Saluric
	Chlorthalidone	Hygroton
Hydrallazine	Hydrallazine	Apresoline

The 'Pill'

Sensitivity to suxamethonium in patients taking the contraceptive pill, is a theoretical possibility in view of the reduction in cholinesterase observed in these patients. There is also an interference with pethidine breakdown, an increased quantity of the drug being excreted unchanged in the urine. There is no valid pharmacological or clinical evidence of adverse reactions between the 'Pill' and methohexitone or any other intravenous anaesthetic agent.

Drugs of Addiction

The combination of drug addiction (particularly heroin) and dental sepsis is well recognized, but many of these patients will not seek or accept dental treatment, particularly under local anaesthesia.

Addiction to stimulants such as amphetamine leads to apparent 'resistance' to general anaesthetic drugs—probably due to the raised level of cerebral activity. Instability of blood pressure may also require special attention. Heroin, morphine and pethidine addicts are generally excitable and very resistant to inhalation methods when they are deprived of their drugs. When allowed to 'premedicate' themselves, they become tranquil, cooperative patients. There is apparently no development of cross tolerance to barbiturates, which can be administered in normal dosage, but inability to perform venipuncture may be an insuperable difficulty in ex-'main-liners' who have succeeded in thrombosing all their superficial veins. Paradoxically, many heroin addicts have an aversion to 'the needle' and insist upon inhalation induction, although the true reason for this preference may be simply the desire for a new 'experience', or even an unwillingness to sacrifice their veins for inessential purposes!

Alcoholics are notoriously anaesthetic resistant—particularly to inhalation induction. 'Self-premedication' is often helpful, but beer, because of its bulk and slow absorption, must be avoided.

Patients addicted to large doses of the barbiturates develop 'tolerance' (page 27) and one might therefore expect them to be unduly resistant to barbiturate anaesthetic agents. In practice, however, we find that normal induction doses of the intravenous barbiturates suffice. This observation can be explained by the fact that the total anaesthetic effect of these drugs is dependant almost entirely on redistribution rather than metabolic breakdown (page 183). It would, however, be reasonable to expect complete recovery from such an induction agent to be accelerated.

3. Pregnancy

All surgical procedures—particularly if performed under light general anaesthesia—should be avoided in the first 12 weeks of pregnancy. The risk of abortion during this period as a consequence of operative stimulation may be theoretical rather than real, but should such an abortion occur spontaneously and fortuitously, the operative stimulus will almost certainly be cited as having been causative. In the final weeks of pregnancy, the increased intra-abdominal pressure predisposes to respiratory embarrassment and gastric regurgitation, so that general anaesthesia must be undertaken with care, and the supine posture avoided (page 165). There is also some risk—possibly only theoretical—of inducing premature labour.

Between 12 weeks and 30 weeks, there is no contraindication to general anaesthesia, which should be tranquil and adequate in depth to obtund reflex response to painful stimulation; pregnant women require some increase in dosage of all anaesthetic drugs, owing to their increased blood-volume. Liberal oxygenation is indicated.

During the early weeks of pregnancy it is not permissible to administer any drug, unless it has been established that it is free from ill-effects on the foetus; particular care should be taken in respect of the tranquillizing agents.

B. CHOICE OF LOCATION FOR OPERATION

It should be appreciated by the dental anaesthetist that, when working in the limited environment of a dental surgery (office) or a school clinic, he carries far more individual responsibility than when working in a well equipped hospital operating theatre. He may have no skilled assistant to double-check his apparatus and drugs, and help him in an emergency. For this reason, the anaesthetist working in the isolation of a dental surgery should be at least as experienced as his counterpart in hospital practice. There is, of course, no level of experience which justifies either dentist or doctor acting as both operator and anaesthetist. However trivial the nature of the operation, general anaesthesia can never be regarded as a minor procedure, requiring anything less than the undivided attention of one professional practitioner.

The scope of anaesthesia will not necessarily be the same in a private dental surgery or school clinic as in a fully equipped hospital operating theatre; thus, the choice of anaesthetic and the type of dentistry to be undertaken will be governed by the general facilities available, and these will be described under three headings.

1. Dental Surgery (office) or School Clinic

Many dental surgeries and clinics today are adequately equipped to satisfy the demands of modern dental anaesthesia, in which case they may be considered as equivalent to hospital out-patient clinics. Some, however, are only equipped for the simplest dental procedure under general anaesthesia. The following minimum basic equipment and personnel are obligatory.

(i) An apparatus for administering oxygen, with equipment for inflation of the patient's lungs under pressure. This is usually automatically provided by the standard anaesthetic machine (page 51). It must be stressed that every machine should contain a reservoir bag, as this is the only wholly satisfactory manual method of inflating the lungs. Such a machine will also provide a supply of anaesthetic gases and vapours which will greatly widen the scope of work which can be undertaken.

(ii) An adequate supply of spare oxygen or some means of inflating the lungs with air (page 155).

(iii) A fully reclining dental chair, the mechanism of which will enable rapid lowering of the patient's body from the sitting to the horizontal position (page 71). In addition to the operating chair, it is desirable to have either a recovery couch or at least a second dental chair which can be fully reclined. These facilities will avoid blocking the main surgery from further use whilst also providing adequate recovery time for the patient.

(iv) An efficient suction apparatus which can be either of the high vacuum or high velocity type; the saliva ejector is not considered an adequate substitute (page 74).

(v) In addition to the routine dental equipment, props, gags and packs are essential (page 80).

(vi) An operator, an anaesthetist, and a nurse in attendance.

2. Hospital Out-patient Department and Fully Equipped Dental Surgery

Under this heading it is assumed that all required equipment for anaesthesia and resuscitation is available and that recovery facilities and nursing care are adequate.

In addition to the basic equipment mentioned in the last section, this clinic should have:

(i) Recovery beds or couches where patients can remain under supervision for as long as is required.

(ii) All the necessary equipment required for endotracheal intubation and full resuscitation.

(iii) A suitable room for full preoperative examination of the patient.

With these facilities, the majority of dental operations not involving excessive tissue trauma can be carried out, and prolonged anaesthesia can prove safe and practical, provided there are no indications for preoperative rest or sedation, or special postoperative care.

3. Hospital In-patients

The decision to admit a patient to hospital for dental treatment will almost certainly depend upon one or more of the following three reasons.

  (i) The degree of tissue trauma resulting from the operation is likely to necessitate pro-
      longed rest and nursing after-care.
 (ii) The physical condition of the patient is such that a period of either preoperative or
      postoperative special nursing or medical care is indicated.
(iii) The home conditions are unsuitable for the operation to be undertaken as an out-
      patient.

There are occasionally anaesthetic considerations (page 254) which make it
desirable to admit a patient for dental treatment. If the patient is admitted and can
stay for at least 24 hours, the anaesthetist has a wider scope in his choice of anaesthetic method. The patient can be suitably and adequately premedicated, a deeper
plane of anaesthesia can be maintained throughout, and adequate postoperative
sedation and rest assured.

C. NATURE OF ANAESTHETIC

The following brief summary will serve to remind the dental practitioner, in his
initial assessment of the case, of some of the features of any intended general
anaesthetic.

Induction of anaesthesia may be inhalational or intravenous. Intravenous induction may delay recovery in the short case, but if methohexitone or propanidid is used
in optimal dosage, recovery is rapid and does not demand elaborate facilities.
Inhalation induction with nitrous oxide and oxygen, supplemented with halothane or
trichlorethylene, is often the method of choice with children who either do not want
an injection or have poor veins. The intravenous route for induction is usually
preferred by adults and there is every reason for the experienced anaesthetist to comply
with these wishes, provided there are no specific contraindications. Many simple
extractions can be carried out under a single dose of methohexitone or propanidid,
but reliance should not be placed on this. Inhalation agents should always be available
for maintenance of anaesthesia in case the operation takes longer than expected, or
good operating conditions prove unobtainable with the unsupplemented intravenous
agent—even when intermittent administration has been selected as the method of
choice.

Maintenance of anaesthesia with nitrous oxide, oxygen and halothane through a
nasal mask is the method of choice in the majority of patients, owing to the smooth
and controllable anaesthesia that can be achieved. Maintenance with nitrous oxide,
oxygen and Trilene will give good conditions at a much lower cost, but the establishment of stable anaesthesia may prove more difficult, the recovery slightly longer, and
the incidence of post-anaesthetic sequelae greater. The use of intermittent injections
of methohexitone and propanidid is sometimes advocated for the maintenance of
anaesthesia for exodontia. This method has certain advantages but in normal
circumstances inhalation maintenance is the method of choice (page 211).

The essential requisite of anaesthesia in the ordinary dental surgery, apart from
the production of safe and satisfactory operating conditions, is a rapid recovery so
that the patient can go home accompanied, within half an hour of completing treat-

ment. Although the duration of the anaesthetic, and the nature of the agents used, will influence the rate of recovery, the practitioner must ensure that the patient fully understands and accepts the inevitable restrictions involved following any general anaesthetic.

D. PREPARATION OF THE OUT-PATIENT FOR GENERAL ANAESTHESIA

1. Preoperative Visit

General assessment of the patient should, whenever possible, be made at the patient's preoperative visit to the surgery. All relevant advice and instructions can be given at the same time.

(i) *Food and Drink*

A full stomach constitutes a serious risk in general anaesthesia, because vomited stomach contents may be inhaled into the lungs under conditions in which either the patient's voluntary protective actions, or his involuntary protective reflexes, are impaired. There is no arbitrary starvation time which can guarantee an empty stomach under all circumstances, and common sense must be the chief guide. Injured, shocked, ill, pregnant or nervous patients have delayed stomach emptying. A non-milk drink will usually leave the stomach rapidly, a heavy meal slowly. Thus all rules must be sufficiently flexible to fit the circumstances of the case. Prolonged pre-anaesthetic starvation is usually unnecessary and may be harmful, especially in small children who develop hypoglycaemia and dehydration very readily, particularly in hot weather. If, therefore, a rigid routine of at least 6 hours starvation is observed, this may well lead to deprivation of all solids and fluids for some 18 hours, the child not having been allowed to eat or drink from 6 p.m. until midday the following day. The practitioner must make it quite clear to parents that such a situation is not intended. Moreover prolonged starvation—especially in a nervous patient—will often result in an accumulation in the stomach of resting gastric juice which, if vomited and inhaled, may prove more injurious than stomach contents diluted with a small quantity of bland fluid. A heavy meal should not be taken on the day of a proposed anaesthetic, nor the previous night if that anaesthetic is administered in the morning. A light snack (e.g. cup of sweet tea and a biscuit) may be allowed up to 3 hours preoperatively; a few sips of water up to $1\frac{1}{2}$ hours, thus rendering oral premedication permissible. If a heavy meal has been eaten and the anaesthetic cannot be postponed until the following day, 6 or 8 hours delay is advised. Large quantities of beer taken within 2 hours are notoriously associated with vomiting under anaesthesia. Simple commonsense instructions based upon these principles can easily be devised, but no set of rules guarantees an empty stomach under all circumstances.

(ii) *Escorts, Driving and Work*

Every patient who receives a general anaesthetic must be accompanied. Likewise, such patients should not drive vehicles—motor or otherwise propelled—or 'ride pillion'. Work, particularly that involving potentially dangerous machinery or demanding mental acuity and judgement, should be avoided.

These restrictions apply for the remainder of the day on which the anaesthetic has been administered, and all patients must be fully aware of them before treatment is arranged.

(iii) *Consent*

It is not customary to obtain special written permission to administer a general anaesthetic in dental practice, but it is very important to ensure that the parent or guardian of a minor approves any proposed procedure.

If written instructions are issued to patients on the preoperative visit, which we strongly recommend, then this card may be used as a consent form and signed by the patient or parent. (Table IV).

(iv) *Practical Technique of Preoperative Assessment*

This clinical assessment is best made at the preoperative visit, and it is necessary to devise a simple routine of examination and questioning, which will focus attention on significant factors without involving patient and practitioner in a lengthy and largely irrelevant discussion. The full implications of a limited physical examination are discussed on page 257.

(a) *Examination and Observation*

Pallor—generalized, indicating fear or possibly anaemia
   —of conjunctivae and mucous-membranes, indicating anaemia
Dyspnoea
Cyanosis
Oedema
Cough
Nicotine stains
Clubbing of fingers
Pulse rate and rhythm
Congestion of neck veins
Race—(n.b. sickle-cell disease and porphyria)
Smell of alcohol, or puncture marks of drug addiction.
General build.

(b) *Questioning*

Have you had an anaesthetic (or 'gas') before?
Are you quite fit?
Are you attending your doctor for anything?
Do you take any medicine, tablets, drugs or injections?
Have you had any serious illness in the past, such as rheumatic fever, St Vitus's Dance, heart or lung trouble?
Do you suffer with coughs, colds, sinus trouble, fainting attacks, black-outs, allergies, travel-sickness?
Can you breathe through your nose?

The foregoing account should enable the practitioner to make a sensible decision as to the best method of dealing with any particular patient, including of course, the instigation of any further clinical investigation or the administration of premedication.

TABLE IV.—*Instructions for Patients Receiving Dental Treatment under General Anaesthesia*

Your appointment is at .... a.m./p.m. on ....

For your own safety it is essential that you follow the instructions below.

BEFORE THE ANAESTHETIC

1. You may have a light meal before .... a.m./p.m.
2. You may have a cup of tea or fruit juice and one biscuit before .... a.m./p.m.
3. You may swallow any tablet ordered with a sip of water up to .... a.m./p.m.
4. You must be accompanied by a responsible adult who will escort you home.
5. Immediately before your appointment you should go to the toilet.
6. When you enter the surgery do not forget to tell the doctor or dentist about your general health and any medicines you may be taking.

AFTER THE ANAESTHETIC

1. Under no circumstances must you drive any vehicle or operate machinery until the day following the anaesthetic.
2. You should not return to work or school until the day following the anaesthetic.
3. If you feel unwell on returning home, go to bed and rest for a while. If you do not improve you should either contact the surgery or your own doctor.
4. Alcohol should not be consumed until the day following the anaesthetic.

I have read and understood the above instructions and agree to the operation and anaesthetic advised.

Signature of patient or parent/guardian.............................

Date.......................19....

(v) *Premedication (in Out-patient)*

The main objectives of premedication are six-fold:
(a) To reduce salivation and respiratory secretions.
(b) To protect the heart against reflex vagal over-activity.
(c) To produce a sedative or calming effect on the anxious patient.
(d) To produce a degree of analgesia which may be of value both during the anaesthetic and postoperatively.
(e) To produce amnesia to the events immediately prior to the induction of anaesthesia.
(f) To reduce the incidence of postoperative nausea and vomiting.

With the exception of the first two, these objectives are achieved only at the expense of early ambulation of the patient; therefore, in the out-patient, premedication should only be used after the disadvantages of impaired recovery have been carefully weighed against the benefits achieved.

In the techniques of anaesthesia described in chapters 5 and 10 for exodontia without intubation, we do not consider it necessary routinely to use drugs such as atropine or hyoscine for the specific purpose of drying secretions, since the anaesthetic agents described are non-irritant to the respiratory mucosa. However, the vagolytic action of atropine is often used to protect the heart against bradycardia and even cardiac arrest. If the heart-rate is extremely slow (i.e. the pacemaker depressed), there is an increased opportunity for ectopic beats (extra-systoles) to arise within the ventricular muscle. On the other hand, if vagal tone is reduced by the use of atropine, it is possible that dyshythmias initiated by catecholamine release are more likely to occur (page 166). A rapid heart-rate can also be undesirable by interfering with cardiac filling and hence output; moreoever, tachycardia may be subjectively unpleasant to the patient if produced before the induction of anaesthesia. On balance, therefore, we feel that the use of atropine preoperatively in the dental out-patient is seldom justified in the unintubated patient.

When considering sedation of the nervous patient, the aim should be to achieve a maximum calming effect with minimal depression of those areas of the brain not directly concerned with anxiety; therefore the tranquillizers, the actions of which are mainly confined to the reticular system (page 31), are generally recommended in preference to the purely sedative drugs (e.g. barbiturates). This preference does not normally apply to young children. When the tranquillizers are used, it is often advisable to commence treatment a day or two prior to the proposed operation.

We consider that the use of the powerful narcotic analgesics is seldom, if ever, justified in premedication of the out-patient; however, a further discussion of their use in the 'Jorgensen' technique appears on page 247. Patients with a history of distressing nausea following a previous anaesthetic, or severe travel sickness may benefit by taking one of the anti-emetic drugs discussed on page 39.

To sum up, we find it seldom essential to premedicate the dental out-patient, although in certain specific circumstances it is advisable to do so. Whether or not the routine use of atropine to protect the heart against vagal overactivity is justified, is at present controversial and a final judgement must await the results of further research. It may also be claimed that the current small incidence of postanaesthetic nausea could be further reduced by the routine administration of an anti-emetic drug (e.g. perphenazine 2 mg orally) about 2 hours before the expected appointment. Such a routine would also produce mild sedation, but would be unlikely to interfere significantly with normal recovery.

(vi) *Clothing*

At the preoperative visit, patients should be advised to wear warm, loose clothing which will allow ready access to the veins at the elbow, and the upper, outer quadrant of the buttock for intramuscular injection if this is anticipated.

2. Immediate Pre-anaesthetic Rules

Immediately before treatment, the following matters should receive attention.

(a) Check recent health, food and drink.

(b) Toilet.

(c) Remove dentures and other removable appliances. Check on position of crowns, etc. Note any loose teeth or fillings.

(d) Remove or protect watches, jewellery, etc.

(e) Deal tactfully with cosmetics, including wigs and false eye-lashes and also any unduly tight clothing which may interfere with comfortable breathing. Heavy mascara can act as a conjunctival irritant under anaesthesia.

Whilst the medical assessment carried out at the preoperative visit should usually ensure the patient's overall suitability for general anaesthesia, it is the anaesthetist who must make the final assessment in the light of his special training and the particular anaesthetic technique indicated. We believe that satisfactory assessment can be achieved by an experienced practitioner without routinely conducting a full physical examination of the patient. Indeed, should the necessity for such an examination be suggested by the history, it is not usually possible to carry it out satisfactorily in the average dental surgery. This matter is more fully discussed on page 257.

RECOMMENDED READING

1. Danger List for the Anaesthetist.
GROGONO, A. W., LEE, P. (1970) *Anaesthesia*, **25**, 518.

2. Monoamine Oxidase Inhibitors.
BOAKES, A. J. (1971) *Prescrib. J.*, **11**, 105.

3. Sickle Cell Anaemia.
SEARLE, J. F. (1973) *Anaesthesia*, **28**, 48.

CHAPTER TWO

PREOPERATIVE AND POSTOPERATIVE DRUGS

Drugs used preoperatively may be divided into two groups; those used by the anaesthetist as premedicants, and those already being taken by the patient for a purpose unconnected with the operation or anaesthetic. In this chapter we will discuss only those drugs used specifically for premedication and postoperative sedation and analgesia.

A. PREMEDICANTS

These drugs constitute a clinical rather than a pharmacological group, since they may be given to achieve a number of widely different pharmacological effects. For convenience, these effects and the drugs which produce them, will be considered under the same headings as were used in the clinical discussion of premedication (page 17).

1. Antisialogogues

Inhibition of secretory activity in the upper respiratory and alimentary tracts is best achieved by the use of drugs which block the muscarinic action of acetylcholine. The most commonly used are atropine and hyoscine, both of which have other pharmacological actions which are generally considered desirable during anaesthesia.

Atropine

Hyoscyamine sulphate—chemical name
Atropine sulphate (B.P.)
Atropine sulfate (U.S.P.)

Pharmacological Properties

(a) **Central Nervous System.**—The initial central effect of atropine is that of stimulation which, with increasing dosage, may be followed by depression; thus in therapeutic dosage, atropine has central stimulant rather than sedative properties. Initial stimulation of the vagal centre may result in temporary slowing of the pulse, before its peripheral cardiac accelerator effect becomes predominant. This paradoxical bradycardia is unlikely to be pronounced unless the dose is low.

(b) **Autonomic Nervous System.**—The autonomic nervous system comprises sympathetic and parasympathetic divisions. In the main, parasympathetic activity results in the liberation of acetylcholine at its nerve endings, and it is the muscarine-like properties of this substance which are responsible for the following effects:

 (i) Salivation and other secretomotor activity
 (ii) Sweating and lacrimation
(iii) Smooth muscle contraction (e.g. bronchioles and intestines)
(iv) Slowing of heart, and vasodilatation in some areas of the body
 (v) Constriction of pupil

Atropine blocks these muscarine effects of acetylcholine, and it is for its anti-sialogogue and cardiac effects that it is used in premedication.

(c) **Cardiovascular System.**—As already explained, atropine increases the heart-rate by peripheral vagal blockade. Initial slowing may result from temporary stimulation of the vagal centre, particularly if the dose is small. The blood pressure is normally unchanged, unless it has been previously reduced as a result of vagal overactivity, when atropine can be expected to restore it to normal.

(d) **Respiratory System.**—Minute volume may be increased slightly due to central stimulation. The bronchial secretions are reduced and the musculature relaxed, the latter resulting in an increase in anatomical and physiological dead space.

Route of Administration and Fate in the Body

Atropine is usually administered by intramuscular or intravenous injection but, as it is rapidly absorbed from the gastro-intestinal tract, may also be given by mouth. When administered orally or intramuscularly, the optimum effect is produced in 30–60 minutes. Whilst with intravenous injection the result is rapid, 5 minutes should be allowed to ensure the full antisialogogue effect. Atropine is mainly broken down in the liver and other tissues, but some is excreted unchanged in urine, sweat and breast milk. Its duration of effective action is about 2 hours.

Effects of Overdose

These include dry mouth resulting in dysphagia, blurred vision with dilatation of the pupil, hot dry skin, hyperpyrexia, restlessness and finally delirium. In the elderly patient with prostatic enlargement, its administration may precipitate an attack of urinary retention.

Presentation and Dosage

Tablets: Soluble B.P.C. 0·5 mg. Particularly suitable for use in children.
Ampoules: Colourless fluid. (*Normal strength **in heavy print***) 1 ml may contain 0·4, **0·6**, 0·8, or 1·2 mg. Suitable for any route of injection.
Dosage: The following scheme is suggested as a guide to premedication:—

    Under 2 years — 0·3 mg (injection)
    2–10 years   — 0·5 mg (tablet)
    Over 10 years — 0·5 mg–0·8 mg
                        (tablet or injection)

NB.—The above doses are those adjudged to be clinically safe. The full cardiac vagal blocking dose is in the range of 2–3 mg.

Hyoscine

    Hyoscine hydrobromide—chemical name
    Hyoscine hydrobromide (B.P.)
    Scopolamine hydrobromide (U.S.P.)
    (Kwells—trade name)

Hyoscine is an alkaloid of similar origin to atropine. The actions of hyoscine differ from those of atropine chiefly in respect of their central effects, and in one peripheral aspect.

Central

Hyoscine depresses the cerebral cortex from the outset, especially in the motor areas, and it is this latter property which renders it valuable in the control of Parkinsonism. It also produces marked amnesia and euphoria, and only rarely (in the elderly) restlessness. Its anti-emetic effect is superior to that of atropine, hence its popularity in the control of motion sickness.

Peripheral

The peripheral effects of hyoscine and atropine are identical, but in the generally accepted equivalent dosage judged by antisialogogue activity, hyoscine does not produce tachycardia, and is therefore not considered to give adequate protection to the heart against vagal overactivity.

Route of Administration and Fate in the Body

The routes of administration do not differ from those appropriate to atropine, but there is evidence that hyoscine is more completely broken down in the body, since only 1 % is excreted unchanged in the urine.

Presentation and Dosage

Tablets: B.P. **0·3**, 0·4, 0·6 mg
Ampoules: Colourless fluid
            1 ml contains **0·4** or 0·6 mg
Dosage: 0·2–0·4 mg

Certain drugs which are not primarily anticholinergic in action, e.g. chlorpromazine and promethazine, exhibit mild antisialogogue activity and are fully described under the appropriate headings.

2. Drugs used to Reduce the Irritability of the Cardiovascular System

The place of atropine in cardiac protection from parasympathetic overactivity has already been discussed. Certain drugs, which may serve to protect the heart from the effects of sympathetic overactivity, will now be described. Sympathetic stimulant effects are produced through two different types of receptor mechanism (alpha and beta) and those effects which are responsible for increased cardiac irritability are mediated through the beta receptors, and thus prevented by drugs called adrenergic beta-blocking agents, of which propranolol and practolol are the most commonly used.

Propranolol (Inderal)

Propranolol can be administered orally (10–40 mg), or by slow intravenous injection (1–10 mg). The indications for its use are complicated, and beyond the scope of this book to discuss in detail, but it should be pointed out that cardiac dysrhythmias associated with halothane respond readily to the action of propranolol. Many anaesthetists recommend that this drug should be administered prophylactically when it is anticipated that halothane will accompany, or follow, any injection (e.g. local) containing adrenaline. For this purpose a dose of 1 mg (intravenous) will suffice. The drug should never be given in the presence of heart failure, pregnancy, or asthma, and in any event has no place in the management of dental out-patients, other than in the hands of an experienced physician-anaesthetist.

Practolol (Eraldin)

Like propranolol this drug is a beta-receptor blocking agent; however, in therapeutic dosage it is said to effect only the beta-receptors in the heart, and thus it is claimed to be safe when used on patients suffering from obstructive respiratory disease (asthma).

The indications for its use are the same as those described under propranolol.

3. C.N.S. Depressants

The classification of drugs which act as depressants on the central nervous system has led to much confusion and it is necessary to define carefully the terms used.

Narcotic.—The most common confusion concerns this term, since the classification is sometimes a pharmacological one, and sometimes a legal one. The pharmacological classification includes sedatives, hypnotics, analgesics and general anaesthetics, or indeed, any drug which depresses the central nervous system. It is thus a term carrying little specific meaning. However, according to American federal and state laws and the World Health Organization, the term narcotic denotes a wide range of drugs of addiction, including cocaine and marijuana which are central stimulants.

General Anaesthesia.—General anaesthesia is a state of unconsciousness of such depth that the subject is unable to perform a simple co-ordinated movement in response to a command. At this level of unconsciousness surgical stimulation will neither produce arousal nor be remembered, but may provoke reflex response. At all levels of anaesthesia, the normal mechanisms of protection and maintenance of the airway are jeopardized.

Hypnotic.—A hypnotic is a drug which has a general depressant effect on the central nervous system thus inducing sleep, provided insomnia is not due to severe pain.

Sedative.—A sedative is a drug which is used to calm the emotions. If given in large dosage, it will act as a hypnotic and produce sleepiness.

Tranquillizer.—The distinction between a sedative and a tranquillizer is not clear-cut. Sedatives produce sleep more readily than tranquillizers when used in large dosage. Tranquillizers have a more specific action in allaying anxiety and controlling behaviour disorders. It is probable that the sedatives and hypnotics act mainly on the cerebral cortex, whereas the main site of action of the tranquillizers is subcortical, in the mid-brain reticular formation and hypothalamus.

Analgesic.—An analgesic is a drug which has a specific action in the relief of pain without producing loss or clouding of consciousness.

Amnesic.—An amnesic is a drug which specifically produces a loss of memory.

Euphoria.—A sense of well-being.

Basal Narcosis.—Basal narcosis is a state of deep hypnosis, bordering on light anaesthesia.

HYPNOTICS AND SEDATIVES

It is convenient to divide these drugs into barbiturates and non-barbiturates.

Barbiturates

General Pharmacology

Although certain of the barbiturates exhibit specific individual characteristics, their overall pharmacological actions are sufficiently similar to warrant the general description which follows. In high dosage they produce a general depressant effect on all tissues, but in therapeutic dosage their actions are attributable to specific effects on various systems of the body.

Central Nervous System.—The barbiturates have a generalized depressant effect on the central nervous system with a predominant action on the cerebral cortex and reticular activating system. However, the latter also contains an inhibitory component which might become depressed by small doses of barbiturate, thus leading to excitement and confusion. The medullary centres are depressed from the outset, but the safety margin of these drugs is such as to allow sedation, hypnosis and anaesthesia to be produced without undue depression of the vital cardiac and respiratory centres.

The type of sleep produced by the barbiturates is similar to natural sleep as evidenced by electro-encephalogram studies, but it is noticeable that the rapid eye-movement phase (dream) seen in natural sleep is greatly reduced.

The presence of a phenyl group in the barbiturate molecule often denotes specific anticonvulsant properties which result from depression of the motor cortex.

The barbiturates are known to have no true pharmacological analgesic properties; that is to say, they will not relieve severe pain without a concomitant depressant effect on overall cerebral function. Indeed, it is often evident that, if barbiturates are given in the presence of severe pain, they may produce restlessness; this observation is in keeping with the experimental evidence that in low blood concentrations they may act as anti-analgesics. However, to deny the claim that barbiturates may be of value in the overall control of pain, is to take altogether too facile a view of the mechanism of pain appreciation; for, it is well recognized that fear and anxiety may convert physical discomfort into intolerable pain. It is in this context that the barbiturates may appear to act as analgesics.

Finally, it should be noted that the degree of central depression does not depend only upon dosage, route, speed of administration and circulatory dynamics, but also on the state of excitability of the central nervous system at the time of administration of the drug. Moreover, previous experience (tolerance) may produce a relative resistance to the action of the drug.

Cardiovascular System.—In normal sedative dosage the barbiturates have little, if any, effect on the cardiovascular system, but may produce a small fall in blood pressure in the normal subject. A more striking fall in blood pressure may be produced in the hypertensive subject if anxiety is the dominant causative factor. This effect is assumed to be the result of the normal sedative action of the drug. In larger dosage there may be a considerable fall in both blood pressure and cardiac output due to a reduction in sympathetic tone, and direct depression of the myocardium.

Respiratory System.—The barbiturates produce direct depression of the respiratory centre which is associated with decreased sensitivity to the initial stimulant effects of carbon dioxide. Clinically, this depression is characterized by shallow breathing which may be normal in rate, in contrast to the effects of the powerful analgesics which produce breathing which is slow but of normal amplitude.

Ciliary action is depressed, thus reducing the efficiency of normal bronchial drainage; also, the inhibitory action of the sympathetic nervous system, in respect of bronchial tone, is reduced, thus rendering bronchial spasm the likely response to any stimulus which is irritant to the respiratory mucosa.

Metabolism.—Metabolic rate, and thus oxygen consumption, is reduced.

Fate in the Body.—The barbiturates are distributed throughout all the tissues of the body and, in the blood, variable amounts are bound to the plasma albumin fraction. Absorption into the fat depots is a particular characteristic of those barbiturates commonly used intravenously, e.g. thiopentone and methohexitone.

All the barbiturates, with the possible exception of barbitone, are to some extent broken down in the liver and other tissues, and it is the extent of this breakdown, as opposed to simple unchanged renal excretion, which will in part determine the length of action of the drug. However, some barbiturates give rise to breakdown products which are themselves hypnotically active (e.g. the thiobarbiturates) thus leading to prolonged hypnotic action despite a considerable degree of breakdown. The ultimate elimination of all the barbiturates, including their breakdown products, is by renal excretion. It will thus be seen that any serious degree of impairment of renal function

A.A.D.—2

will delay recovery, to a greater or lesser extent, irrespective of the barbiturate used. So far as liver disease is concerned, those barbiturates which rely primarily on breakdown for their limitation of hypnotic action (e.g. pentobarbitone) should be avoided, or their dose reduced; in any event, their use should be restricted to the in-patient.

Routes of Administration.—These drugs, especially their sodium salts, are readily absorbed from the gastro-intestinal tract, thus rendering them suitable for both oral and rectal administration, with the exception of thiopentone and methohexitone which are not recommended for oral use.

The soluble salts of many barbiturates can be given by deep intramuscular injection. This includes methohexitone but not thiopentone or any other of the thiobarbiturates, as they produce intense tissue irritation.

The soluble salts may also be administered by intravenous injection.

Complications and Special Precautions

(a) Idiosyncrasy

(i) **Natural.**—Natural idiosyncrasy is rare, but occasionally subjects are met in whom restlessness, excitement and even vertigo, vomiting, diarrhoea and muscular pain may be produced by normal dosage.

(ii) **Acquired.**—This is likely to occur in subjects with a tendency to allergy. Symptoms include the usual allergic phenomena, such as swelling of the eyelids, erythematous skin reactions, and bronchospasm. The symptoms will rapidly respond to treatment which consists of discontinuation of the drug and the administration of an antihistamine (e.g. Piriton).

Severe allergic reaction, following the use of an intravenous barbiturate may rarely give rise to acute anaphylaxis. The treatment of this serious condition should be as follows:—

(i) The administration of oxygen.

(ii) The intravenous administration of an antihistamine, e.g. Phenergan 25 mg, Piriton 10 mg (page 40).

(iii) The intravenous administration of hydrocortisone 100 mg–300 mg (page 151).

(iv) Should these measures not prove immediately effective, then 1:1000 adrenaline must be administered by slow intramuscular injection, e.g. 0·5 ml stat., followed by 0·5 ml every 5 minutes, until the required effect has been achieved (page 151).

(b) Porphyria

Porphyria is a rare familial metabolic disease found chiefly in people of Dutch descent. In these subjects there is a defect in the regulation of the enzyme synthetase, which is concerned in the synthesis of porphyrins. An acute attack is characterized by the appearance of large quantities of porphyrins in the urine, associated with abdominal pain and sometimes neurological changes which may lead to paralysis and death. The attacks are characteristically intermittent and during an attack, if the urine is left exposed to light, it will become a dark port wine colour.

It is known that the barbiturates stimulate the production of enzymes responsible for their own destruction—hence the development of tolerance. Moreover, it has been recently shown that they are also responsible for stimulating the production of many other enzymes, one of which is the enzyme already referred to, synthetase. For this reason the barbiturates have a bizarre and important significance in relation to porphyria. The administration of any barbiturate during the latent phase of porphyria may precipitate an acute attack with a possible fatal result. Therefore a history of porphyria in a patient or any member of his family is a strict contraindication to the use of barbiturates. It is unlikely that, in the absence of a family history, a diagnosis will be made in the latent phase of the disease, but the active phase of acute intermittent porphyria (the commonest type encountered) may be characterized by abdominal pain, hysterical behaviour, hypertension and the development of the characteristic urine change. Inadvertent precipitation of an acute attack will necessitate hospitalization, where immediate treatment, often needing artificial respiration, may be necessary.

(c) Chronic Toxicity and Tolerance

Patients accustomed to taking large doses of a barbiturate may develop a so-called tolerance to the entire group of drugs. This is the result of the ability of barbiturates to stimulate the production of self-destructive enzymes. In spite of the development of tolerance, the cumulative effects of the drug can result in chronic toxicity with symptoms such as drowsiness, lethargy, mental depression, confusion and even vergito, ataxia, convulsions, and other neurological disorders.

Barbiturates should be considered as drugs of addiction, since their sudden restriction after prolonged use may lead to withdrawal symptoms.

(d) Overdose

Overdose with a barbiturate may occur as the result of accidental excessive dosage as in automatism, attempted suicide, or errors in therapeutic administration.

Irrespective of cause and route, if the overdose leads to significant respiratory or cardiovascular depression, treatment must be directed towards the appropriate supportive therapy, including, of course, adequate ventilation of the lungs (page 152).

Clinical Classification

For clinical descriptive purposes the barbiturates may be divided into the following groups.

1. *Long acting*—i.e. those which rely mainly on renal excretion.
2. *Short acting*—i.e. those which rely on both breakdown in the liver and tissues, and renal excretion.
3. *'Ultra short acting'*—i.e. those which are given intravenously and rely upon redistribution within the body, followed by chemical breakdown. This group will be fully discussed in Chapter 9.

1. Long Acting (8–12 hours)

These drugs are not normally used as hypnotics because of their hangover effect, but may be of use in small dosage for their prolonged sedative action, or in the specific control of epilepsy.

(i) **Barbitone Sodium B.P.**—(Trade name—Medinal). This is said to be the only barbiturate which is eliminated entirely in the urine and therefore carries the strongest risk of accumulation. It has no selective depressant action on the motor cortex and is therefore not used in the control of epilepsy.

Dosage.—Sedative—200 mg daily
            Hypnotic—300 mg–600 mg

(ii) **Phenobarbitone B.P.**—(Trade name—Gardenal/Luminal, and their sodium salts)
Phenobarbitone Sodium B.P.
Phenobarbital
Phenobarbital Sodium U.S.P.
N.B.—The sodium salt of this drug is soluble and can therefore be used for injection.
In addition to its general depressant properties, phenobarbitone specifically depresses the motor cortex, thus exerting a powerful anticonvulsant action which is utilized in the management of epilepsy. Part is broken down by the liver and other tissues, but most of the drug is excreted unchanged in the urine.

Presentation and Dosage
Tablets—15 mg, **30 mg**, 60 mg, 100 mg
Elixir—15 mg in 5 ml
Ampoules—Phenobarbitone Sodium 220 mg
Dosage—Sedative—30 mg b.d.
            Hypnotic—200 mg

2. **Short Acting (4–8 hours)**

The drugs comprising this group are partly broken down by the liver and other tissues, and partly excreted in the urine. They are used to produce hypnosis or sedation, and are normally administered by mouth, the optimum sedative effect being achieved within $1-1\frac{1}{2}$ hours after administration. They may also be administered by the rectal route, and the soluble sodium salt may be given by intravenous or intramuscular injection.

The following are the more commonly used drugs of this group.

(i) **Amylobarbitone**—(Trade name—Amytal/Dorminal)
Amylobarbitone Sodium B.P.
Amobarbital U.S.P.
Average adult hypnotic dose 100–200 mg

(ii) **Butobarbitone B.P.**—(Trade name—Soneryl)
Available only in tablets
Average adult hypnotic dose 100–200 mg

Sonergan
Sonergan is a tablet which contains
    Promethazine 15 mg
    Butobarbitone 75 mg

Sonalgin
Sonalgin is a tablet which contains
    Butobarbitone 60 mg

Phenacetin 225 mg
Codeine Phosphate 10 mg

(iii) **Cyclobarbitone Calcium tablets B.P.**—(Trade name—Phanodorm)
Average adult hypnotic dose 200–400 mg

(iv) **Pentobarbitone Sodium B.P.**—(Trade name—Nembutal)
Pentobarbital Sodium U.S.P.
Presentation and Dosage
Yellow capsules—100 mg, 30 mg
Yellow/white capsules—50 mg
Elixir—20 mg in 5 ml
Average adult hypnotic dose 100–200 mg
N.B.—Ampoules containing 250 mg of powder to be dissolved in 5 ml of water, are available
for intravenous use (page 247).

(v) **Quinalbarbitone Sodium B.P.**—(Trade name—Seconal Sodium)
Available as capsules and tablets
Average adult dose 100–200 mg
N.B.—May be prescribed as a suppository for rectal use.

Tuinal
Tuinal is a capsule which contains 100 mg of quinalbarbitone sodium and 100 mg of
amylobarbitone sodium.
The following barbiturates, used primarily for intravenous anaesthesia, are discussed in
Chapter 9.

Thiopentone
Methohexitone
Buthalitone Na (Transithal)
Hexobarbitone Na (Evipan)
Thialbarbitone Na (Kemithal)
Thiamylal Na (Surital)

Non-barbiturate Sedatives

(i) **Alcohol.**—Alcohol, in the form of an ordinary alcoholic drink (ethyl alcohol), may be
successfully used as a pre-anaesthetic sedative, provided that both its bulk and total
quantity is sensibly limited. The characteristics and side effects of the drug, taken in
this way, are too well-known to merit any pretentious pharmacological description.

(ii) **Methylpentynol**—(Trade names—Atempol, Insomnol, *Oblivon*, Somnesin)
Capsules—250 mg
Elixir—250 mg in 4 ml
Dose—250 mg–1000 mg
This once popular mild sedative has now been superseded by more reliable agents.

(iii) **Chloral Hydrate**
Chloral Hydrate B.P.C.
Chloral mixture—1 g in 10 ml

Chloral elixir—200 mg in 5 ml
(Paediatric)
  Dose—Chloral mixture up to 2 g.
          Chloral elixir (paediatric) 100–200 mg per year.
Because of its unpleasant taste and smell and gastric irritant properties, this drug has been mainly replaced by the related compounds mentioned below.

Dichloralphenazone—(Trade name—Welldorm)
Tablets—650 mg
Elixir—225 mg in 5 ml
Dose—Adults 1300 mg, children 20 mg per kg

Triclofos Sodium—(Trade name—Tricloryl)
Tablets—500 mg
Elixir—500 mg in 5 ml
Dose—500–1000 mg

The action of all three compounds is due to the trichlorethanol into which they are all converted following absorption from the stomach and small intestine. Cerebral depression resulting in hypnosis is produced and the therapeutic safety margin is large, so that cardiovascular and respiratory depression are seldom, if ever, produced. Thus, these drugs are suitable for the very young and elderly.

Welldorm contains phenazone which possesses mild analgesic properties but has been known, very rarely, to cause blood dyscrasias.

These compounds have a duration of action of 6–8 hours with little hangover.

(iv) **Glutethimide B.P.**—(Trade name—Doriden).
Tablets—250 mg
Dose—250–500 mg for night sedation
        125 mg for day sedation t.d.s.
This is a general purpose mild hypnotic which is relatively non-toxic and therefore of particular value in the elderly subject. It acts within 30–40 minutes of administration and lasts for six hours.

(v) **Meprobamate**—(Trade names—Equinal, Mepavlon, Miltown)
Tablets—200 mg and 400 mg
Dose—400 mg t.d.s.
Meprobamate is a sedative which is said to possess mild anticonvulsant and muscle relaxant properties.

'Equagesic'
Equagesic is a tablet which contains
    Meprobamate 150 mg
    Aspirin 250 mg
    Ethoheptazine 75 mg
    (Ethoheptazine is a mild analgesic)

(vi) **Methaqualone**—(Trade name—Melsedin)
Tablets—150 mg

Dose—150–300 mg

Methaqualone is a hypnotic which can be used as an alternative to the barubitrates.

'Mandrax'

Methaqualone—250 mg
Diphenhydramine hydrochloride—25 mg
Tablets or capsules.

This hypnotic mixture is of special interest owing to the claim that the sleep which it induces is, in contrast to that produced by the barbiturates, indistinguishable in E.E.G. characteristics from natural sleep. It is also claimed to possess antitussive qualities similar in potency to those of codeine.

(vii) **Methyprylone.**—(Trade name—Noludar)

Tablets—200 mg
Capsules—300 mg
Dose—Adult hypnotic dose 200–400 mg
       Children—10 years old—up to 200 mg

The drug is a piperidine compound capable of exerting a moderate hypnotic action comparable to that of the short acting barbiturates. It acts within sixty minutes and lasts about six hours with minimal depressant effects on the cardiovascular and respiratory systems.

TRANQUILLIZERS

By definition, a tranquillizer is a drug which produces calmness and sedation without undue sleepiness or impairment of consciousness.

It must be remembered that when prescribing any drug in this group, the tranquillizing effect will depend as much on the dose used as the drug itself, as most of these drugs will produce sedation and even unconsciousness when given in a large dose. Indeed, many of them are also used as hypnotics. There is a wide variation in response between individuals. A dose which will produce little subjective effect on one patient may render another uncontrollably sleepy.

Care should always be taken when prescribing these drugs to warn patients of the potentiating effect of alcohol, and the dangers associated with driving and operating machinery.

An important clinical characteristic of any particular member of the tranquillizing group of drugs is its tendency to produce symptoms of extrapyramidal disturbance when used in high or prolonged dosage. It is convenient to classify the drugs according to the chemical group to which they belong, i.e. Phenothiazines, Butyrophenones, and Benzodiazepines.

Clinical Use of Tranquillizers in Dentistry

The tranquillizing drugs have been mainly studied in relation to the long term control of emotional disturbances. In dentistry the problem usually becomes one of an isolated, frightening episode, and thus the dose regime used must be adjusted accordingly.

Ideally, medication should begin at least 24 hours prior to the dental appointment and end with a preoperative dose 1–2 hours before treatment. This dose should consist of the total dose given in the last 24 hours and may be given orally or, if maximum effect is required, intravenously. For example,

Diazepam. 2–5 mg t.d.s. day prior to appointment
6–15 mg 1–2 hours preoperatively *or*
6–15 mg intravenously immediately preoperatively.

The Phenothiazines

This is a large group of more than twenty allied compounds, all of which produce extrapyramidal side effects in large dosage. Only a few of these are likely to be used in dental practice—the properties of the most useful being presented in Table V.

TABLE V.—*Properties of Selected Phenothiazines*

Chemical name	Proprietary name	Tranquillizing Dose mg	Extra-pyramidal effects	Anti-emetic effects	Sedative effects	Hypotensive effects
Chlorpromazine	Largactil	75–150	Moderate	High	High	Moderate
Promazine	Sparine	25–50	Moderate	Moderate	Moderate	High
Perphenazine	Fentazin	4–8	High	High	Low	Low
Trifluoperazine	Stelazine	5–10	High	High	Moderate	Low
Prochlorperazine	Stemetil	5–25	High	High	Moderate	Low
Promethazine	Phenergan	10–25	Low	Moderate	High	Moderate
Trimeprazine	Vallergan	30–40	Low	Moderate	High	Moderate
Pecazine	Pacatal	5–10	Moderate	Moderate	High	Low

All the phenothiazines have certain common properties. They tame wild animals, abolish sham rage in cats, and diminish restlessness. They lower the response to most sensory stimuli, but some have been shown to be anti-analgesic in low dosage. They inhibit activity in the hypothalamus and reticular formation, and depress the vomiting centre in the medulla. They have strong anti-adrenergic and weak anticholinergic effects which may result in hypotension, peripheral vasodilatation and hypothermia.

Chlorpromazine—(Trade name—Largactil)
Tablets—10 mg, 25 mg, 50 mg, 100 mg
Ampoules—25 mg in 1 ml, 50 mg in 2 ml
    Should be protected from light
Syrup—10 mg per teaspoon (5 ml)
Dose—Tranquillizer 25–100 mg
    Anti-emetic 25–50 mg by intramuscular injection.

This drug may be given orally, rectally or by injection. The intramuscular injection may be painful, but can be administered in a 2% procaine solution. Intravenous administration may result in pronounced hypotension, since the drug produces blockade of the alpha sympathetic receptors.

Promazine Hydrochloride—(Trade name—Sparine)
Tablets—25 mg, 50 mg, 100 mg
Injection—50 mg per ml

Syrup—2 mg per ml
Dose—Tranquillizer 25–50 mg orally up to a daily dose of 400 mg

The drug is usually given orally but may be given by the intramuscular or intravenous route for deep sedation. If given intravenously, it should be diluted with an equal volume of saline. The drug is liable to produce postural hypotension, so that the patient should lie down for at least half an hour after intravenous administration.

Promethazine Hydrochloride (Trade name—Phenergan)

Tablets—10 mg, 25 mg
Syrup—5 mg in 5 ml
Ampoules—25 mg in 1 ml
Dose—Tranquillizing dose 10 mg in divided doses, up to 50 mg daily.

The drug may also be used as a sedative, and is commonly prescribed for premedication in children as a syrup—in a dose of 0·5 mg–1 mg per kg of body weight.

This drug has an anti-emetic and sedative action. It has less alpha-blocking action than chlorpromazine and is therefore less likely to produce hypotension.

It relaxes bronchial musculature and produces some inhibition of secretions (atropine-like action).

It has a marked antihistamine action, thus making it useful for the treatment of acute allergy, for which it may be given intravenously in a dose not exceeding 50 mg.

It has been claimed to reduce the analgesic action of pethidine and other analgesics.

Promethazine Theocolate—(Trade name—Avomine)

Tablets—25 mg
Dose—25 mg as required.
N.B.—This drug is used as an anti-emetic and cannot be given intravenously or intramuscularly.

Perphenazine B.P.—(Trade names—Fentazin, Trilafon U.S.P.)

Tablets—2 mg, **4 mg**, 8 mg
Syrup—3 mg per ml
Ampoules—5 mg in 1 ml
Dose—It is a potent tranquillizer and may be given by mouth in doses of 4 mg–8 mg three times a day. This dose should not be exceeded owing to its depressant action on the bone marrow. It should not be given during early pregnancy.

It is a powerful anti-emetic, and is used for this purpose by intramuscular injection of 2·5 mg, or intravenous injection of 1 mg. Extrapyramidal symptoms have been reported following a single dose.

Trifluoperazine Hydrochloride B.P.—(Trade name—Stelazine)

Tablets—1 mg
Spansule capsules—2 mg
Syrup—1 mg in 5 ml
Ampoules—1 mg in 1 ml
Dose—2 mg–4 mg a day; excessive dose will produce extrapyramidal symptoms.
It is a potent tranquillizer with only moderate sedative effects.

A.A.D.—2*

It is a powerful anti-emetic and should be administered in 1 mg dose by intramuscular injection.

Trimeprazine Tartrate B.P.C.—(Trade name—Vallergan, Alimemazine)
Tablets—10 mg
Syrup—7·5 mg per 5 ml
Syrup Forte—6 mg per 1 ml
Injection Solution—25 mg in 1 ml
Dose—Tranquillizer 30 mg–40 mg up to 100 mg daily
       Premedication in children—2 mg–5 mg per kg.

This drug is one of the most useful phenothiazines in dental practice, since it has marked sedative and antihistamine properties; however, its anti-adrenergic activity is sufficient to give some cardiovascular depression when used in large doses; thus, caution must be exercised to keep the patient lying down for several hours after administration, when doses greater than 2 mg/kg are used.

Pecazine Hydrochloride—(Trade name—Pacatal)
Tablet—25 mg
Injection—Pecazine acetate
Dose—25 mg–100 mg daily.

Prochlorperazine Maleate B.P., U.S.P.—(Trade names—Stemetil, Compazine)
Tablets—5 mg, 25 mg
Syrup Forte—25 mg per 5 ml
Injection Ampoules—12·5 mg in 1 ml
Suppositories—5 mg, 25 mg
Mainly used as an anti-emetic
Dose—12·5 mg by intramuscular injection
5 mg–10 mg by mouth
5 mg suppositories for children
10 mg suppositories for adults

The Butyrophenones

The most important drugs in this group are Haloperidol and Droperidol. These two drugs are usually classified as neuroleptics, having a markedly selective action on the central nervous system which produces a state of mental calm with very little sedation. In fact, they are often antisoporific. It is said that the mode of action is by stimulating the caudate nucleus, which in turn depresses the reticular formation. This action may be responsible for the extrapyramidal side-effects.

These drugs have powerful anti-emetic action and virtually no anti-adrenergic activity, thus producing very little change in the blood pressure.

The butyrophenones should not be given to patients with lesions of the basal ganglia, and thus should be avoided in the elderly patient with arteriosclerosis.

Droperidol—(Trade name—Droleptan)
Tablets—2·5 mg, 10 mg
Ampoules—10 mg in 2 ml
Dose—Premedication—10 mg by mouth or 5 mg intramuscularly

(Premedication in children—0·2 mg–0·6 mg per kg)
Neuroleptanalgesia—5 mg–15 mg intravenously, followed ten to twenty minutes later by a powerful analgesic such as phenoperidine.

Haloperidol—(Trade name—Serenace)
Tablets—1·5 mg
Ampoules—5 mg in 1 ml
Dose—Premedication—5 mg intramuscularly one to eight hours preoperatively.

This drug has a longer action than droperidol and lasts up to twenty-four hours.

The Benzodiazepines

The benzodiazepine group of drugs has been in wide clinical use since the early 1960's. The chief therapeutic actions of these drugs are:

(a) Tranquillization (b) Sedation and hypnosis (c) Muscular relaxation

There are at present five commonly used members of the group, namely diazepam (Valium), chlordiazepoxide (Librium), nitrazepam (Mogadon), metazepam (Nobrium), and oxazepam (Serenid D).

TABLE VI.—*The Benzodiazepines*

Diazepam   Chlordiazepoxide   Nitrazepam

Oxazepam   Metazepam

Although the clinical and pharmacological properties of these drugs are similar, the predominant action in each case is different. Thus chlordiazepoxide and oxazepam find their main usage as pure tranquillizers, nitrazepam as a 'night sedative', and diazepam as a tranquillizer, a muscle relaxant, anticonvulsant, and finally to induce 'heavy' sedation or even full anaesthesia. This multiplicity of usages in the case of diazepam is a consequence not only of its relatively high potency as an anticonvulsant, but also of the fact that it is the only one of the five drugs readily available in both tablet and injection form. When any drug is administered by intravenous injection, it is, of course, possible for a relatively high temporary cerebral level to be achieved with a comparatively small total dose. Thus, of this group of drugs, it is diazepam which has aroused great interest in the sphere of out-patient dentistry, and it is diazepam which will here be described in some detail.

Diazepam—(Trade name—Valium)
Tablets 2 mg (white)
Tablets 5 mg (yellow)
Tablets 10 mg (blue)
Syrup 2 mg in 5 ml
Ampoules for injection—10 mg in 2 ml

Physical Properties

Diazepam is insoluble in water, the solution for injection being made up with an organic solvent in light-protected ampoules. The resultant solution is moderately irritant to the tissues, and venous thrombosis is not uncommon following its use. If used undiluted, the solution should be injected into a large (antecubital) vein (page 249). Some authorities recommend that the 2 ml ampoule should be diluted to 5 ml or 20 ml or more (*not* to 10 ml) with 5% dextrose.

Pharmacology

Central Nervous System.—Diazepam is thought to exert its tranquillizing effect by virtue of its depressant action upon the limbic system and, in particular, the amygdala, which is that part of the limbic system responsible for the relay of 'emotional' impulses via the hypothalamus, pituitary and autonomic system to their ultimate expression.

The well marked muscle-relaxant and anticonvulsant properties are related to its inhibitory action on polysynaptic spinal reflex pathways.

Although the most striking pharmacological property demonstrable in animals is that of muscular relaxation and generally diminished locomotor activity, there is nevertheless a well-marked and quite distinct 'taming' or tranquillizing effect, and thus the drug has become established in clinical practice as both an anticonvulsant and a tranquillizer. Diazepam administered intravenously is now considered by many to be the treatment of choice in the control of convulsions (e.g. status epilepticus). The relaxant properties of diazepam are utilized not only in the control of convulsions, but also in the relief of pain and spasm associated with various musculo-skeletal disorders. The relaxant effect is exerted on uterine as well as skeletal muscle, and this property has been found of value in the control of dysmenorrhoea. The daily dose of diazepam administered orally in these conditions has varied widely from 10 to 60 mg, and the establishment of a satisfactory dosage regime appears to be very much a question of individual response.

Diazepam has been widely used as a tranquillizer, the usual adult dose being of the order 2–5 mg six or eight hourly, administered orally. In psychiatry, the drug has also been used successfully in the treatment of severe phobias, and for this purpose 10 mg is administered intravenously—followed, of course, by the appropriate psychotherapy. If dosage by the intravenous route is large enough, consciousness will ultimately be lost, and the drug has indeed been used as an induction agent. The dosage required for this purpose varies widely from 0·1 to 0·8 mg per kg depending upon the physical and emotional status of the patient, his age, and the nature or absence of premedication. In particular the elderly show extreme sensitivity to intravenous injection. The drug has also been employed both orally and by injection, as a routine premedicant.

In dentistry, diazepam has been used successfully by the oral route in order to allay anxiety in the moderately nervous patient. Its administration by the intravenous route to the extremely nervous patient has aroused great interest, and is fully discussed on page 249. Antegrade amnesia commonly results from moderately high dosage.

Cardiovascular System.—Experimental evidence in cats and dogs shows that even large doses of diazepam, given intravenously to the anaesthetized animal, do not cause a significant alteration in blood pressure, although the heart rate is reduced; there is, however, a considerable reduction in 'pressor response' as a result of quite small doses. In man, large doses administered intravenously do not appear to interfere seriously with the basic integrity of the cardiovascular system. There is usually a moderate fall in blood pressure under stable conditions, but in the previously anaesthetized subject this fall is usually small. The significance of the larger fall observed in the nervous, conscious subject must obviously be interpreted with care, since it may represent a return from elevated to normal rather than a serious reduction from normal. The drug does seem, in man, to interfere with the pressor reflexes, and postural hypotension is likely to occur following a moderate intravenous dose, although the observed fall in blood pressure is seldom accompanied by symptoms indicative of any serious cardiovascular deficiency.

Respiratory System.—Animal experiments indicate that diazepam does not produce any reduction in respiratory activity other than that to be expected from the reduced metabolic demands of the tranquillized state; nor does it interfere with the normal respiratory response to carbon dioxide. In man, some workers have noted a slight rise in respiratory rate, but on the whole, diazepam, even when used as an anaesthetic induction agent, produces remarkably little alteration in respiratory activity, and for practical purposes cannot be classified as a respiratory depressant.

Metabolism.—Initial clinical recovery from a single dose of diazepam is largely due to the high degree of protein-binding, and hence temporary inactivation, which occurs. Long-term recovery is, however, dependant upon a process of de-methylation and hydroxylation leading to break-down into oxazepam, which itself is pharmacologically active (see page 39). This final product is ultimately excreted by the kidney in the form of the glucimonide. It is thought that some 50% of the administered dose of the drug is excreted in man within ten hours, and the drug persists in the plasma for at least forty-eight hours following a single dose. It will thus be apparent that total clinical recovery from diazepam may take many hours, but also may be preceded by a misleading 'apparent recovery' possibly due to the high degree of protein-binding. Although there is no evidence to suggest that diazepam is contraindicated in the first trimester of pregnancy, we are of the opinion that, owing to its comparatively short association with anaesthetic practice, it is best avoided in the present state of knowledge.

Summary of Actions

Diazepam is an efficient tranquillizer when administered orally, and in effective dosage has a very wide margin of safety, unpleasant side-effects being extremely uncommon. When administered in larger dosage and in particular by the intra-venous route, deep tranquillization, heavy sedation, hypnosis, muscular relaxation, and even anaesthesia may be achieved with minimal cardiovascular and respiratory depression. The chief disadvantages are postural unsteadiness, postural hypotension, prolonged recovery, an increased sensitivity to other central nervous system depressants (e.g. anaesthetic agents, alcohol, etc.), and local venous thrombosis. The drug is likely to prove invaluable in out-patient dentistry, particularly for conservation in the nervous patient, which subject is discussed fully in Chapter 12.

Chlordiazepoxide—(Trade name—Librium)

Capsules—5 mg, 10 mg
Tablets—5 mg, 10 mg, 25 mg
Injection—100 mg dry powder with 2 ml solvent

Physical Characteristics

Chlordiazepoxide is a colourless crystalline substance highly soluble in water, the resultant solution being, however, unstable.

Pharmacology

Chlordiazepoxide is similar in all its actions to diazepam. Its tranquillizing potency is one fifth, its anticonvulsant potency one tenth that of diazepam. It is particularly useful in the treatment of pruritis. Its side-effects are similar to those of diazepam, and it is very widely used as a simple oral tranquillizer. It is not thought to exert any harmful effects during pregnancy. It is broken down in the body, the end-products being excreted partly in the urine, partly in the faeces.

Nitrazepam—(Trade name—Mogadon)

Tablets—5 mg
Syrup—5 mg in 5 ml
Dose—2·5 mg–10 mg

Pharmacology

Nitrazepam is utilized almost exclusively as a night sedative. The pattern of sleep produced approximates more closely to normal, in terms of E.E.G. activity, than does that associated with barbiturate sedation. It is said to act by screening the wake system from emotional and sensory stimuli rather than by directly depressing it. The sleep produced is characterized by satisfactory duration together with almost complete freedom from 'hangover'. The margin of safety is very large, an attempted suicide having taken 300 mg without harmful sequelae.

Oxazepam—(Trade name—Serenid D)

Tablets 10 mg and 15 mg

Pharmacology

This is similar to other members of the group, and the drug is used solely as an anxiolytic agent. Its safety in pregnancy has not been established.

THE ANTI-EMETICS

Vomiting may occur as a reflex response either to stimuli arising within the gastro-intestinal tract, or to various other stimuli including those produced by drugs known to exert an emetic effect. The central mechanisms involve two closely related, but functionally different, areas within the medulla oblongata. The so-called emetic centre, situated in the region of the fasciculus solitarius, is thought to be activated primarily by gastro-intestinal stimulation, and appears to have little importance in anaesthesia-induced nausea and vomiting, except when blood has been swallowed during the recovery period. The chemoreceptor trigger zone which is situated on the surface of the medulla, close to the vagal nuclei is thought to be the site of action of the central emetic drugs such as apomorphine and morphine, and also the area concerned with motion-sickness. It has been shown that destruction of this area prevents vomiting due both to the emetic drugs and to motion-sickness. Clinically, this relationship is supported by the observation that post-anaesthetic or drug-induced nausea and vomiting is frequently encountered in patients known to suffer from motion-sickness. Indeed, drugs which are most effective in the prevention of motion-sickness, are also the most efficient in preventing post-anaesthetic nausea and vomiting. Thus a history of motion-sickness should indicate the advisability of administering an anti-emetic prior to anaesthesia, and the final choice of drug should be dictated by the patient's previous experience in the control of his motion-sickness. To be effective these anti-emetics, if given orally, must be administered at least sixty minutes before the anaesthetic. If nausea is already established, the drug is best administered by the intramuscular or intravenous route.

Many of the most powerful anti-emetics belong to the phenothiazine group, the pharmacology of which has already been discussed (page 32). Table VII lists the anti-emetics most commonly used.

TABLE VII.—*Anti-emetic Drugs*

Name	Proprietary name	Oral dose	Comments
Hyoscine	Kwells	0·6 mg	See page 22
Cyclizine	Marzine	50 mg	50 mg Suppositories for children
Meclozine	Sea-legs	50 mg	—
Dimenhydrinate	Dramamine	100 mg	—
Promethazine theoclate	Avomine	25 mg	See page 33
Promethazine	Phenergan	25 mg	See page 33
Chlorpromazine	Largactil	50 mg	See page 32
Perphenazine	Fentazin	4 mg	See page 33
Prochlorperazine	Stemetil	10 mg	See page 34
Trifluoperazine	Stelazine	5 mg	See page 33
Metocloptamide	Maxolon	10 mg	See below

Maxolon

Maxolon exerts a powerful anti-emetic action on the afferent visceral nerves which run to the emetic centre. In addition, it acts centrally on the chemoreceptor trigger zone, and is thus effective in both vomiting due to gastric irritation, and that caused by central emetic factors. Like all drugs, maxolon should not be given during the first 3 months of pregnancy, until proven to be devoid of risk.

Since nausea is a common side-effect of the powerful analgesic agents, certain proprietary mixtures contain a combination of analgesic and anti-emetic drugs. Examples of these are given on page 42.

ANTIHISTAMINES

The antihistamines comprise a group of drugs which reverse the effects of histamine release, by competitive action. In dentistry they are of significance for the following reasons:

1. They may be of value in the treatment of allergic reactions.
2. Their sedative and anti-emetic properties render certain members of the group useful in pre and post medication.
3. The administration of other central nervous system depressants to patients being treated with antihistamines should be undertaken with caution.
   Table VIII lists a few of the many drugs in common use.

TABLE VIII.—*The Antihistamines*

Name	Proprietary name	Dose	Comments
Mepyramine	Anthisan	100–200 mg oral	
Promethazine	Phenergan	25–50 mg oral 25–50 mg I.V. or I.M.	See page 33
Phenindamine	Thephorin	25–50 mg oral	Does not cause sedation
Dimenhydrinate	Dramamine	25–100 mg oral	Sedation marked, mainly in motion sickness
Chlorpheniramine	Piriton	4–16 mg oral 10–20 mg I.V. or I.M.	The injection is of particular value in acute allergy

ANALGESICS

An analgesic is a drug which has a specific action in the relief of pain. The interpretation of any particular stimulus as painful is dependent not only upon the character and intensity of the afferent impulses which it engenders and transmits to the thalamus, but also upon the individual's interpretation of those impulses at cortical level. Thus it is, that drugs which cannot be shown experimentally to possess specific analgesic properties, nevertheless can be utilized to modify the individual's ability to tolerate any particular painful situation. It is generally accepted that anxiety and many other emotional disturbances lower the pain-threshold, and therefore any method of allaying that anxiety, including the administration of sedative drugs, will contribute greatly to the ultimate control of pain. This simplified account of the complex mechanism of pain appreciation is not at variance with either the theory of Central Summation or Gate Control, the details of which lie beyond the scope of this book. With this broader concept in mind, it is however necessary to consider those drugs the actions of which are known to be primarily analgesic. It is convenient to describe them under two headings, namely the powerful naturally occurring and synthetic narcotic analgesics, and the mild non-narcotic analgesics.

Powerful Analgesics

This group consists of the naturally occurring opiates, of which morphine is the most important, and various synthetic substances. All members are drugs of addiction, and produce depression of the central nervous system, affecting particularly the respiratory centre.

1. The Opiates and their Synthetic Derivatives

Opium, which is extracted from the opium poppy seed, contains many alkaloids of which the two most important are morphine and codeine.

Morphine (D.D.A.)

Morphine Hydrochloride B.P.
Morphine Sulphate B.P., U.S.P.

Pharmacology

(i) **Central Nervous System.**—The actions of morphine on the central nervous system are both depressant and stimulant. The depressant activity leads to analgesia, slowing of the respiratory rate, depression of the cough and laryngeal reflexes, and a reduced ability to concentrate and deal with complex thought processes. This may ultimately result in sleep. Its stimulant effects are evidenced by both its action on the chemo-receptor trigger zone which may lead to vomiting, and its action on the oculomotor nucleus producing constriction of the pupil which may become pin-point with over-dose. It produces a characteristic change in mood, inducing a state of relaxation, tranquillity and euphoria, which may however be disturbed by the nausea and vomiting which occasionally occurs, particularly if the patient is ambulant. On account of this euphoric effect, morphine and its derivatives are widely used as premedicants, often accompanied by an anti-emetic drug. In view of its other desirable premedicant proper-ties, hyoscine is often the anti-emetic of choice, and thus a combination of an opium alkaloid and hyoscine has rightly retained its popularity in premedication.

(ii) **Alimentary Tract**.—Although morphine increases smooth muscle tone, in the gut its predominant action is to depress co-ordinated peristalsis, although sphincteric tone is increased. Constipation is often the result.

(iii) **Bronchial Muscle.**—The tone in the bronchial smooth muscle is slightly increased; theoretically therefore the drug should be avoided in asthmatic and bronchitic subjects.

(iv) **Fate in the Body.**—About 90% of any dose is excreted by the kidneys after conjugation in the liver has taken place; thus, the drug should be used with caution in severe renal and liver disease. The usual duration of action is 4–6 hours. The drug and all its deriva-tives are relatively contraindicated in patients receiving M.A.O.I.s (page 8).

(v) **Addiction.**—The relation of morphine to this tragic phenomenon is well known and its special relevance in dentistry is discussed on page 11.

Presentation.—Ampoules of 1 ml–10 mg, 20 mg, 30 mg

Dose—5 mg to 15 mg by subcutaneous and intramuscular injection.
If given intravenously great care must be exercised in order to avoid undue respiratory depression.

Mixtures containing morphine

1. *Cyclimorph* 10
    Morphine 10 mg
    Cyclizine 50 mg

2. *Cyclimorph* 15
    Morphine 15 mg
    Cyclizine 50 mg

3. *Morpha*
    Morphine 30 mg
    T.H.A. 15 mg
    This mixture is used for the treatment of intractable pain

Papaveretum (D.D.A.)—(Trade names—Omnopon, Pantopon)

Ampoules of 1 ml–20 mg
Dose—10 mg–30 mg by subcutaneous and intramuscular injection
    Papaveretum is a mixture containing the water soluble alkaloids of opium, standardized to contain 50% anhydrous morphine. Its therapeutic efficacy is mainly due to its morphine content, although it is claimed that the other alkaloids present reduce the incidence of side-effects such as vomiting.

Nepenthe (D.D.A.)

    Nepenthe contains 0·91% of total opium alkaloids of which 0·84% exists as anhydrous morphine. The drug is effective both by mouth and by injection, and is a convenient way of prescribing morphine for children.
Dose—The traditional dosage is 1 minim per year of age plus 1 minim, but modern metric prescribing demands a standard of 1 ml as the adult dose with the appropriate weight adjustment for children. 1 ml contains 8·4 mg morphine.

Codeine Phosphate B.P.

Tablets B.P.—15 mg, **30 mg**, 60 mg
Linctus Codeine B.P.C.—15 mg in 5 ml
Dose—60 mg by mouth
    This naturally occuring alkaloid of opium is weaker in its actions than morphine, but has a relatively powerful depressant action on the cough reflex, thus being used mainly as an antitussive and mild analgesic. Sedation is poor, and nausea, vomiting and addiction are rare.

Di-hydrocodeine Bitartrate B.P.C.—(Trade name—DF118)

Ampoules—50 mg in 1 ml
Tablets B.P.C.—30 mg
Dose—30 mg–60 mg orally
        20 mg–50 mg by injection
    It is related chemically to codeine and its analgesic potency lies between that of codeine and morphine. (30 mg di-hydrocodeine is said to be equivalent in analgesic potency to 10 mg morphine.)
    Sedative effect, duration of action, respiratory depression, and nausea and vomiting are claimed to be less than that associated with morphine, but we have found nausea to be troublesome, particularly in the ambulant patient.

Diamorphine Hydrochloride B.P.C.—(Trade name—Heroin Hydrochloride)

    This is a very powerful analgesic with the main disadvantage that it is very likely to cause addiction; for this reason its use is forbidden by law in some countries. We consider that it has no place in dentistry.

Oxymorphone Hydrochloride (D.D.A.)—(Trade name—Numorphan (A.N.)

Dose—1 mg = 10 mg morphine

This is a morphine derivative which appears to have no clear-cut advantage over morphine.

2. Other Synthetic Analgesics

Pethidine Hydrochloride *B.P.* (*D.D.A.*)
Meperidine Hydrochloride U.S.P.
(Trade names—Demerol, Dolantal)

Pethidine shares many properties with both morphine and atropine, but is chiefly used as an alternative to morphine, and the main differences will be stressed in the following account of its action.

(i) **Central Nervous System.**—In equivalent analgesic dosage (100 mg pethidine = 10 mg morphine), pethidine does not exert so profound an hypnotic or euphoric effect as morphine; however, respiratory depression is equally marked. The stimulant effect on the vomiting centre is similar to that seen with morphine, but the pupils are not constricted in the same way—possibly due to its atropine-like action. Similarly, these atropine-like qualities render it particularly effective in pain associated with spasm of smooth muscle.

(ii) **Alimentary Tract.**—Unlike morphine it does not produce constipation.

(iii) **Respiratory System.**—Owing to its relaxant effect on established bronchospasm, it is the analgesic of choice in asthma, bronchitis, and emphysema. The cough reflex is not specifically depressed, but there is some decrease in secretions from the respiratory tract.

(iv) **Cardiovascular System.**—Pethidine is said to have a quinidine-like action on the heart, thus reducing irritability, but sometimes producing tachycardia. When given intravenously, pethidine may produce vasomotor depression leading to a fall in blood pressure; also the intravenous route is likely to produce local histamine release leading to a striking erythema superficial to the course of the vein. This effect may be considerably reduced by diluting the drug five to ten times before injection.

(v) **Fate in the Body.**—The drug is broken down in the liver prior to excretion. The rate of breakdown is reduced during pregnancy and in women on the 'pill'. However, far more serious from the practical point of view is the interference in breakdown and the adverse reaction which occurs with patients on monoamine oxidase inhibitors. Pethidine should not be administered to patients on these drugs (page 8).

(vi) **Addiction.**—The problem of addiction is serious, as with morphine and the other powerful narcotic drugs.

Presentation (D.D.A.)

Ampoules—50 mg in 1 ml. 100 mg in 2 ml
Tablets B.P.—25 mg, 50 mg
Dose—50 mg–150 mg by injection
        50 mg–150 mg by mouth

Pamergan

These preparations contain Promethazine and Pethidine, with or without Scopolamine or atropine, and are popular preparations for premedication.

(a) *P 100*
    Pethidine 100 mg
    Promethazine 50 mg

(b) *P 100/25*
    Pethidine 100 mg
    Promethazine 25 mg

(c) *AP 100/25*
    Pethidine 100 mg
    Promethazine 25 mg
    Atropine 0·6 mg

(d) *SP 50*
    Pethidine 50 mg
    Promethazine 50 mg
    Scopolamine 0·43 mg

(e) *SP 100*
    Pethidine 100 mg
    Promethazine 50 mg
    Scopolamine 0·43 mg

Fentanyl (A.N.), (D.D.A.)—(Trade name—Sublimase)

Ampoules—2·15 ml containing 0·05 mg per ml
Multidose vials—10 ml containing 0·05 mg per ml
Dose—0·05 mg–0·15 mg intravenously or intramuscularly

This drug is chemically similar to pethidine, 0·15 mg being equipotent in terms of analgesia to 100 mg pethidine. The drug can be usefully employed as a short acting intravenous analgesic agent, but facilities for counteracting respiratory depression should always be available.

Levorphanol Tartrate B.P. (D.D.A.)—(Trade name—Dromoran)

Ampoules—2 mg per ml
Tablets—1·5 mg
Dose—1·5 mg–4·5 mg orally

It has morphine-like analgesic properties with little sedative action and is therefore said to be suitable for the ambulant patient. The incidence of nausea and vomiting is claimed to be low.

Methadone Hydrochloride B.P., U.S.P. (D.D.A.)—(Trade name—Physeptone)

Ampoules—10 mg per ml
Tablets—5 mg
Linctus—2 mg in 5 ml

Dose—5 mg–10 mg by injection
   5 mg–10 mg by mouth 4 hourly

A synthetic analgesic at least as potent as morphine but producing less sedation. Its cough depressant action is well marked.

N.B.—Dextramoramide (Palfium) and Dipipanone (Pipadone) are both methadone derivatives.

Pentazocine (A.N.)—(Trade name—Fortral)

Ampoules—1 and 2 ml, 30 mg per ml
Tablets—25 mg (yellow film coated)
Dose—30 mg by injection

It is a strong analgesic (30 mg being equivalent to 10 mg morphine).

Clinical trials suggest that there is little liability to addiction, and the drug is claimed to exert less respiratory depressant effect than the other powerful analgesics; this effect cannot however be reversed by nalorphine or levalorphan. Clinical use of the drug, particularly when given intravenously, has shown consistent evidence of sympathetic stimulation—producing an occasional rise in systolic blood pressure of about 30 mm Hg. In addition, several cases of disorientation following its use have been reported.

Phenoperidine Hydrochloride (A.N.)—(Trade name—Operidine)

Ampoules—2·5 ml, 1 mg per ml
Dose—up to 1 mg by intravenous or intramuscular injection.

Long acting powerful analgesic similar to pethidine, with pronounced respiratory depressant effect.

B. POSTOPERATIVE DRUGS

Many of the drugs described under 'Premedicants' will be of value in the postoperative period. In addition, there is a special need in dentistry for mild analgesics.

Mild Analgesics

The majority of these analgesics also have antipyretic and anti-inflammatory properties. Their main sphere of usefulness is in the treatment of rheumatism and related conditions. Whatever the precise mechanism of pain relief, the main site of action appears to be peripheral at the site of the inflammatory process or injury, rather than central.

In this section we will deal with only those drugs which are of particular relevance in dentistry.

Acetyl Salicyclic Acid B.P., U.S.P.—Aspirin

Aspirin Soluble B.P. *Tablets* 300 mg
Dose—1–3 tablets four hourly

The actions of aspirin will be described in some detail, owing to its wide and sometimes prolonged use in the control of dental pain. It is not uncommon for dental patients to present for emergency treatment having taken large doses of aspirin over the preceding few days. Likewise, attempts to control the chronic pain from conditions such as 'dry socket' may result in the development of toxic side-effects, which therefore have a particular relevance in dentistry. The following are the main effects and side-effects of aspirin.

(i) **Analgesic Effect.**—The analgesic effect is particularly valuable in the treatment of headache, and the relief of pain from teeth, bones, joints, muscles and all inflammatory lesions. Relief from visceral pain is, on the other hand, poor. Analgesia is confined to a specific dose range, above which toxic side-effects occur, unaccompanied by any increase in pain relief.

(ii) **Antipyretic Effect.**—In febrile conditions, the action of aspirin on the temperature-regulating centre results in vasodilatation and sweating, associated with an increase in heat-loss through the skin, with a consequent lowering of body temperature.

(iii) **Anti-inflammatory Effect.**—This effect is well recognized and much utilized, but the precise mechanism is complex, controversial, and beyond the scope of this book.

(iv) **Metabolic Effects.**—Salicylates interfere with various enzyme actions and produce an increase in oxygen consumption. Respiration may be stimulated, and respiratory alkalosis sometimes results. The blood-sugar level may be lowered by moderate dosage, a fact to be borne in mind when treating the patient who has not been able to eat normally owing to severe dental pain. With high dosage, the blood-sugar level may be raised. Uric acid excretion is increased with high dosage.

(v) **Hypoprothrombinaemia.**—When dosage is in excess of 5 g daily, the risk of haemorrhage due to lowered prothrombin activity must be considered. Should such haemorrhage occur, it may be treated by Vitamin K, which may be administered as Phytomenadione (Konakion) 10 mg by intramuscular or intravenous injection.

(vi) **Gastro-intestinal Disorders.**—The tendency of aspirin to cause damage to the gastric mucosa, and bleeding which is usually gastric in origin, is well known. These effects are particularly pronounced in some 5–10% of the population, and aspirin-containing compounds should be avoided in subjects known to be sensitive and also in haemophiliacs (page 285). The incidence of these side-effects is reduced if the soluble form is used, well diluted.

(vii) **Overdose and Sensitivity Reactions.**—In addition to any of the above side-effects, the following signs and symptoms may be considered indicative of overdose: nausea, vomiting, tinnitus, deafness, headache, restlessness, mental confusion, sweating and hyperpnoea. Specific sensitivity, unrelated to dosage, may occur in some subjects, causing bronchospasm, urticaria, angioneurotic oedema and rhinorrhoea.

The chief aspirin-containing compounds are listed at the end of this chapter.

Mefenamic Acid (A.N.)—(Trade name—Ponstan (Kapseals))

Dose—250 mg–500 mg

This drug is similar in analgesic potency to aspirin, and also possesses anti-inflammatory and antipyrexial properties. Side-effects are rare, the drug being less likely than aspirin to cause gastrointestinal disturbances, with the exception of diarrhoea, which may contraindicate its use in susceptible subjects.

Prolonged treatment should be avoided owing to its long term depressant effect on bone marrow.

Phenacetin B.P., Acetophenetidin U.S.A.

Tablets—300 mg

Dose—300–600 mg

Phenacetin is an aniline derivative which possesses mild analgesic and anti-pyrexial properties. It is less liable to cause gastric irritation than aspirin, but occasionally results in renal damage, anaemia and methaemoglobinaemia. As a result of these rare, but serious complications, it is generally considered that para-cetamol (its active metabolite) should be used in its place.

Paracetamol B.P.—(Trade name—Panadol)

Tablets—500 mg

Elixir Paediatric B.P.C.—120 mg in 5 ml

Dose—0·5–1 g

Paracetamol is the active metabolite of phenacetin, does not cause methaemo-globinaemia, and is generally thought to be less toxic.

Mild Analgesic Mixtures and Preparations

The following list is not comprehensive, but most of the commonly used (U.K.) products are included.

(a) B.P.C. Mixtures

  (i) **Aspirin and Phenacetin Tablets B.P.C.**
     Aspirin (225 mg), phenacetin (150 mg)

 (ii) **Aspirin Compound Tablets B.P.C.**
     Aspirin (225 mg), phenacetin (150 mg), caffeine (30 mg)

(iii) **Aspirin, Phenacetin and Codeine Soluble Tablets B.P.**
     (Tabs. Cod. Co.)
     Aspirin (250 mg), phenacetin (250 mg), codeine phosphate (8 mg)

(b) Proprietory Preparations

  (i) **Analgin.**—Aspirin (194 mg), phenacetin (233 mg), codeine (4·85 mg), caffeine (9·7 mg)

 (ii) **Codis.**—Aspirin (500 mg), codeine phosphate (8 mg)

(iii) **Distalgesic.**—Dextropropoxyphene—a methadone-like analgesic (32·5 mg), para-cetamol (325 mg)

(iv) **Norgesic.**—Orphenadrine (35 mg) has specific action in the relief of muscle spasm and is said to produce euphoria and act as a mild anti-histamine.
     Paracetamol (450 mg)

 (v) **Paynocil.**—Aspirin (600 mg), glycine (300 mg)

(vi) **Solprin** (soluble aspirin).—Aspirin (300 mg), calcium carbonate (100 mg), citric acid (30 mg)

(vii) **Veganin.**—Aspirin (250 mg), phenacetin (250 mg), codeine (10 mg)

C. ANTIDOTES TO THE RESPIRATORY DEPRESSANT DRUGS

These antidotes can be considered in two distinct groups. Firstly, those which have a specific competitive action against morphine and most of the powerful synthetic analgesics including pethidine; this group also, to some extent, interferes with the analgesic action of the drugs involved. Secondly, those drugs which are non-specific central cerebral stimulants.

Specific Morphine (and Synthetic Analgesic) Antagonists

Levallorphan Tartrate B.P., U.S.P.—(Trade name—Lorfan)
Dose—1 mg–2 mg by intravenous or intramuscular injection

Levallorphan is related chemically to levorphanol (dromoran), and when used alone has both analgesic and respiratory depressant properties. However, when given to a patient who has respiratory depression as a result of morphine or certain other analgesics, the drug acts as a powerful specific antidote, both reversing the respiratory depression, and modifying the analgesic action. The practice of premixing pethidine and levallorphan (as in 'Pethilorfan') appears to be unwarranted.

Nalorphine Hydrobromide B.P.—(Trade name—Lethidrone)
Dose—2 mg–5 mg by intravenous injection

Nalorphine is chemically related to morphine, and when used alone has a respiratory depressant, but little analgesic action. The respiratory depression which follows morphine and pethidine overdose usually takes the form of a marked reduction in respiratory rate; this depressant effect is dramatically reversed by the intravenous administration of nalorphine.

Non-specific Respiratory Stimulants

Amiphenazole Hydrochloride (A.N.)—(Trade name—Daptazole)
Dose—150 mg intravenously

Amiphenazole was at one time thought to minimize the depressant effect of morphine, but it is now recognized that it is purely a cerebral stimulant, restoring wakefulness and temporarily reversing respiratory depression—irrespective of the cause of that depression.

Bemegride B.P.—(Trade name—Megimide)
Dose—25 mg–50 mg intravenously

Bemegride is a non-specific central stimulant similar to daptazole.

Nikethamide B.P.—(Trade names—Anacardone, Coramine, Corediol, Corvotone)
Dose—250 mg–1 g (i.e. 1–4 ml) intravenously.

Nikethamide is a cerebral stimulant and analeptic. Its stimulant effect on the respiratory centre is thought to be mediated through the chemoreceptors in the carotid and aortic bodies. It is probably the least likely of the analeptics to produce convulsions, and is thus generally considered to be the safest.

Vanillic Acid—(Trade names—Vandid, Ethamivan)

Dose—5–10 ml of 5% solution intravenously

Vanillic acid is a respiratory stimulant and analeptic similar to nikethamide.

Tacrine Hydrochloride (A.N.) —(Trade names—Romotal, T.H.A.)

Dose—30 mg–60 mg

Tacrine has been used as an antidote to the depressant effect of morphine, but is properly classified as a non-specific respiratory stimulant with marked anticholinesterase activity, thus prolonging the action of suxamethonium. It may produce vomiting.

RECOMMENDED READING

1. Pharmacology

(*a*) LAURENCE, D. R. (1966) *Clinical Pharmacology*. London: Churchill.

(*b*) WALTON, J. G., & THOMPSON, J. W. (1970) *Pharmacology for the Dental Practitioner*. London: B.D.A.

(*c*) WOOD-SMITH, F. G., STEWART, H. C. & VICKERS, M. D. (1968) *Drugs in Anaesthetic Practice*. London: Butterworth.

2. Theory and Management of Pain

KATZ, J. (1970) *Scientific Foundations of Anaesthesia*, Section II., Ed. C. Scurr and S. Feldman. London: Heinemann. p. 226.

CHAPTER THREE

EQUIPMENT

In this chapter we propose to describe the equipment which we routinely use, rather than attempt to provide a comprehensive survey of all the equipment available.

ANAESTHETIC MACHINES

Introduction

All anaesthetic machines—other than those in common use in out-patient dentistry—are of the continuous flow variety. That is to say that gases are delivered to the patient via accurate flow-meters, the flow being continuous and measured in litres per minute. The traditional dental anaesthetic machine is of the intermittent or demand type, but recently a fuller appreciation of the drawbacks and inaccuracies commonly inherent in many of these traditional machines has led to the increasing popularity of various models of continuous flow apparatus in dentistry. In the following account, we will describe the broad principles governing the design and intelligent use of each type of machine and also an example of one such machine in detail. Our choice is arbitrary, and not based upon any alleged superiority over other similar designs.

Intermittent Flow Machines

Gases, that is to say nitrous oxide and oxygen, which are stored in cylinders under considerable pressure (pages 93, 98) are led from these cylinders via reducing valves to a mixing chamber and hence to the patient. The relative proportions of the constituent gases in the resultant mixture depend upon the setting of the mixture-control by the anaesthetist, and the accuracy of the mixture-control mechanism. The rate of total gas flow to the patient is, however, only partly under the anaesthetist's control, being also dependent upon the patient's own respiratory activity. The typical intermittent flow machine is designed in such a way that, if the nitrous oxide and oxygen cylinders are turned on and the gas delivery pressure lever or dial is set at zero, no gases will flow from the mixing chamber unless a patient is attached to the outflow end of the machine, and then only when that patient applies a negative pressure to the outlet, i.e. breathes in. Thus, the machine used in this way, can properly be described as a 'demand' system, for gases are supplied to the patient only on demand, and only in such quantities as the patient's respiratory activity dictates. All flow ceases during expiration, the expired gases escaping into the atmosphere through a one-way expiratory valve situated on the outlet limb of the machine, close to the patient. The proportions of nitrous oxide and oxygen delivered to the patient are controlled by a lever or dial which adjusts the relative proportions in the mixing chamber. Such a machine, if used in the way described, would in many ways represent the ideal system for the patient breathing spontaneously, economy being maximal since the total gas flow is always sufficient for, but never exceeds, the patient's needs. Unfortunately, in practice, no intermittent flow machine can be satisfactorily used in this ideal manner at all times. There are two major drawbacks.

(a) The resistance of all the working parts, including the outlet tubing and nasal mask, is so great that if the gas delivery (pressure) control is set at zero, the inspiratory effort required for the machine to satisfy the patient's demand is considerable; too great, in fact, to allow comfortable spontaneous respiration to proceed. Thus, in practice, the gas delivery control is never set at zero, but rather at a setting which would provide a positive flow of gases from the machine when not attached to the patient. If a patient is now attached, the flow-rate of gases will increase during inspiration, and decrease during expiration, so that the sytem is now one in which the flow of gases is continuous, but waxes and wanes with the patient's respiratory cycle, being maximum during inspiration and minimal (or possibly ceasing) during expiration. The machine is thus commonly used in a manner which combines continuous with intermittent flow. The economy of such a system depends upon the setting of the gas flow control. These controls are traditionally calibrated in millimetres of mercury pressure which, of course, is a scale with which it is neither possible nor meaningful to attempt to measure the flow-rate of gases. Thus the traditional calibration system provides the administrator with no accurate information as to the flow-rate of gases, and in practice almost always results in the use of excessive flow-rates, so that the intermittent method is usually a wasteful one—far removed from the economy envisaged in the theoretical concept of a true demand system. The method must, perhaps, also be criticized for having allowed the purely 'dental' anaesthetist to be brought up to believe that gas flows are measured in millimetres pressure of mercury rather than in litres per minute.

(b) The mixture-control mechanism is inaccurate—sometimes wildly so—in the majority of intermittent flow machines manufactured earlier than the Walton Five A setting of, say, 20% oxygen may result in the delivery of a mixture containing 20% oxygen at a given setting of the gas flow pressure control, but either decreasing or increasing that pressure will often result in considerable variation of the oxygen content at the same mixture-control setting. Thus it is never possible for the administrator to be certain whether he is actually delivering to the patient more, less or the intended percentage of oxygen. Such a situation is clearly not acceptable in the context of modern—possibly prolonged—dental anaesthesia, and whilst it is true that most of the older machines 'over-deliver' oxygen, the reverse is sometimes the case, and the results could be dangerous.

Since the intermittent flow machine is capable of delivering very large flow-rates, it is not necessary to incorporate a reservoir bag in the circuit, the machine itself being able to meet the patient's peak inspiratory needs. For reasons discussed on page 212 we believe, however, that it is advantageous to use such a bag, but in any event, no anaesthetic machine should be marketed or supplied which does not enable the anaesthetist readily to inflate the patient's lungs; since the most satisfactory way of doing this is by manual compression of a reservoir bag, we deprecate the supply of any anaesthetic machine in which the bag is presented as 'an optional extra' rather than as an essential component of the machine, albeit one which may be switched out of circuit when not required. At low pressure settings, the presence in circuit of a reservoir bag might be expected to lead to rebreathing, but in practice a pressure-setting of 5 mmHg or more appears to prevent it.

The gases may be passed through a vaporizer containing a volatile liquid anaesthetic such as halothane or trichlorethylene, and such vaporizers are usually sited between the machine and the reservoir bag.

There are many models of intermittent flow machines available for purchase, and we will here describe only the Walton Five as being representative of a modern version of this type of machine. We choose the Walton Five because it has been subjected to the most rigorous series of performance tests by an independent observer, and because it is the most widely used in the United Kingdom.

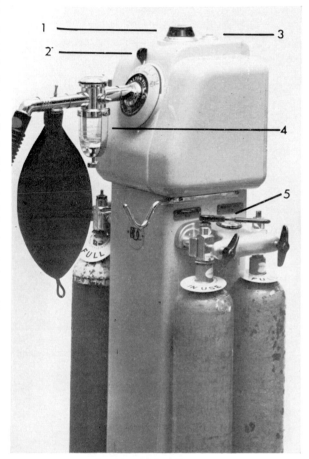

FIG. 1.—Walton Five

1 Pressure control.
2 Mixture control.
3 Emergency oxygen.
4 Goldman vaporizer.
5 Ratchet spanner.

The Walton Five (B.O.C.) (Figs. 1 and 2.)

(a) *Cylinders and Spanner*

The machine normally carries two oxygen cylinders of 24 cu. ft. (0·68 m³) capacity each and two nitrous oxide of 400 gallons (1818 litres). The apparatus may, however, be coupled without modification directly to a piped gas supply, using special yoke-adaptors. A ratchet-type spanner for opening and closing cylinders easily, is recommended. (Fig. 1.)

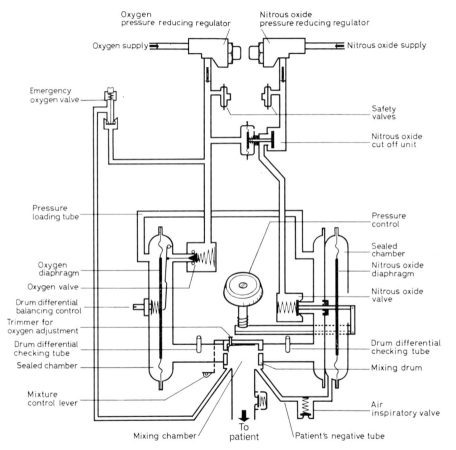

Fig. 2.—Schematic presentation of Walton Five apparatus

Oxygen and nitrous oxide pressure gauges are built in to their respective cylinder yokes. The oxygen gauge gives an accurate indication of the cylinder contents, since the pressure falls *pari passu* with the diminishing quantity of gas. The nitrous oxide pressure gauge, in contrast, only commences to fall on exhaustion of the entire liquid contents of the cylinder, and thereafter the cylinder will become rapidly exhausted.

TABLE IX.—*Walton Five Flow-rates*

PRESSURE INDICATION mmHg	FLOW-RATE Litres per Minute	
	Oro-nasal attachment	Corrugated tubing with face mask
5	20	40
10	50	100
15	80	130
20	110	140

(b) *Pressure (Flow-Rate) Control*

The range of the pressure control is from 0–20 mmHg, and Table IX gives some indication of the flow-rate at various pressure settings.

(c) *Mixture-Control Lever*

This lever is operated on a scale extending from 0 to 100% oxygen content of the delivered mixture.

(d) *Reservoir Bag*

This is mounted with a short lever which enables it to be switched in or out of circuit, but it should always be on the machine for the purpose of resuscitation.

(e) *Safety Devices*

(i) *Automatic Cut-Off Valves.*—If the oxygen pressure, as indicated by the gauge, falls to zero, the nitrous oxide supply is automatically cut off, thus preventing the inadvertent administration of 100% nitrous oxide. The gas mixture delivered by the apparatus remains constant until the moment of cut-off. It should be noted that if the mixture control is set to 100% nitrous oxide, the oxygen pressure inside the apparatus will keep the nitrous oxide cut-out valve open and operative even though the oxygen cylinder itself is exhausted or turned off. In such circumstances, it would be possible to draw 100% nitrous oxide from the apparatus. However, as soon as the mixture control is moved away from the 100% nitrous oxide position, the oxygen is gradually used up at the indicated mixture percentage setting until it is exhausted, at which point the nitrous oxide supply is automatically shut off.

The oxygen supply likewise cuts out in the event of nitrous oxide supply failure although the emergency oxygen control continues to function. This arrangement could prove to be a disadvantage under circumstances in which nitrous oxide was not available, but in which a continuous supply of oxygen was required without recourse to the high flow-rate associated with the emergency by-pass.

(ii) *Emergency Air Inspiratory Valve.*—An air inspiratory valve, adjusted to open at negative pressures slightly in excess of those normally required to draw gas from the apparatus, operates to admit air if, for any reason, the gas mixture is cut off.

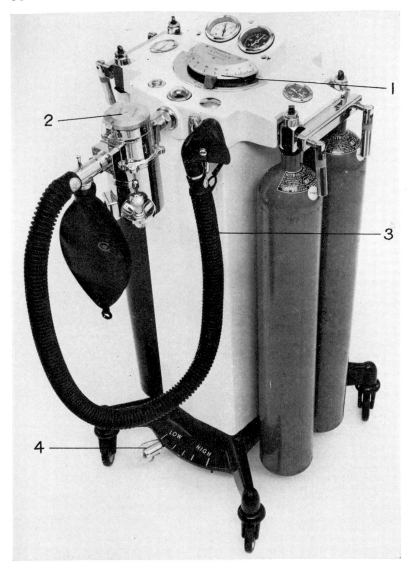

FIG. 3.—The A.E. (Cyprane) intermittent flow machine. 1. Mixture control. 2. Cyprane fluothane vaporizer. 3. Elephant tubing carrying Goldman nasal mask. 4. Foot operated pressure control

NOTE.—This machine is normally supplied without reservoir bag. We recommend that a bag should always be attached between outlet and tubing before use

(iii) *Emergency Oxygen Control.*—A button marked 'Emergency Oxygen' is situated on the top of the head casing behind the pressure control knob. When this button is pressed, a copious flow of oxygen passes to the breathing attachment regardless of mixture or pressure control settings.

The mechanism of these safety devices is illustrated in the circuit-diagram. (Fig. 2)

The A.E. (Cyprane) (Fig. 3)

This machine is similar in principle to the Walton V, but the pressure control may be either hand or foot operated. A non-return valve to prevent rebreathing is incor-

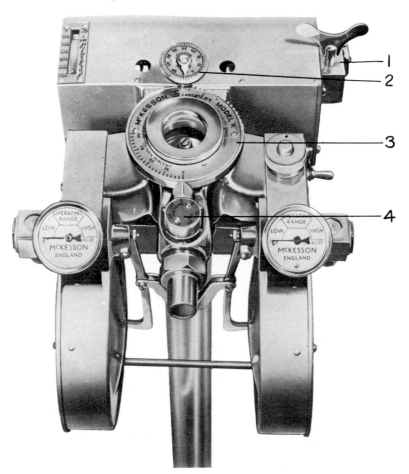

FIG. 4.—The McKesson Simplor. 1. Casement enclosing partial rebreathing bellows. 2. Fine oxygen percentage control. 3. Coarse oxygen percentage control. 4. Pressure Control

porated in the circuit, and the machine is regrettably supplied without a reservoir bag unless one is specially requested.

The McKesson Range (Figs. 4 and 5)

These machines operate in a similar manner to other intermittent flow models, but are characterized by the fact that the operating range of gas pressures is regulated at 60 lb/sq. in as compared with the Walton Five range of 7–11 lb/sq. in. We believe that in practice this influences neither the efficiency nor the clinical usage of the machines. Some of the older models carry proportional rebreathing devices, the use of which we do not recommend.

Continuous Flow Machines

Gases such as nitrous oxide, oxygen, carbon dioxide, cyclopropane, helium, ethylene are led from cylinders, through appropriate reducing valves when necessary,

A.A.D.—3

to accurate flow-meters where the exact flow-rate to the patient is under the manual control of the anaesthetist. These gases may also be passed through a vaporizer, or series of vaporizers, containing volatile liquid anaesthetic. The flow-rate of gases to the patient is, under normal conditions, entirely within the control and continuous observation of the anaesthetist, and it is therefore his responsibility to ensure that an adequate total flow-rate to satisfy the patient's demands under varying conditions is, at all times, supplied. Flow-rates in excess of the patient's needs are wasteful but not harmful. In addition to ensuring an adequate total flow-rate, the anaesthetist has also to arrange that the mixture of gases delivered to the patient at no time contains less than 20% oxygen.

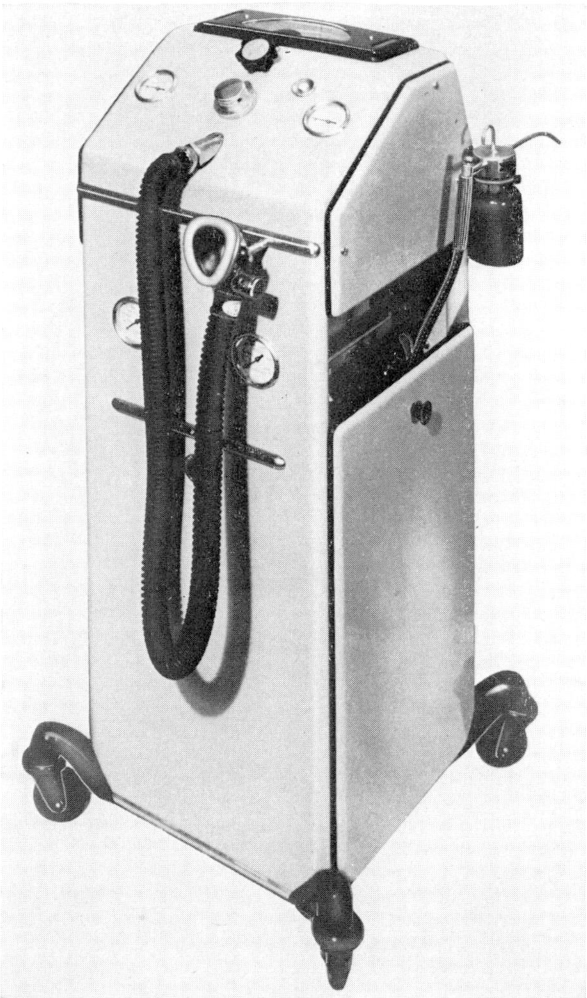

In order to assess the minimum permissible flow-rate, it is necessary to have some knowledge of elementary respiratory physiology. The normal resting adult inspires— and thus expires also—some 500 ml of air with each breath; this quantity is known as the *Tidal Volume*. The respiratory rate of such a subject is some 16 breaths per minute. Thus the total fresh gas needs over one minute are $500 \times 16 = 8000$ ml, and in this case the *Minute Volume* would be said to be 8 litres per minute. (See page 273 for children's chart). If the subject is allowed to breathe only from a system of fresh gas supply, into which supplementary air cannot be drawn from the atmosphere, on

Fig. 5.—The McKesson "Anesthesor Special"

superficial consideration, it would appear essential to provide him with a total flow of fresh gases at least as great as his minute volume. For if his minute volume exceeds the fresh gas supply, only part of the subject's expired gases will be blown off to atmosphere through the expiratory valve, for part will be expired into the anaesthetic circuit and rebreathed together with the inadequate fresh gas supply at the next breath. In practice, however, when a patient breathes spontaneously under stable anaesthetic conditions, using a standard Magill (Mapleson 1) circuit (e.g. from the Salisbury machine—page 61), it has been observed that a fresh gas flow of only two thirds the patient's measured minute volume suffices to maintain both the arterial oxygen and carbon dioxide tensions at normal levels. This observation is explained by the postulate that the first one third of the expiratory volume consists of dead space air (which is non-respiratory) and is breathed back into the circuit, whilst the last two thirds represents true alveolar air and is blown into the atmosphere via the expiratory valve, provided that valve is correctly designed as regards spring loading. The next inspiration results in the inhalation of a mixture containing two thirds fresh gases and one third dead space contents of acceptable gaseous composition. In the dental anaesthetic of short duration, the administrator would be well advised to ignore these theoretical considerations, and at all times ensure a fresh gas flow-rate greater than the patient's minute volume. Rebreathing in excess of that described above is always undesirable unless special measures are taken to compensate for its three peculiar characteristics. Firstly expired air contains carbon dioxide, so that unless a soda lime cannister is incorporated in the circuit to absorb this gas, the concentration of carbon dioxide in the circuit—hence in the lungs—hence in the blood-stream will build up insidiously and eventually exert its characteristic harmful, and finally fatal effects (page 161). Secondly, since the subject is continuously inspiring a mixture containing fresh gases and expired air, the concentration of oxygen inspired will be less than that delivered in the fresh gas mixture. This potential source of hypoxia must be eliminated by an appropriate increase over and above 20% in that fresh gas mixture. Thirdly, if a powerful volatile supplement such as halothane is in use, it must be remembered that, since the expired air will contain halothane, a slow but considerable build-up of that agent's concentration within the circuit is possible. With these special considerations in mind, we believe that anaesthetic techniques which encourage or allow rebreathing have no place in routine out-patient dental anaesthesia, unless the administrator possesses very special skill and experience in their use. Thus, the first requisite when using a continuous flow machine is that the total flow of fresh gases per minute should be in excess of the patient's expected minute volume. This principle is sound, but represents an oversimplification, for the subject's respiratory needs fluctuate within the time period of a minute. Let us assume, for the sake of arithmetical simplicity, that a particular subject has a tidal volume of 500 ml, a respiratory rate of 20 breaths per minute, and hence a minute volume of 10 litres per minute. Each breath, therefore, occupies 3 seconds, of which approximately one second is spent in inspiration, two in expiration. The gases are flowing into the lungs only during inspiration, so that although the flow-rate required to supply these needs is 10 litres during one whole minute, in each 3-second period there will be no flow of gases into the lungs during the 2-second expiratory phase, so that during that one-second inspiratory phase, gases will flow into the lungs at the rate, not of 10, but of 30 litres per minute. The one-second inspiratory flow does not even take place at a steady rate, so that for a fraction of a second, gases will have to flow into the lungs at a rate in excess of 30 litres per minute in order to satisfy the needs of the peak inspiratory flow. Fortunately, a reservoir bag provides a simple method of making these large flow-rates available for short periods of time, without the overall minute volume requirements of the subject being exceeded. The bag is incorporated in the circuit between the flow-meters and vaporizer on the one hand, and the expiratory valve and patient on the other (Fig. 6). Thus, during expiration, there being no demand for fresh gases, these enter the reservoir bag at the steady rate of 10 litres per minute, so that during the ensuing inspiration there are available to the patient not only gases flowing at a steady rate of 10 litres per minute from the machine, but also the reservoir of fresh

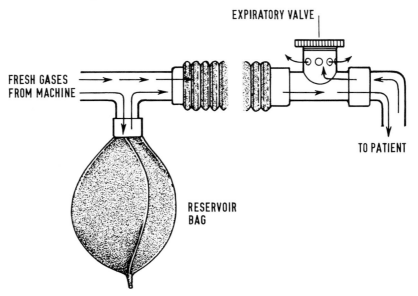

FIG. 6.—Semi-open Magill (Mapleson 1) Circuit

gases which has accumulated in the bag during expiration. So long as the reservoir bag offers no resistance to the entry of fresh gases into it during expiration, and the total flow-rate of these gases is adequate to prevent rebreathing of alveolar air, the continuous flow machine is quite capable of meeting the patient's fluctuating demands, but the foregoing account must make clear the absolute necessity for the incorporation of a reservoir bag in any continuous flow circuit.

All anaesthetic machines in common use outside dentistry are continuous flow in type. Many of them are too bulky and unnecessarily complex for routine use in the dental surgery, and recently several models have been marketed which can be conveniently used in the dental out-patient environment. First of these was the Salisbury, which we will now describe in detail.

The Salisbury (M. & I. E.) (Fig. 7)

In the unmodified dental model the rotameter control unit is linked by a cross line indicating flow-rates in 5 positions, each of which will ensure a 75%/25% nitrous oxide/oxygen mixture at the appropriate flow-rate. The maximum flow-rate able to be achieved is 12 litres/min (9 litres nitrous oxide/3 litres oxygen). The flow of both nitrous oxide and oxygen is fed into the rear of the rotameter control unit via copper tubing assemblies, from pre-set reducing valves.

A separate fine adjustment control is provided to regulate the exact flow of each

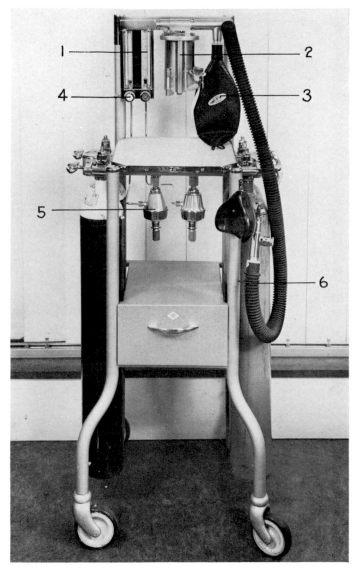

FIG. 7.—The Salisbury dental anaesthetic machine incorporating modified flow-meter block as described in text giving oxygen 5 litres, nitrous oxide 15 litres. 1. Rotameter control unit. 2. Fluothane vaporizer. 3. Reservoir bag. 4. Emergency oxygen lever. 5. Oxygen reducing valve. 6. Elephant tube carrying expiratory valve and face-mask

gas. An emergency oxygen lever which, when in the horizontal position, will deliver an oxygen flow of 20 litres per minute is available for use. It must be appreciated that the nitrous oxide and halothane units should be turned off when this device is in use.

A temperature compensated vaporizer for the administration of halothane as an inhalational supplement is fitted to the outlet of the rotameter control unit. The original vaporizer has no intermediate control position; it is either ON or OFF. In the ON position a 2% concentration of halothane will be delivered to the patient and this 2% concentration is accurate over a wide variation in room temperature.

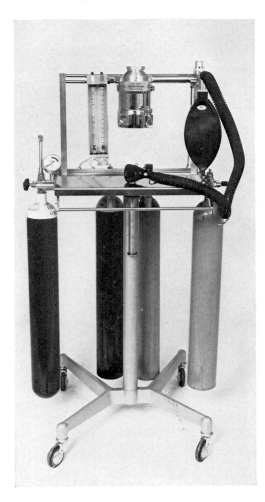

FIG. 8.—The Mini-Boyle with Fluotec Mark 3

The halothane vaporizer is actuated by a thermostat which ensures that over a temperature range of 40–100°F (3–38°C) a consistent concentration of 2% throughout the entire range of flow-rates is made possible. The capacity of the halothane vaporizer is 150 ml and the contents can be observed from a sight glass window after filling through the removable filler situated at the front of the unit. A drain plug is fitted at the base of the vaporizer to facilitate the removal of halothane after use.

The foregoing description relates to the original standard model. We recommend the following modifications on the grounds that they will widen the scope of the machine.

(a) *Flow-Meters*

A maximum total flow-rate of 12 litres per minute will occasionally be insufficient to meet the minute volume requirements of a large, nervous adult during inhalation induction. Moreover, higher flow-rates are sometimes useful when using the 'air replacement' method of inhalation induction described for children (page 225). Indeed, an observant parent might well notice that the anaesthetist has set flow-meters well above the 'Child' marking on the facing. We therefore recommend that the flow-meter block should be replaced by one without markings and able to deliver 15 litres/minute nitrous oxide, and 5 litres/minute oxygen.

(b) *Vaporizer*

A vaporizer which delivers either 0% or 2% halothane is unsatisfactory, and it is essential to have 0·5% gradations. Also, a vaporizer which enables the experienced anaesthetist to use up to 4% halothane is of value.

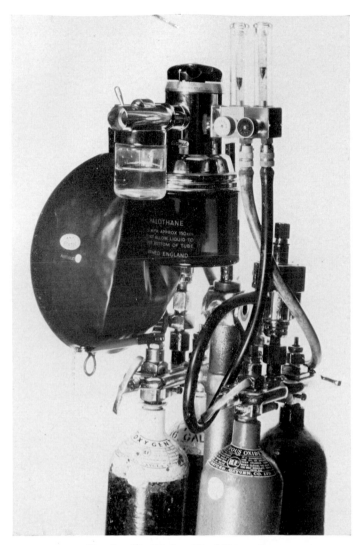

FIG. 9.—The Medrex Head (Airmed)

NOTE.—The Rowbotham vaporizer replaces the Medrex bottle when in general use

The other continuous flow machines commonly used in the dental surgery are the following.

The Mini-Boyle (B.O.C.) (Fig. 8)

The Mini-Boyle has similar characteristics to the Salisbury, and if supplied with a 4% halothane vaporizer and rotameters to deliver 15 litre of nitrous oxide and 5 litre of oxygen, it is very suitable for dental anaesthesia. It is, however, slightly more bulky than the Salisbury, which may be a disadvantage in a small dental surgery.

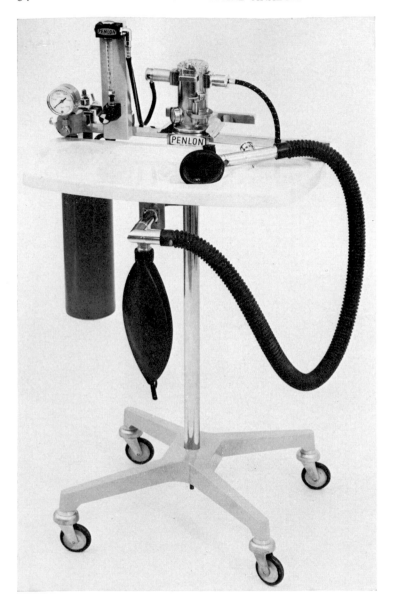

FIG. 10.—The Latham Entonox machine *Note*: Oxford Vaporizer

The Medrex (Airmed) (Fig. 9)

The Medrex Head is a compact, portable continuous flow machine, which can be mounted on any convenient cylinder stand. We recommend that the circuit is not used with the vaporizer set at 'Patient's Breath Only' in the manner described in the manufacturer's literature, unless due attention is paid to the serious disadvantages which may be associated with the prolonged use of a rebreathing technique. We suggest that the large vaporizer bottle supplied should be kept out of the circuit and replaced by a small vaporizer as in Fig. 9.

The Latham 'Entonox' (Penlon) (Figs. 10 and 11)

This machine is adapted for use with 'Entonox' cylinders (page 101), so that patients may be anaesthetized with 50% nitrous oxide/50% oxygen, delivered from a single cylinder through a single flow-meter. The machine incorporates an Oxford Miniature Vaporizer, which can be calibrated for use with either halothane or trichlorethylene.

Wall-Mounted Anaesthetic Head (Fig 12)

Bulky cylinders within the dental surgery can be avoided by the use of suitable wall mountings for most of the standard rotameter (flow-meter) blocks. Fig. 12 illustrates one such example, the gaseous inflow being piped from large cylinders sited outside the surgery.

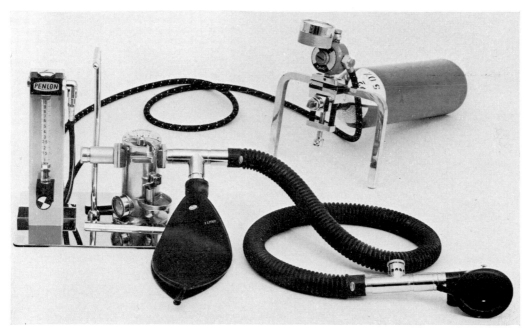

FIG. 11.—Entonox Machine Portable Model

The Quantiflex (Cyprane) (Fig. 13)

This machine, which was originally designed for the administration of 'Relative Analgesia' (page 252), has now been successfully modified to provide anaesthesia, and incorporates the following usefultur feaes:—

(a) The oxygen control valve is adjusted to give a minimum oxygen flow of 3 l/min; and the nitrous oxide valve to give a maximum flow of 10 l/min; thus the minimum oxygen concentration obtainable is approximately 23%.

(b) A single ON and OFF switch supplies both oxygen and nitrous oxide to the flow-meters. This means that the gas flows can be pre-set and turned on and off when required.

(c) An oxygen 'fail safe' system prevents gases from flowing unless oxygen pressure is

A.A.D.—3*

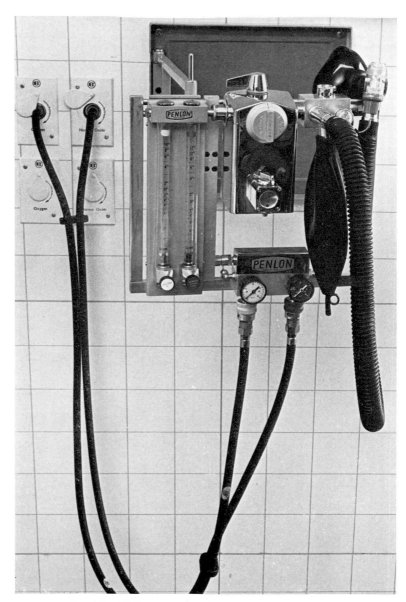

FIG. 12.—Wall mounted machine using piped gas supply
Note:—Abingdon Halothane Vaporizer

available. As the oxygen pressure falls, the nitrous oxide is automatically reduced so as to maintain the pre-set oxygen percentage.

(d) An air intake valve provides the patient with air should the gas flow fail.

VAPORIZERS
Low Efficiency

These vaporizers are designed to deliver low concentrations of volatile agents, but the precise concentration will vary with the flow-rate and temperature. It should be noted that as the administration proceeds, the temperature of the vaporizer and liquid anaesthetic within it will fall, and thus at a given control setting, the vapour concentration delivered will gradually decrease. This effect may be minimized by the use of some form of water jacket, as in the Oxford Miniature Vaporizer (Figs. 10 and 11).

Goldman (Fig. 14)

This vaporizer is designed to deliver both halothane and trichlorethylene in safe concentrations. The approximate concentrations delivered are shown in Tables X and XI.

TABLE X.—*Goldman Vaporizer. Halothane*
Halothane percentages by volume (approximate)
Nominal liquid temperature 20° C

Drum position	Gas flow-rate		
	2 litres/ minute	8 litres/ minute	30 litres/ minute
1	0·1%	0·1%	0·1%
2	0·5%	1·0%	1·0%
ON	1·5%	2·5%	1·5%

Rowbotham (Fig. 15)

This vaporizer was originally designed for the administration of trichlorethylene, but may be used for halothane, in which case it is advisable to calibrate each vaporizer individually. Table XII shows the results of one such calibration.

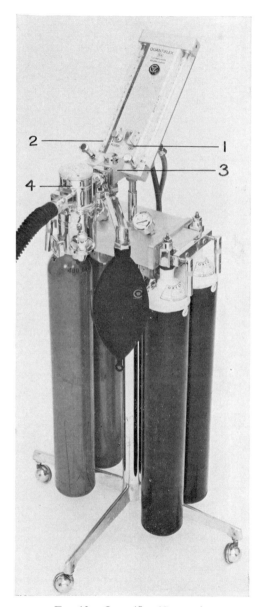

FIG. 13.—Quantiflex (Cyprane)
Note:—1. Switch controlling flow of gases to both flow-meters. 2. Emergency oxygen button. 3. Air intake valve. 4. Cyprane vaporizer

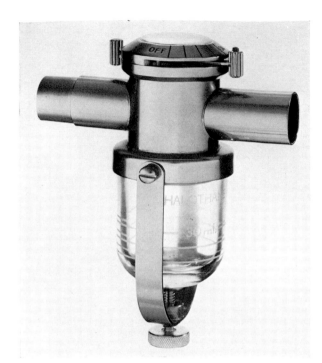

FIG. 14.—The Goldman Vaporizer

FIG. 15.—The Rowbotham Vaporizer

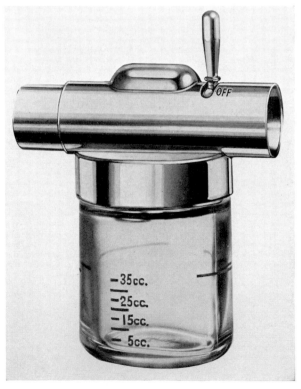

TABLE XI.—*Goldman Vaporizer. Trilene*

Trichloroethylene percentages by volume (approximate)
Nominal liquid temperature 20° C

Drum position	Gas flow-rate		
	2 *litres/minute*	8 *litres/minute*	30 *litres/minute*
1	0·1%	0·1%	0·1%
2	0·2%	0·5%	0·5%
ON	0·5%	1·0%	0·5%

TABLE XII.—*Rowbotham Vaporizer* (*Example for halothane*)

10*l/min* flow-rate at 25·5° C

Setting	1	2	3	4	5	ON
% Halothane	0	0	1	2·5	3	3·2

McKesson (Fig. 16)

Table XIII shows the approximate concentration of halothane delivered.

The Oxford Miniature Vaporizer (Figs. 10 and 11)

This vaporizer is incorporated in the Latham Entonox machine. It is calibrated for either halothane or trichlorethylene, a maximum concentration of 3·5% halothane being obtainable. The vaporizer is not temperature-compensated, but contains in its base a small sealed water filled compartment which acts as a heat reservoir and buffer, thus ensuring minimum fall in vapour concentrations during prolonged use.

TABLE XIII.—*The McKesson Halothane Vaporizer Mark II*

The figures quoted below describe the average concentrations of halothane vapour obtained with flow-rates of around 8 litres per minute which corresponds approximately to 5 mm pressure on the McKesson machines. The figures are given with the vaporizer dial knob at the various settings.

Dial Reading	Halothane percentage
1	0·05%
2	1·05%
3	1·84%
ON	2·8%

High Efficiency

These vaporizers are fully compensated to deliver a consistent percentage of halothane at each control setting, irrespective of the prevailing temperature and flow-

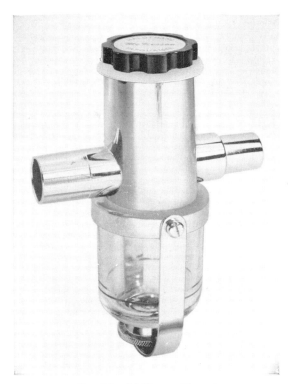

FIG. 16.—McKesson Vaporizer

rate, within the limits of normal usage. They can be constructed to deliver very high concentrations of halothane, but in practice the highest upper limit is 10%.

The Fluotec 3 (Fig. 8)

The dial setting shows accurately the concentration delivered at flow-rates as low as 250 ml/min and up to well over 10 l/min.

The M. & I. E. (Fig. 7)

The dial is normally calibrated up to 4% halothane.

The Abingdon Vaporizer (Fig. 12)

The Cyprane Vaporizer (Figs. 3 and 13)

This vaporizer incorporates a non-return valve at its exit.

CYLINDERS

Table XIV shows the British Standard Colour Code for medical gases. The individual characteristics of cylinders are described in Chapter 4. It should be noted that both nitrous oxide and oxygen are available in Pin-Index fittings suitable for direct attachment to the anaesthetic machine, and also in Bull-Nose cylinder valve fittings for bulk storage supply.

TABLE XIV. — *British Standard Colours for Medical Gas Cylinders*

Gas	Cylinder Body	Cylinder Neck
Oxygen	Black	White
Nitrous Oxide	Blue	Blue
Cyclopropane	Orange	Orange
Carbon Dioxide	Grey	Grey
Entonox	Blue	White/Blue
Air	Grey	White/Black
Helium	Brown	Brown

DENTAL CHAIRS

In general, dental chairs fall into two categories.

1. The conventional chairs which are designed primarily for the upright or reclining posture.
2. The contoured chairs which are designed primarily for low seated dentistry.

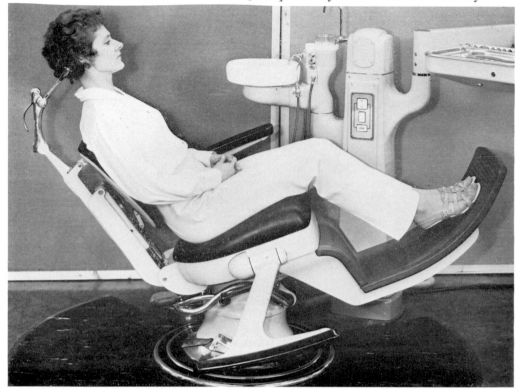

FIG. 17.—Ash Conventional chair. Note that arm-rest can be lowered if required.

1. The Conventional Chair (Fig. 17)

This type of chair is designed to give the maximum range of mobility, and is therefore particularly suitable for most general anaesthetic purposes. The wide range of independent adjustment of back-rest and head-rest provides the anaesthetist with the flexibility required for safe control of the airway under a variety of circumstances. It does, however, carry the disadvantage that when used in the horizontal posture (Fig. 18), the support afforded the patient is not optimal for prolonged procedures, nor is the operator able to work in the true 'low-seated' position on account of the bulk of the head-rest and back-rest controls. This type of chair must incorporate a mechanism whereby it can be lowered from upright to horizontal posture with the minimum delay. For children, either a fixed or a removable child's seat is essential (page 223). We strongly recommend the routine use of a leg support as shown in Figs 18 and 19 (pages 164 and 181).

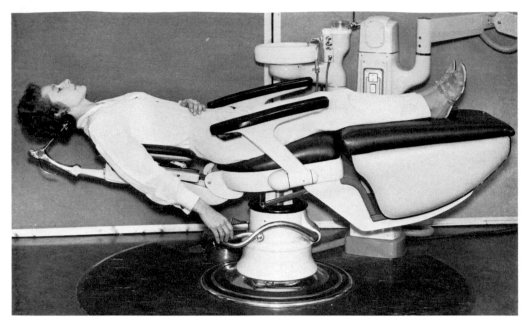

FIG. 18.—The same chair as in fig. 17 used in the horizontal posture with a Murray Laxer leg support
Note poor back support, and difficulty in retaining arms in safe position.

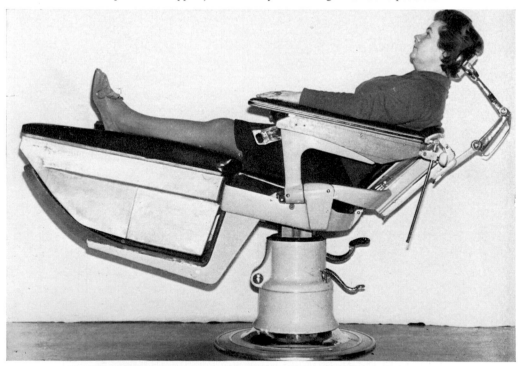

FIG. 19.—Ritter Conventional chair with leg support showing reclining posture
Note:— Armboard for intravenous administration.

72

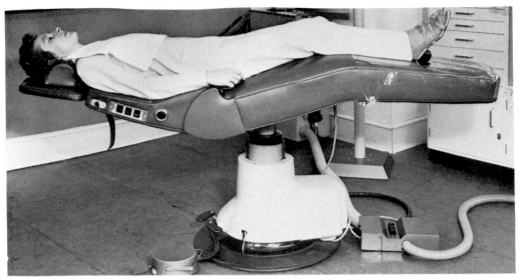

FIG. 20.—Ash contoured fully electrically operated chair showing horizontal posture with slim head-rest suitable for low-seated dentistry. Note good support for arm afforded by adequate width and design of back-rest. (Right arm-rest removed).

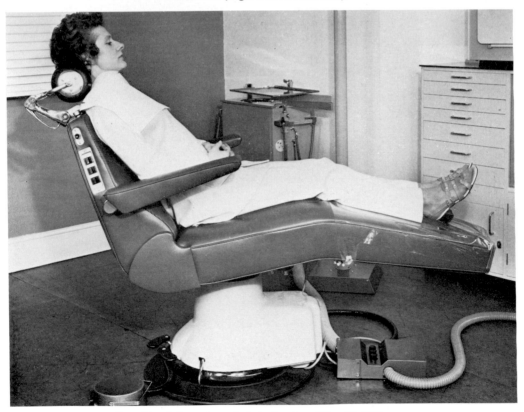

FIG. 21.—Ash contoured chair showing sitting posture
Note:—Adjustable head-rest suitable for exodontia.

2. The Contoured Chair

There is available a wide variety of contoured chairs which are particularly suitable for low-seated dentistry. These chairs, however, present the anaesthetist with certain difficulties in the unintubated patient, since the solid one piece head-rest is non-adjustable, hinders manual support of the mandible, and renders the use of twin tube nasal mask more difficult. Figs. 20, 21 and 22 illustrate a chair in which the needs of most situations can be met by changing or removing the head-rest.

Many modern chairs are electrically operated. It is important that the mechanism which lowers the patient from upright to horizontal is either rapid in action or, for

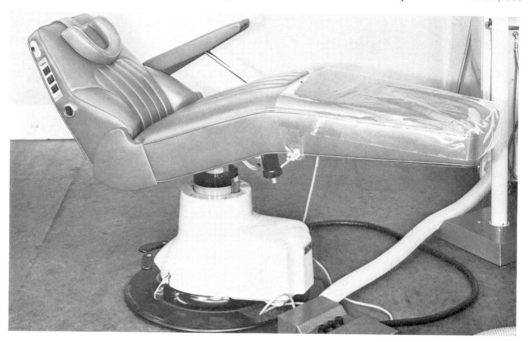

FIG. 22.—Ash contoured chair with head section removed and head ring attached. Suitable for children.

preference, has an over-riding manual control. In addition there may be some increased risk of catching patients' limbs during changes of posture.

Some chairs incorporate armboards for intravenous work. Removable armboards are, however, available and Figs. 23 and 24 illustrate two varieties.

Finally, it should be borne in mind that the well-upholstered chair may provide a too resilient surface for cardiac resuscitation (page 172).

SUCTION APPARATUS

Wherever general anaesthesia is employed, it is essential that efficient, powerful suction apparatus should be available; the conventional saliva ejector is totally inadequate in this context. Modern suction apparatus is of two main types.

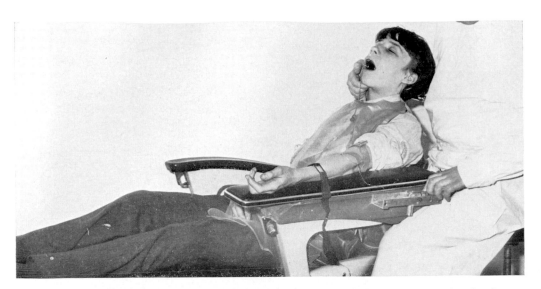

FIG. 23.—The detachable Bae armboard shown in this figure can be fixed to most conventional and some contoured chairs. Note the apparatus in use for the administration of methohexitone intermittently.

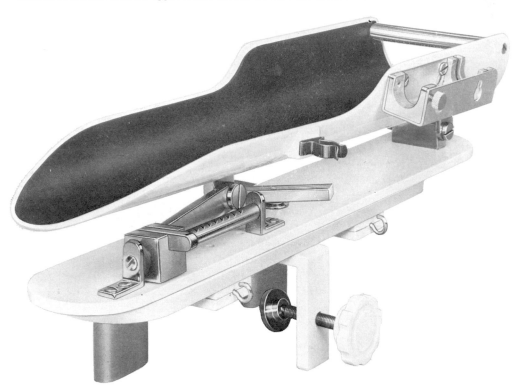

FIG. 24.—Detachable Ash Intravenous Armboard (Wilkinson Pattern).

1. **High Vacuum Suction** (Fig. 25)

This type of apparatus should develop a negative pressure of 30 cm water. Those models suitable for use in an operating theatre incorporate a bacterial filter and conform to the standard anti-explosion requirements. They are fitted with non-collapsible pressure tubing which can carry either a surgical end, or a perforated atraumatic attachment (Fig. 26) for use in the pharynx.

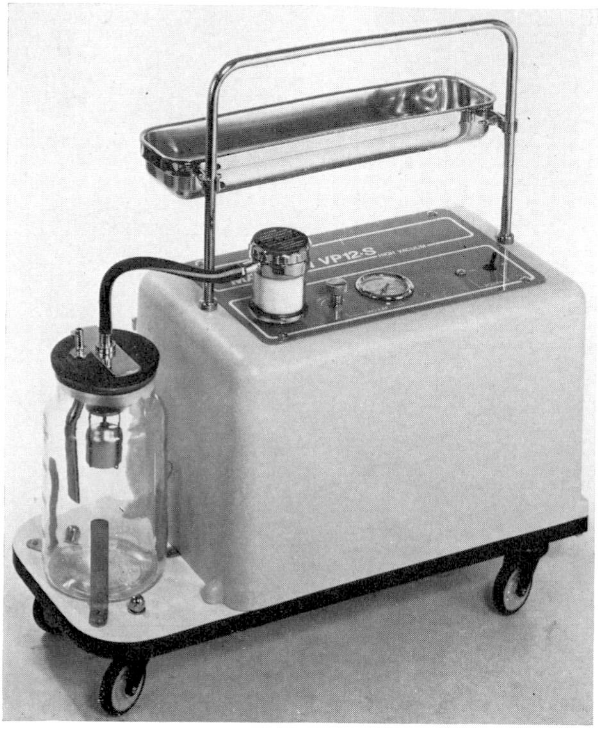

2. **High Velocity Aspirator** (Fig. 27)

This type of apparatus is part of the standard equipment in most dental surgeries, since it constitutes the best method of controlling the large volumes of water currently used with the high-speed drill. Most models are designed to clear 0·5 litre of water in one second, and do so at low vacuum—high velocity. The advantages claimed in dentistry are that fluid can be removed across an air gap of about 0·5 inch (13 mm), and that the design provides a combination of maximum fluid clearance with minimal tissue trauma. A wide variety of aspirator 'tips' is available (Fig. 28) and several can be used synchronously.

Fig. 25.—High vacuum suction apparatus.

(*Matburn V.P.12-S. Courtesy Eschmann Bros. & Walsh Ltd.*)

This apparatus is invaluable for the maintenance of a dry operating field—and hence airway—particularly in conservative dentistry, but is less than satisfactory for the performance of pharyngeal toilet for the following reasons. The tubing is usually too readily kinkable and of insufficient length to reach the pharynx during laryngoscopy; neither is there a suitable 'tip' for this purpose, and great care has to be exercised using the conventional 'tips' in order to avoid trauma to the soft palate, uvula and epiglottis. It is hoped that in future the apparatus will incorporate the small modifications necessary to meet these requirements.

FACE-MASK (Fig. 29)

A face-mask attached by the appropriate angle-piece to an expiratory valve mount (Fig. 30) should always be available for resuscitation purposes. It may also be used to anaesthetise the persistent mouth breather.

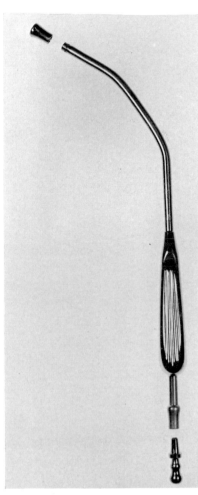

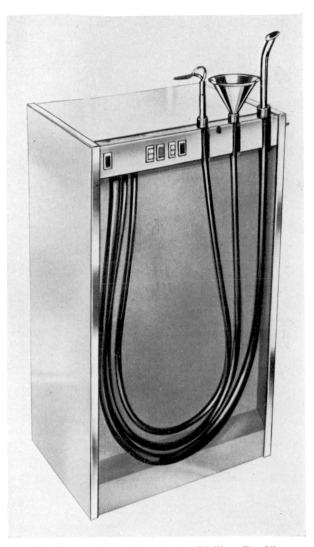

FIG. 26.—Jankauer's atraumatic
suction end.

FIG. 27.—High velocity aspirator. Virilium Dry View.

NOSE-MASKS

There are two main types of nasal mask, but no design is completely satisfactory.

1. Twin Tube Conventional (Fig. 31)

This type is well-shaped and can be readily fixed to the patient's head. There is a tendency for the rubber variety to become soft, and thus unmanageable, with use. This may be counteracted by incorporating a metal stiffener, but care must be taken not to damage the face by pulling such a mask on too tightly. The all-metal variety

77

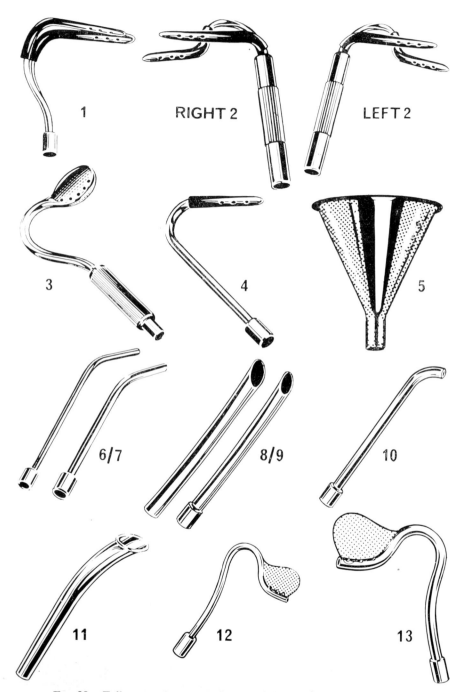

FIG. 28.—Full range of aspirator tips for Virilium high velocity aspirator.

78

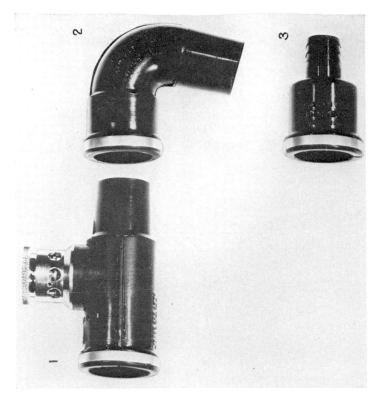

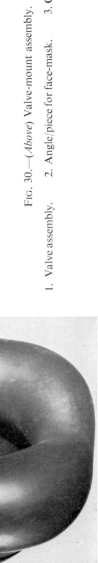

FIG. 30.—(*Above*) Valve-mount assembly.

1. Valve assembly. 2. Angle/piece for face-mask. 3. Catheter mount.

FIG. 29.—(*Left*) Flat-pad face-mask.

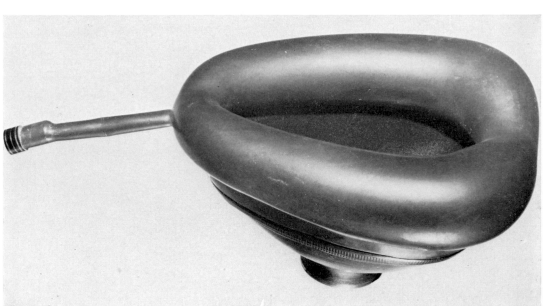

will not, of course, collapse, but perhaps lacks the necessary resilience and temperature for comfort.

The narrow bore and length of the twin tubing renders the resistance to inspiration undesirably high when total flow-rates little in excess of the patient's minute volume are used. It is generally held to be unsuitable for use with a continuous flow machine, but we have found that in practice, provided a generous flow-rate is employed, the apparatus is satisfactory.

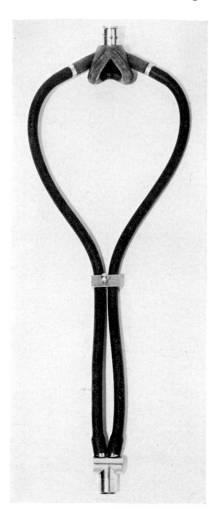

FIG. 31.—Conventional twin-tube nasal mask.

2. **Goldman** (Fig. 32)

Although the description 'wide bore' is often applied to this mask, the diameter of the inlet is only about 1·4 cm. However, the direct attachment of mask to wide bore elephant tubing results in a lower inspiratory resistance than that associated with the twin tube variety. The mask cannot readily be fixed on the patient's face, although a home-made harness (canvas and elastic) can partially overcome this inconvenience. The present manufactured harnesses are unsatisfactory. The convex lower border of the mask tends to impede access to the upper front teeth.

Neither the twin tube nor the Goldman mask is wide enough to enclose the negroid nares, and it is to be hoped that the manufacturers will produce a set of nasal masks incorporating all the desirable features we have mentioned.

Mouth-Cover

The ideal mouth-cover, which is not at present manufactured, should incorporate the following features:

(a) A bore of comparable diameter to the nasal assembly.

(b) An expiratory valve.

(c) A simple on/off switch close to the patient. The standard swivel device at present manufactured is most unsatisfactory.

Mouth-Props (Fig. 33)

There exists a multitude of mouth-props, and Fig. 33 illustrates the three designs which we find meet all our needs.

1. *Devonshire.*—This prop is supplied in three sizes. It is wedge-shaped, and is the most comfortable and satisfactory for use in patients with normal regular dentition.

2. *McKesson.*—Similar in principle to the Devonshire, but with flanges on buccal and lingual aspects, so that the teeth or gums lie within a trough. The lingual flange is shallower than the buccal, and the prop is less comfortable but more stable than the Devonshire, thus rendering it preferable for use on the edentulous gum, or in any situation where the Devonshire tends to slip out of position.

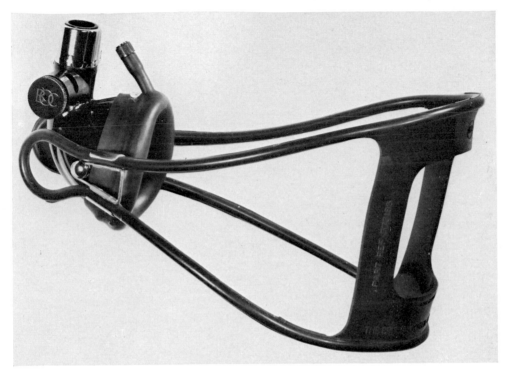

Fig. 32.—Goldman mask and harness.

3. *Hewitt.*—In spite of many modifications of the original design, we find this prop useful in the edentulous patient for whom the buccal flange of the McKesson is uncomfortable. The prop and latex cap must be cleaned and sterilized separately, and reassembled dry.

Mouth Gags

Fergusson (Fig. 34).—This gag is characterized by a ratchet locking mechanism, which is easier to control than the original Mason, with its screw device.

The early straight jaw ratchet-type gag has been modified to facilitate opening the tightly closed mouth. Thus, the present-day Fergusson gag is characterized by long handles to provide maximum leverage and, if required, single plane blades (Ackland) for ease of insertion between the teeth; in spite of the existence of right and left sided Ackland blades, we find that whichever way round it is used, the gag becomes unstable and is therefore suitable only for the initial opening of the mouth. Since the long handles are frequently impeded by the modern head-rest, we consider that the present day Fergusson gag is not strictly suitable as an alternative to the prop.

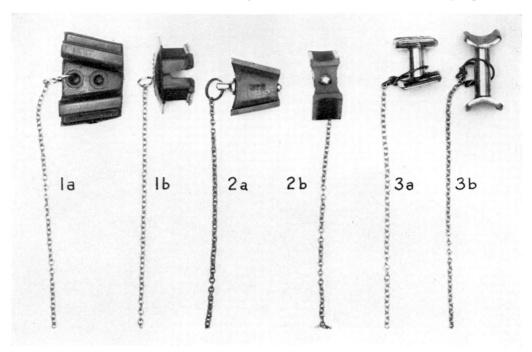

FIG. 33.—Mouth props
1. McKesson   (a) Right side, lingual view.   (b) Left side, posterior view.
2. Devonshire   (a) Lateral,   (b) Posterior view.
3.   Hewitt, Latex caps removed.   (a) Lateral,   (b) Posterior view.

Doyen Gag (Fig. 35).—This gag is designed not only to open the mouth when it is relatively relaxed, but also to act as an alternative to the prop in maintaining mouth opening.

Rubber Protection for Gag Blades

Both types of gag described are made of stainless steel, and there is therefore a risk that the teeth or gums may be damaged during mouth-opening. It is thus common practice to cover the blades with protective rubber or plastic. This carries the following disadvantages.

(a) There is a real danger of the rubber slipping off during use, and being lost in the mouth and possibly inhaled into the lungs. It is therefore essential that any covering should fit firmly and extend well beyond the curve of the gag jaw as illustrated. (Fig. 36).

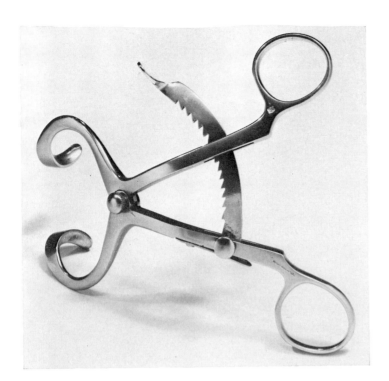

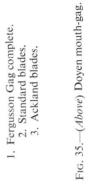

Fig. 34.—(*Left*) Fergusson Gag.

1. Fergusson Gag complete.
2. Standard blades.
3. Ackland blades.

Fig. 35.—(*Above*) Doyen mouth-gag.

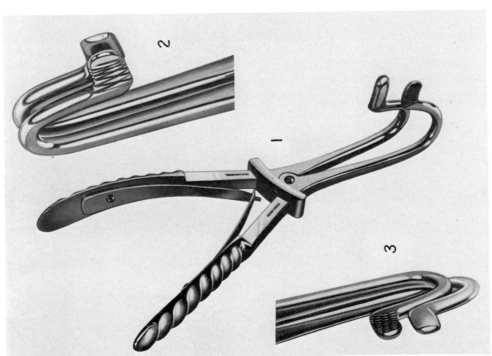

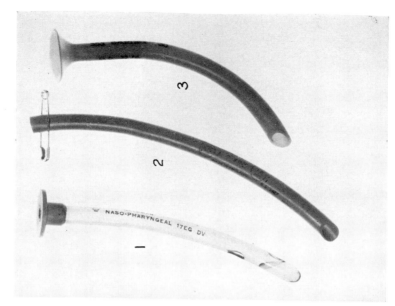

FIG. 37.—Nasopharyngeal airways.
1. Flanged blunt-ended Portex (Goldman).
2. Cut nasotracheal tube with safety pin.
3. Flanged open-ended Latex.

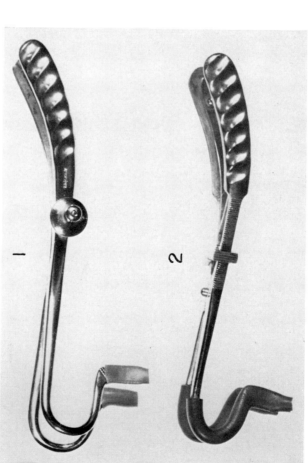

FIG. 36.—Mouth gags with rubber protection.
1. Wrong way to apply rubber (Mason's gag).
2. Correct way to apply rubber (Fergusson's gag).

(b) The presence of a cover makes the gag more difficult to clean adequately, and ideally it should be sterilized with the covering removed.

(c) If the rubber is not changed frequently, there is a tendency for it to disintegrate into fragments which may be inhaled.

(d) The presence of rubber inevitably increased the thickness of the blades, so that a greater degree of initial mouth-opening is required before the gag can be inserted between the teeth.

Whether or not the gag blades are covered, the greatest possible care must be exercised to ensure that the lips are not caught between the gag and the teeth.

MOUTH PACKS

This subject is fully discussed on page 127.

ORAL AIRWAY

Fig. 77 illustrates the two main varieties. The subject is fully discussed on page 153.

NASOPHARYNGEAL AIRWAY

Fig. 37 illustrates several types of naso-pharyngeal airway, and the subject is discussed on page 142.

MONITORING EQUIPMENT

It has not, in the past, been customary to monitor the dental out-patient with complex equipment. However, with growing anxiety related to the high incidence of cardiac irregularities (page 163), there is an increasing awareness amongst dental anaesthetists of the need for simple and reliable cardiovascular monitoring devices.

1. Pulse Monitor

There is a wide variety of these instruments on the market. Fig. 38 illustrates one variety which not only indicates the pulse rhythm by means of a flashing light, but also records the rate. The standard method of digital recording carries the disadvantage that the instrument is sensitive to outside interference, particularly movement, and is unreliable in the presence of peripheral vasoconstriction. We have found the San-Ei finger attachment gives the least interference.

2. Oscillotonometer

Fig. 39 illustrates two types of apparatus commonly used in operating theatres in order to obtain a peripheral blood pressure reading without the use of a stethoscope. It carries the disadvantage that any external pressure on the cuff will interfere with the accuracy of the recordings obtained.

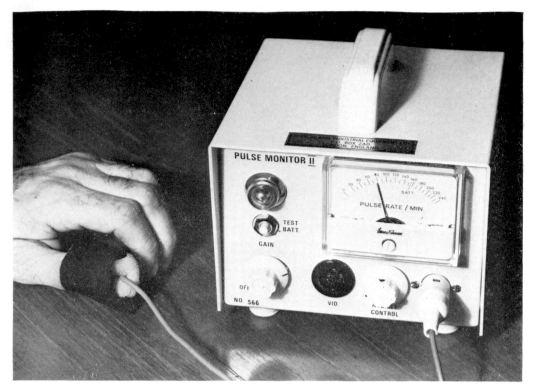

Fig. 38.—M. & I.E. Pulse Monitor. Flashing light and pulse-rate dial.

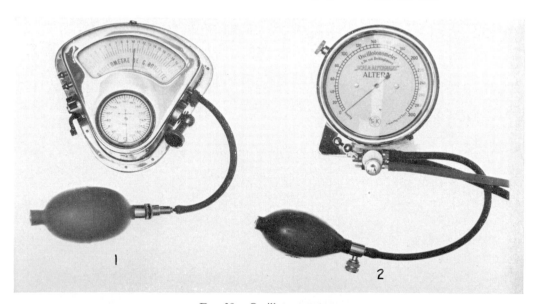

Fig. 39.—Oscillotonometer.
1. Boulitte.   2. Scala Alternans Altera.

86

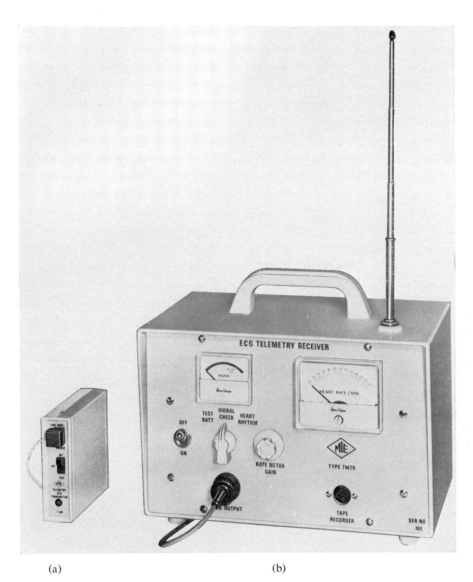

FIG. 40.—M. & I.E. Telemetric Cardiac Monitor.
(a) The transmitter, (b) The receiver with E.C.G. and tape recorder outlets.

3. Electrocardioscopic Monitoring

Fig. 40 shows a radio-telemetric device which is particularly suitable for direct cardiac monitoring in the dental chair and during recovery.

Equipment for endotracheal intubation is discussed on page 264.
Equipment for resuscitation is discussed on pages 156 and 174.

RECOMMENDED READING

1. Apparatus for Dental Anaesthesia.

THOMPSON, P. W. (1971) In *General Anaesthesia for Dental Surgery*, Ed. A. R. Hunter and G. H. Bush. Altrincham: Sherratt, p. 7.

2. The Performance of Walton Five.

SMITH, W. D. A. (1961) *Br. J. Anaesth.*, **33**, 440.

3. Some Hazards of Dental Gas Machines.

NAINBY-LUXMORE, R. C. (1967) *Anaesthesia*, **22**, 595.

CHAPTER FOUR

THE INHALATION AGENTS

It is our purpose in this chapter to discuss in detail only those drugs, the use of which we advocate in Chapter 5, i.e. nitrous oxide, halothane and trichlorethylene. Many other inhalation agents are available which have been, and still may be, used to produce anaesthesia in dentistry. These agents will receive mention, but readers are referred to other books for a detailed account of their properties.

In addition to these anaesthetic agents, it is necessary to describe the gases involved in normal breathing, i.e. oxygen, nitrogen and carbon dioxide, and to discuss the behaviour of both physiological and inert gases in the body.

Normal Breathing and Behaviour of Gases Involved

Room air, which contains approximately 80% nitrogen and 20% oxygen, when inhaled reaches the pulmonary alveoli where the gases equilibrate with those in solution in the adjacent capillary blood. This blood comes from the right ventricle via the pulmonary artery, but is, of course, venous in character, since it contains the gaseous product of metabolism, namely carbon dioxide, and has also had abstracted from it the oxygen requirements of the body. The nitrogen content of the inhaled air acts merely as a supporting gas and takes no part in the metabolic processes. During equilibration, oxygen diffuses into the blood and carbon dioxide out of it, thus determining the composition of the alveolar air, which contains approximately; nitrogen 80%; oxygen 14·5%; carbon dioxide 5·5%. Expired air is inevitably a mixture of alveolar air and the air in the non-respiratory portion of the air passages (dead space air) which is in direct continuity with room air. The composition of expired air is approximately: nitrogen 80%; oxygen 16%; carbon dioxide 4%. From the viewpoint of gaseous exchange in the body, it is the partial pressure exerted by a gas, rather than its actual volume percentage which is of direct significance. If the total dry gas pressure of room air is 740 mmHg, i.e. barometric pressure (760 mm) minus water vapour pressure at room temperature, and its percentage composition is 80% nitrogen and 20% oxygen, then the partial pressure of oxygen in that air is:

$$\frac{20}{100} \times 740 = 148 \text{ mmHg}$$

and the partial pressure of nitrogen is:

$$\frac{80}{100} \times 740 = 592 \text{ mmHg}$$

The same concept is applicable to gases in solution in physiological fluids such as blood, the tension of the gas in solution being determined by the partial pressure of the gas to which that solution is exposed across the alveolar capillary membrane. Let us assume that the inspired room air containing the partial pressure distribution of gases indicated above, is brought into contact with the venous blood within the pulmonary artery, containing in solution in its plasma, oxygen at 40 mmHg tension, carbon dioxide at 46 mmHg and nitrogen at 570 mmHg. The pressure gradient between the gases in solution and those in the alveolar air will allow rapid diffusion of oxygen from the alveoli through the thin pulmonary epithelium into the plasma, and a like diffusion of carbon dioxide in the reverse direction. Equilibrium will be rapidly achieved, so that the resultant gaseous partial pressure content of the alveolar air will approximate closely to the tension of gases in solution in the plasma leaving the lungs.

So far we have confined our remarks to the influence of gas tension in solution. It must be remembered that each gas has a specific solubility in any particular solvent, and that it is this characteristic which determines the actual amount of gas in solution at any given tension or partial pressure. For example, carbon dioxide is twenty times more soluble than oxygen in plasma, so that plasma exposed to carbon dioxide at a partial pressure of 100 mmHg would absorb twenty times as much carbon dioxide as it would of oxygen presented to it at the same partial pressure of 100 mmHg. The tension of either gas in solution would be 100 mmHg although the actual amount of gas so dissolved would differ greatly. If the tension of either gas were doubled, then the concentration of that gas in solution would also be doubled (Henry's Law).

Understanding of the principles outlined above is essential for the appreciation of the physical processes involved in the distribution of gases within the body, and in the case of nitrogen, it is only physical principles which are involved. But it must be clearly understood that both oxygen and carbon dioxide participate actively in metabolism, and are therefore subject to physiological as well as physical influences.

Oxygen and Carbon Dioxide Carriage in the Body

Oxygen.—Owing to the low solubility of oxygen in plasma, the blood is capable of carrying only 0·3 ml per 100 ml *in solution* when the subject is breathing air at atmospheric pressure, and this amount represents only a small proportion of the body's resting metabolic needs. However, the actual oxygen carrying capacity of blood under the same conditions is 19·3 ml of oxygen per 100 ml, 19 ml being carried in chemical combination with haemoglobin. If the subject breathes 100% oxygen for a considerable length of time, the oxygen in solution could theoretically rise to about 2 ml/100 ml of blood. The haemoglobin saturation, however, would only increase from 95% to 100%, that is to say from 19 ml to 20 ml oxygen per 100 ml blood. Thus the maximum oxygen carrying capacity of normal blood, with the subject breathing pure oxygen at atmospheric pressure is 22 ml of oxygen per 100 ml of blood. Whilst under normal physiological conditions, there is little advantage in breathing mixtures containing more oxygen than is present in air, under certain abnormal circumstances, found in both disease and anaesthesia, the benefits may be very great. In the maintenance of anaesthesia, and in recovery, it has been found that some degree of haemoglobin desaturation is common when breathing mixtures containing 20% oxygen. It is therefore both customary and often advisable to administer higher than atmospheric concentration of oxygen during these phases of anaesthesia. In particular, during recovery from prolonged nitrous oxide anaesthesia, an abnormally low alveolar oxygen partial pressure may occur owing to the release of large quantities of nitrous oxide from the blood and tissues into the alveolar air. This effect is observed in subjects with a normal minute volume breathing air, and is known as diffusion hypoxia or the Fink Effect.

The capacity of the haemoglobin to take up and release oxygen is dependent upon both the tension of oxygen in solution in the plasma to which the haemoglobin is

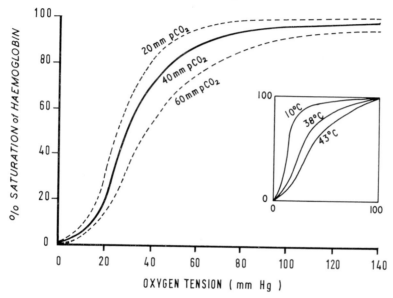

FIG. 41—Oxygen dissociation curve of haemoglobin (After Samson Wright)
Effects of CO_2 tension and temperature

exposed, and also the immediate environmental pH and temperature. These characteristics are best illustrated by the well known oxygen dissociation curves shown in Fig. 41.

It will be noted that haemoglobin saturation only begins to fall steeply at an oxygen tension of 35 mmHg which is the normal resting tissue tension, so that increased tissue activity gives rise to a rapid release of oxygen from oxyhaemoglobin.

Cyanosis.—Cyanosis is the term used to describe a bluish colour of the skin and mucous membranes, and is due to a change in character of the blood circulating in the capillaries of the cyanosed region. The commonest cause of this change is the presence of an abnormal amount of reduced haemoglobin in the capillary blood, and it is conventionally accepted that 5 g of reduced haemoglobin per 100 ml of blood will result in recognizable cyanosis. Rarely, however, it may be due to the presence of other dark pigments such as methaemoglobin or sulph-haemoglobin. It must also be appreciated that cyanosis may result from a purely local state of circulatory stasis and is not therefore always indicative of generalized hypoxaemia. To appreciate the true basis of this important sign, the following normal standards must be borne in mind. When the subject is breathing room air, the oxygen saturation of arterial haemoglobin is 95%. That is to say, that with a normal haemoglobin content of 15 g per 100 ml blood, $15 \times \dfrac{95}{100} = 14\cdot25$ g haemoglobin are oxygenated and 0·75 g per 100 ml are reduced, in arterial blood. Mixed venous blood is 70% saturated with oxygen in the resting subject, so that $15 \times \dfrac{70}{100} = 10\cdot5$ g of haemoglobin are oxygenated, and 4·5 g haemoglobin are reduced in venous blood. By convention, capillary blood is assumed to be mid-way between arterial and venous in terms of oxygen saturation, so that in the normal resting state, the concentration of reduced haemoglobin in capillary blood may be expressed as follows:

$$\frac{0\cdot75 + 4\cdot5}{2} = 2\cdot63 \text{ g reduced haemoglobin/100 ml blood}$$

This figure is, of course, well below the conventionally accepted cyanosis level of 5 g reduced haemoglobin per 100 ml blood, and thus the normal resting subject appears pink.

If, however, the arterial haemoglobin is only 75% saturated with oxygen, then arterial blood contains $15 \times \dfrac{75}{100} = 11\cdot2$ g oxyhaemoglobin and 3·8 g of reduced haemoglobin per 100 ml blood. Mixed venous blood, under these circumstances, contains $15 \times \dfrac{50}{100} = 7\cdot5$ g oxyhaemoglobin and 7·5 g reduced haemoglobin per 100 ml blood. Thus, the concentration of reduced haemoglobin in capillary blood under these circumstances would be:

$$\frac{3\cdot8 + 7\cdot5}{2} = 5\cdot7 \text{ g per 100 ml blood}$$

Since this is in excess of the conventional figure of 5 g per 100 ml, cyanosis would be apparent.

It will be appreciated from the foregoing account that in the anaemic subject cyanosis will indicate a greater degree of hypoxaemia than in the normal, and indeed, if the haemoglobin content is less than 5 g per cent (33%), cyanosis will not occur even in the presence of complete anoxaemia. Conversely, cyanosis in a subject with a high haemoglobin content (e.g. polycythaemia) may occur unassociated with severe hypoxaemia.

Whilst we have, in accordance with convention, assumed that capillary blood is under observation, in practice the blood in the skin more closely resembles arterial blood in terms of oxygen content, owing to the low oxygen utilization in this region;

on the other hand, peripheral stasis due to gravity or any other cause will allow the blood under observation to become more desaturated than the mixed venous blood in the same patient, thereby giving cyanosis in the absence of generalized hypoxaemia. Thus, the practice of rubbing the skin is frequently used to minimize this source of error (page 135).

In conclusion, it is worth drawing attention to two further factors. Firstly, that the recognition of cyanosis is dependent upon such variables as the visual acuity of the observer and the prevailing lighting conditions. Secondly, recent work has shown that under ideal conditions, cyanosis can be recognized when the quantity of reduced haemoglobin in capillary blood is considerably less than the conventional 5 g%.

Carbon Dioxide.—Carbon dioxide is one of the normal products of metabolism. The arterial blood reaches the tissues with a carbon dioxide tension (PCO_2) of 40 mmHg and comes into contact with a tissue tension of 46 mmHg, equilibrium being reached between tissue and venous blood.

Dissolved carbon dioxide passes readily into the corpuscles where the following reaction $CO_2 + H_2O \rightleftharpoons H_2CO_3$ proceeds to the right, accelerated by the enzyme carbonic anhydrase. The subsequent dissociation of carbonic acid $H_2CO_3 \rightleftharpoons H^+ + HCO_3^-$ proceeds rapidly within the red cell owing to the fact that reduced haemoglobin acts as a H^+ ion acceptor. This dissociation would be very limited in the absence of reduced haemoglobin. Most of the HCO_3^- ions pass out into the plasma in exchange for Cl^- ions which enter the red cell (chloride shift). This is by far the most important mechanism in the carriage of carbon dioxide. A smaller quantity of carbon dioxide combines directly with haemoglobin to form carbamino-haemoglobin, this reaction being facilitated by the simultaneous reduction of haemoglobin.

The physiological effects of carbon dioxide excess and deficiency are fully discussed on page 161.

Physical Characteristics and Supply

Oxygen.—Molecular weight—32; Solubility in water at 37°C—2·4 vol. %; Relative density (air = 1)—1·105.

Oxygen under pressure may cause an explosion if exposed to oil or grease. Oxygen is normally supplied in cylinders at a pressure of approximately 2,000 lb per in² (132 atmospheres), at which pressure it is in a gaseous state at room temperature.

The cylinders are painted black with white shoulders (International standard), and are supplied in the following sizes:

Pin-index: 38 gallons, 74 gallons, 150 gallons
Bull-nose: 300 gallons, 750 gallons, 1500 gallons

The gas can also be piped from a central supply in which the oxygen is usually stored in liquid form.

Carbon Dioxide.—Molecular weight—44; Solubility in water at 37°C–100 vol. %; Relative density (air = 1)—1·50.

Carbon dioxide is non-inflammable. It is stored in the liquid state in cylinders painted grey (International standard) at 750 lb per in^2 (50 atmospheres). It should be noted that when gases are stored in cylinders in the liquid state, the pressure gauge will indicate the pressure of the gas above the liquid and that this will remain constant until all the liquid has been exhausted, after which it will fall rapidly as the cylinder empties. Thus the pressure gauge is not a reliable indication of cylinder content.

Nitrogen.—Molecular weight—28; Solubility in water at 37°C—1·28 vol. %; Relative density (air = 1)—0·967.
Nitrogen is not normally supplied for medical purposes, but its use has been described in dental anaesthesia in order to eliminate the explosion risk when using cyclopropane, oxygen mixtures. This technique is now generally considered obsolete.

Helium.—Molecular weight—4; Solubility in water at 37°C is low; Relative density (air = 1)—0.178.
Owing to the low density of helium, helium/oxygen mixtures (80:20) will flow through a given orifice three times as fast as will air, and thus these mixtures are of value in facilitating respiration through obstructed air passages. If fed through a nitrous oxide flow-meter, the reading must be multiplied by 3·3 to get the approximate rate of flow in litres per minute.

ANAESTHETIC GASES

This subject will be dealt with under two distinct headings.

1. The physiological and physical factors governing the behaviour of these gases in the body.
2. The characteristics of individual agents.

1. Physiological and Physical Factors

The level of anaesthesia produced by an anaesthetic agent is directly dependent upon the concentration of that agent in the brain. This concentration will in turn be determined by the blood concentration and the cerebral blood flow.

Cerebral Blood Flow.—The cerebral blood flow is determined by two main factors—firstly, the mean arterial blood pressure which is the force responsible for driving the blood through the brain; secondly, the cerebrovascular resistance which is the product of all influences tending to impede the flow of blood through the brain. Provided the mean arterial blood pressure is sufficiently high to permit an adequate blood flow, the actual regulation of that flow is determined by the intrinsic mechanisms which control the cerebrovascular resistance. The factors which influence cerebrovascular resistance are the following.

(a) *The Functional Tone of Cerebral Vessels*
This tone is chiefly controlled by alterations in blood PCO_2 and PO_2, which are thought to act directly upon the cerebral vessels. For example, if the subject breathes a

mixture containing 5–7% carbon dioxide, a 75% increase in cerebral blood flow may result. If the subject breathes a mixture containing 10% oxygen the increase in cerebral blood flow will be in the order of 35%. Conversely, a low PCO_2 or a high PO_2 will result in a reduction in cerebral blood flow. The neurogenic control of cerebral vascular tone is of secondary importance to these chemical mechanisms.

(b) *Patency of the Small Cerebral Vessels*

The patency of these vessels may be reduced in cerebral arteriosclerosis, thus leading to an increase in cerebrovascular resistance and therefore a decrease in blood flow.

(c) *Intracranial Pressure*

An increase in intracranial pressure will lead to a restriction in cerebral blood flow.

(d) *Cerebral Arterio-Venous Pressure Difference*

To some extent, the cerebral blood velocity will depend upon the pressure gradient between the cerebral arteries and veins. The cerebral venous pressure is 6–8 mmHg when supine and is reduced to zero in the upright posture. Thus any tendency for the reduced cerebral arterial pressure to give rise to a reduction in cerebral blood flow in the upright position, will be partially compensated by the reduction in venous pressure in this position.

(e) *Viscosity of the Blood*

The greater the viscosity of the blood, the greater will be the resistance to its flow though the brain. Thus, the cerebral blood flow is increased in anaemia and decreased in polycythaemia.

It will be seen that all these factors may influence the speed of cerebral saturation and thus the rate of induction of anaesthesia.

Blood Concentration of Anaesthetic Agent.—The cerebral concentration will of course depend upon the concentration of the agent in the arterial blood supplying the brain and this, in the case of an inhalational agent, will in turn depend upon the alveolar concentration of that agent. Under normal conditions, equilibrium across the alveolar-arterial barrier is virtually instantaneous. It thus becomes necessary to examine the factors which determine the rate of accumulation of alveolar tension of any inspired gas.

For the purpose of clarity, it is convenient to use the 'bellows' analogy described by Kety (1950) and illustrated in Fig. 42. In this analogy the bellows represents the lungs and has a capacity of 2·5 litres; each stroke of the bellows represents a tidal exchange of 500 ml. The neck of the bellows receives the new gas at a constant inspired tension, and through a one-way valve allows the expelled bellows air to be totally eliminated. Thus at each stroke of the bellows, the gas which is inhaled into it, is diluted five-fold with the air already in the bellows. With the first 'breath', the bellows content goes one fifth of the way towards the inspired gas concentration. On the second 'breath' it moves another fifth of the way towards inspired concentration, and so on, never quite achieving complete alveolar washout and equilibrium with the inspired gas tension. These steps may be smoothed out to give an exponential curve

(Fig. 42). It is obvious that either an increase in ventilation (minute volume) or a decrease in 'bellows' volume (lung volume) will result in a faster rate of wash-out. The lungs, of course, cannot accurately be represented by a simple bellows, and it is necessary to imitate the effect of the pulmonary circulation by placing a 'leak' in the

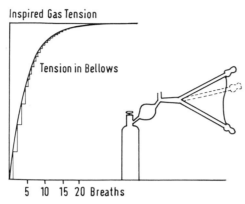

FIG. 42.—Alveolar tension increase ignoring pulmonary circulation (Kety)

bellows as in Fig. 43. Through this leak, fresh air (pulmonary artery blood) enters, and bellows-air (pulmonary vein blood) leaves, in addition to respiration which takes place as already described through the bellows neck. The concentration in the bellows can now never approximate to the inspired gas concentration, for it is continually being diluted by fresh air through the leak. The concentration which can be reached is determined by the ratio of the respiratory minute volume to the size of the 'leak', which represents the combined effect of the pulmonary blood-flow (cardiac output) and the solubility of the gas in blood. The larger the cardiac output and the higher the solubility of the gas in blood, the greater is the effect of the leak, and the lower the bellows (alveolar) concentration able to be achieved.

The pulmonary circulation cannot, however, be accurately represented by a

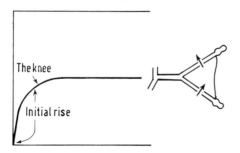

FIG. 43.—Alveolar tension increase modified by pulmonary 'leak' (Kety)

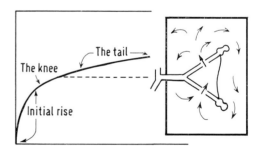

FIG. 44.—Alveolar tension increase modified by pulmonary 'leak' and body saturation (Kety)

'fixed leak', and therefore to complete the analogy, the bellows with its leak must be placed in a hermetically sealed room which represents the body and its tissues (Fig. 44). Under these circumstances, the room itself gradually becomes saturated with the leaking bellows-contents, so that in time more and more of the gas returns to the bellows via the input side of the leak. Eventually, both the gas in the bellows and the gas in the room will reach the inspired concentration. The rate at which this equilibrium is established depends upon:

(a) the size of the leak; that is to say that a large cardiac output, whilst retarding the initial rate of accumulation of alveolar tension, ultimately accelerates the establishment of complete equilibrium.

(b) the size of the room; that is to say that a large body mass will take longer to become saturated with the gas; in addition, the more soluble the gas in body tissue the longer, will the body take to absorb its full complement.

It will now be apparent that the shape of the arteriolar or alveolar uptake curve will depend not only upon the minute volume, lung volume, cardiac output, and body mass, but also to a very significant degree upon the solubility of the gas in both blood and body tissue. The uptake curves of the commonly used anaesthetic gases are shown in Fig. 45.

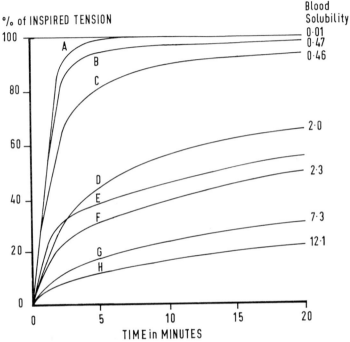

FIG 45.—Effect of blood solubility on alveolar (or arterial) tension of inhaled gases. After Bourne, J. G. Studies in Anaesthetics, 1967).

A. 80% N₂.
B. 80% N₂O.
C. 20% Cyclopropane.
D. 5% Ethyl Chloride.
E. 1% Halothane with 74% N₂O.
F. 1% Halothane with air.
G. 1% Chloroform.
H. 10% di-ethyl ether.

It is hoped that the foregoing account will help to clarify certain of the broad principles governing the speed of uptake of inhaled gases. It must, however, be stressed that many complexities have been artificially simplified in the cause of clarity.

Recovery.—The solubility of the anaesthetic gas in body tissues, particularly fat, will determine the total amount of anaesthetic able to be taken up by the body over a long period. Thus the administration of a very fat-soluble anaesthetic to a fat subject over a long period of time will inevitably lead to delay in its total elimination follow-

A.A.D.—4*

ing discontinuation of its administration. Indeed, in most respects recovery may be considered to be governed by factors similar to those already discussed in relation to induction.

Potency.—From the foregoing account, it can be seen that the solubility of an anaesthetic agent in brain, blood and body tissue will exert a considerable influence upon the speed of induction of anaesthesia. In addition, the solubility of the drug in brain tissue will affect its apparent potency. For example, it is not permissible ever to expose a patient to a concentration of anaesthetic exceeding 80% (i.e. 20% oxygen) of the total inspired mixture. In the case of nitrous oxide this concentration will never produce a deep level of anaesthesia; however, a highly brain-soluble anaesthetic such as ether, if administered in only 10% inspired concentration, will result in profound anaesthesia, the brain being capable of absorbing a much greater total quantity of soluble as compared with insoluble agent. Although brain solubility may not be the sole determining factor in potency, it has been shown that there is a correlation between the lipid solubility (oil/gas partition coefficient) and the potency as judged by the minimum alveolar (and therefore brain) tension required to prevent a muscular response to a skin incision. Finally, the volatility of an anaesthetic agent, by determining the maximum attainable inspired concentration, will indirectly influence its total potency.

2. The Characteristics of Individual Agents

Nitrous Oxide (N$_2$O)

Physical Properties

Molecular Weight—44; Solubility in water—100 vols. %; in plasma—45 vols. %; Solubility Coefficient (oil/water)—3·2; Relative density—1·5 (air = 1). Nitrous oxide is supplied in blue cylinders (G.B.) in which it is compressed to a liquid at a pressure of 650 lb/in^2. The significance of storage in liquid form is described on page 94. It is normally available in cylinders of the following sizes:

Pin-index: 50, 100, 200, 400 gallons
Bull-nose: 800, 2000, 3000, 4000 gallons

The gas is neither flammable nor explosive. It has a characteristic odour, but is non-irritant to the respiratory passages.

Nitrous Oxide Impurities

Nitrous oxide is manufactured by the thermal decomposition of ammonium nitrate at a temperature not exceeding 280°C. During this process small quantities of impurities occur which are removed by a process of scrubbing and then compressed by stages to remove the less easily liquified gases such as nitrogen and oxygen.

Should the thermal process become uncontrolled and the temperature rise above 280°C large quantities of nitric oxide and nitrogen dioxide may be formed and, in consequence, fail to be removed by the normal scrubbing processes. Under these circumstances, when the cylinder is first opened, high concentrations of nitric oxide will be delivered, since it is thirty times more volatile than nitrous oxide. This hazard explains the practice of releasing a small quantity of gas to the atmosphere before attaching the cylinder to the anaesthetic machine—a practice which we feel could well be continued as an additional safeguard against an isolated failure of the manufacturing process. Nitric oxide released into circuit reacts with the oxygen in the anaesthetic mixture so that the gas mixture reaching the patient will contain nitrous oxide, oxygen, nitric oxide, nitrogen dioxide, nitrogen trioxide and dinitrogen tetra-oxide. Such a mixture is highly poisonous to the patient and in 1966 a series of tragedies resulted from this very set of circumstances.

Clinical Features of Poisoning
1. Derangement of acid base equilibrium,
2. Methaemoglobinaemia,
3. A delayed toxicity, resulting from oxidation and nitrosation of hydroxylic-amino and sulphydryl containing compounds in the body, such as vitamin C, lysine and cysteine, thus disrupting many of the normal body processes.
   Death has been reported after a latent period of as long as 4 weeks after exposure to the higher oxides of nitrogen.

Clinical Features which should lead the Anaesthetist to consider
Nitric Oxide Poisoning
1. Immediate hyperventilation and perhaps coughing on administering the gas.
2. The development of cyanosis after only a few minutes of administration, in spite of adequate oxygen in the mixture.
3. Failure to improve the degree of cyanosis, in spite of the administration of 100% oxygen.
4. Circulatory collapse and hypotension following such a period of cyanosis.
5. Ultimate development of pulmonary oedema.

These features are similar to those found following the inhalation of acid gastric contents but in the latter the cyanosis may be expected to improve with the administration of oxygen.

Suggested Treatment
1. Administration of 100% oxygen.
2. Reversal of methaemoglobinaemia with methylene blue, 1–2 mg/kg by intravenous injection over 5 minutes.
3. Prevention and treatment of the pneumonitis by parenteral and possibly endobronchial administration of corticosteroids.
4. Administration of antibiotics.
5. Administration of 250 ml of 8·4% bicarbonate by intravenous infusion to correct acidosis.

6. Artificial ventilation.
7. The administration of dimercaprol.
8. Vasopressors to support circulation.

Pharmacological Properties

1. *Central Nervous System.*—Nitrous oxide has weak anaesthetic properties—that is to say that when administered in the maximum permissible inspired concentration of 80%, only light first plane surgical (3rd stage) anaesthesia can be obtained even after full tissue saturation. Indeed in so-called 'resistant' subjects, i.e. alcoholics, even this light level of surgical anaesthesia may be impossible to achieve, the subject never progressing beyond the 'excitement' (2nd) stage of anaesthesia. There is no depression of respiratory or vasomotor centres.

Nitrous oxide is conventionally accepted as possessing strong specific analgesic properties; thus, if administered in concentration insufficient to produce loss of consciousness, there will result considerable reduction in pain-appreciation—a characteristic which has long been utilized in obstetric and dental practice, and more recently in the field of postoperative analgesia. Details of the levels of analgesia obtainable with nitrous oxide is further discussed on page 139.

2. *Cardiovascular System.*—There is no direct action on the heart, the pulse and blood pressure remaining unaffected in the absence of surgical stimulation.

3. *Respiratory System.*—Respiration is said to be stimulated during induction, but it is difficult to be certain that this is a true pharmacological property of the drug. There is no effect upon bronchial secretions or calibre but, in common with all anaesthetic agents, nitrous oxide depresses ciliary activity.

4. *Miscellaneous.*—There is no significant effect on either voluntary or smooth muscle tone. Neither hepatic nor renal function is disturbed, but prolonged administration depresses bone-marrow function. Provided oxygenation is adequate, post-anaesthetic headache, nausea, vomiting, malaise are rare. Nitrous oxide interferes less with normal physiology and produces fewer toxic side-effects than any other inhalation anaesthetic agent. Its major disadvantage is its lack of potency.

Uptake and Elimination

The low solubility of nitrous oxide in blood as compared with other anaesthetic agents (see Table XV) will result in a rapid build-up of alveolar and hence brain tension, thus allowing rapid induction. Likewise, its low tissue and fat solubility prevents undue prolongation of recovery, irrespective of the length of administration. Nitrous oxide is excreted almost entirely through the lungs, a very small amount being said to diffuse through the skin. The rapid pulmonary elimination of the drug may lead to diffusion hypoxia (see page 91).

TABLE XV.—*Partition Coefficients at 37°C of the Inhalational Anaesthetics*

Nitrogen Values for Comparison

Gas	Blood/gas	Tissue/Blood		Oil/gas
Nitrogen	0·01	Brain	1·1	
		Liver	1·1	
		Fat	5·2	
Cyclopropane	0·46	Liver	1·34	
		Muscle	0·92	11·2
		Fat	20·0	
Nitrous Oxide	0·47	Brain	1·0	
		Heart	1·0	1·4
		Fat	3·0	
Halothane	2·3	Brain	2·6	
		Liver	2·6	224
		Muscle	3·5	
		Fat	60·0	
Trichlorethylene	9·0	Fat	106·7	
Ether	12·1	Brain	1·14	65
Methoxyflurane	13·0	Brain		
		(White matter)	2·34	
		(Grey matter)	1·7	825
		Muscle	1·34	
Teflurane	0·6	Brain	1·9	
		Muscle	3·5	29

This table is compounded from information from the following sources.
BOURNE, J. G. (1967) *Studies in Anaesthetics*. page 14.
GREENE, N. M. (1968) *Clinical Anaesthesia, Halothane*. Oxford: Blackwell.
JONES, G. O. M. *et al.* (1969) Teflurane in Clinical Use. *Anaesthesia*, **24**, 378.

Entonox

Entonox is a mixture of nitrous oxide and oxygen in equal proportions. The mixture is stored in a cylinder in gaseous form at a pressure of 1980 lb per in². The gas will deliver from the cylinder at a constant mixture provided the temperature of the cylinder does not fall below −4°C. Should the cylinder be cooled below this temperature and rewarmed, it must be well agitated before use.

The cylinders are coloured blue, with quartered white and blue collar, and are available in the following sizes:
Pin-index: 500 litres (109 gallons), 2000 litres, 5000 litres.

Halothane and Other Fluorinated Hydrocarbons

The search for a fluorinated hydrocarbon anaesthetic agent began in 1932, when it was appreciated that the anaesthetics in common use carried serious disadvantages. Diethyl ether was, at that time, the only potent agent in constant use, in spite of its irritant properties to the respiratory tract and its inflammability. Chloroform, a potent non-inflammable anaesthetic, had by this time lost its popularity because of its harmful effects on heart and liver. Ethyl chloride was still used, particularly for the induction of anaesthesia in children, but the marked myocardial depression produced, caused considerable misgivings as to its safety; divinyl ether (vinesthene), on the other hand, enjoyed a reputation for safety, but the practical difficulties entailed in its administration, its high inflammability, its unpleasant odour, and its marked salivary secreto-motor properties combined to limit its sphere of usefulness. Cyclopropane was introduced by Waters in 1934; it proved to be a potent and useful drug, but carried the disadvantage of being highly explosive, which led to a number of accidents. It was largely because of this characteristic that the search for a non-explosive agent was further encouraged. The introduction of trichlorethylene into anaesthetic practice by Langton Hewer in 1941 surmounted the explosion hazard, but its slow induction potential and failure to produce muscular relaxation left much to be desired. Thus, the development of halothane may be said to have resulted, in the first instance, from a quest to produce an anaesthetic agent of high potency and low toxicity which was also non-explosive and non-irritant to the respiratory mucosa. By the 1950's it was appreciated that it would be advantageous for any new agent to be characterized by a low solubility in blood, in order to facilitate rapid induction. Likewise, its solubility in fat and other body tissues should be relatively low, so that recovery time would not be prolonged. Both these clinical characteristics are particularly desirable in out-patient dental anaesthesia. Having established these criteria, it appeared logical to develop a hydrocarbon similar to cyclopropane, and to render it non-inflammable by chemical means. It was found that fluorination rendered the hydrocarbon inert from the point of view of not only flammability but also, unfortunately, anaesthetic potency; however, if the fluorine was bonded to a hydrocarbon containing other halogen links, such as bromine and chlorine, then the fluorine acted by stabilizing the links between carbon atoms and other halogens. In this way, the compound retained its anaesthetic potency, and because of its increased stability, it interfered less with body metabolism and was thus less toxic than non-fluorinated compounds, whilst still remaining non-inflammable. Thus, halopropane, halothane, and a number of other fluorinated anaesthetic agents were developed. Three of these compounds remain of interest at present, and there is a possibility that others, even more suitable for dental anaesthesia, may appear in the near future.

Halothane   Methoxyflurane   Teflurane

Halothane—(Trade name—Fluothane)

Physical Properties

Halothane is a colourless liquid, the vapour of which is non-inflammable, non-irritant, and has a sweet odour. Some decomposition occurs on exposure to light, and this is reduced by the addition of 0·01 % thymol, and storage in amber coloured bottles. It is unaffected by soda-lime and may, therefore, be used in a closed circuit.

Molecular weight—197·4; Relative density—6·8; Boiling point—50°C; Vapour pressure (20°C) 243 mmHg; Solubility partition coefficients—(a) Blood/gas—2·3; (b) Brain/blood—2·6; (c) Fat/blood—60·0; (d) Rubber/gas—121.

The main clinical significance of these physical properties lies in the influence which they exert upon the speed of induction and recovery, and will be discussed below.

Blood/Gas Partition Coefficient.—Amongst the anaesthetic agents, the blood solubility of halothane lies between that of nitrous oxide and trichlorethylene (see Table XV), being sufficiently low to allow a fairly rapid build-up of alveolar and hence brain tension. Since the agent is non-irritant, a high inspired concentration is always possible and rapid induction is achieved by ensuring that the inspired concentration exceeds that required for maintenance of surgical anaesthesia. In practice, induction concentrations ranging from 2 % to 10 % (page 70) may be used, but great care should be taken to reduce this concentration to the normal maintenance level of 0·5 %–1 % as soon as the required depth of anaesthesia has been achieved. In dental anaesthesia, the required depth of light surgical anaesthesia can generally be rapidly achieved using an induction concentration of 4 %, provided that the diluent mixture consists of nitrous oxide and oxygen in 75:25 proportions. If oxygen alone is used a higher concentration of halothane will be required in order to achieve an equally rapid induction.

Tissue/Blood Partition Coefficient.—Again, the tissue solubility of halothane lies between that of nitrous oxide and trichlorethylene, but much more closely approximates the latter (see Table XV). This relatively high tissue solubility is responsible for the fact that equilibrium will take a long time to occur, and the rapid rate of tissue abstraction from the blood will serve to slow down the induction. It should be stressed that, because of solubility characteristics, considerable tissue saturation will have occurred by the time a satisfactory level of anaesthesia has been achieved. It is thus important to reduce the inspired concentration to maintenance level as soon as possible, if delayed recovery is to be avoided.

Rubber/Gas Partition Coefficient.—Halothane has a high rubber solubility which could theoretically retard the rate of induction if low gas flow-rates are used, and likewise delay recovery if the patient is allowed to continue breathing from the machine after withdrawal of the halothane. This theoretical possibility is of practical significance only during closed circuit anaesthesia.

Vapour Pressure.—As the saturated vapour pressure of halothane is 243 mmHg at 20°C, it is possible to obtain a vapour concentration of approximately 33% at room temperature. In view of this potentially high concentration it is important that an accurate vaporizing device should be used, and that its position within the circuit should be carefully considered.

(a) *Semi-Open Circuit.*—In the semi-open circuit, the inspired concentration will never exceed the concentration delivered by the vaporizer, provided that no rebreathing is permitted. It is therefore necessary only to ensure that the vaporizer is accurate for any particular flow-rate and ambient temperature, and also that it should automatically compensate for any likely change in these factors. For example, should the room temperature rise from 20°C (68°F) to 30°C (86°F), the saturated vapour concentration will rise from 33% to 50%. The characteristics of individual vaporizers have been discussed in Chapter 3.

(b) *Closed Circuit.*—If halothane is administered within a closed circuit, the vaporizer can be placed either inside the circuit (V.I.C.), or outside the circuit (V.O.C.).

(i) *V.I.C.*

This technique should be practised with caution, for the expired gases will contain an ever-increasing proportion of halothane vapour, and in passing through the vaporizer will pick up more halothane, so that the final inspired concentration may greatly exceed that indicated by the vaporizer setting. Provided the vaporizer is relatively inefficient in respect of its ability to adapt to low flow-rates (e.g. the Goldman and Marrett), as respiratory depression increases, so will vaporization at a given setting diminish—thus a servo-mechanism is achieved. However, when respiration is controlled, and the minute volume therefore maintained, a dangerously high concentration of halothane may be inadvertently achieved within the circuit.

(ii) *V.O.C.*

Placing the vaporizer outside the circuit carries the advantage that under normal conditions the concentration of inspired halothane will never exceed that indicated by the vaporizer setting. Indeed, the rapid tissue uptake of halothane ensures a low expired concentration, which in turn serves to dilute the vapour emerging from the vaporizer. This safety factor applies to both controlled and spontaneous respiration, and it should be noted that a very efficient vaporizer is required in order to function accurately at the low basal flow-rate in use.

For practical purposes in dental anaesthesia, the semi-open circuit is normally advisable owing to the technical difficulty of establishing and maintaining an efficient leak-proof closed system. It should, however, be pointed out that, irrespective of vaporizer position, the closed circuit is much more economical.

Pharmacological Properties

1. *Central Nervous System.*—The pattern of depression of the central nervous system follows that of the other powerful anaesthetic agents, overdose ultimately leading to central respiratory and vasomotor paralysis. Analgesic properties are not well marked.

2. *Autonomic System.*—The sympathetic is depressed more than the parasympathetic, the tone of the latter thus predominating. This effect may be utilized to facilitate venipuncture, particularly in the transfusion of shocked patients.

3. *Cardiovascular System.*—The effects of halothane on cardiovascular function are complex and variable, and thus are the subject of considerable controversy. However, all observers agree that halothane produces a fall in blood pressure if the alveolar concentration is increased above a critical level. This level varies not only from individual to individual, but also in the same individual according to circumstances. Various studies have shown that the average fall in blood pressure with inspired concentrations of 1·4–2% is in the order of 20–30%. Although blood pressure alteration is often the most striking sign of disturbed cardiovascular function, in order to appreciate the significance of any alteration it is necessary to recall that blood pressure is the product of cardiac output (C.O.) and total peripheral resistance (T.P.R.), i.e. B.P. = C.O. × T.P.R.

Halothane exerts an influence on both components and the relevant effects are described below.

(a) *Cardiac Output.*—Cardiac output is the product of stroke volume and heart rate, and under normal circumstances will adjust itself to the venous return.

Thus any drug may affect cardiac output either by exerting a direct influence on venous return or by impairing the heart's ability to respond to any variations in that venous return. There is clearly no way in which the heart is able to distribute more blood than is returned to it, and should the cardiac output fail to keep pace with the returned blood, congestive heart failure will inevitably result.

Cardiac output, in addition to other factors, influences venous return, so that the effects of any drug upon the circulatory dynamics are often complex and variable, thus accounting for much of the controversy which surrounds the cardiovascular action of such drugs.

In the case of halothane the following effects may exert an influence on cardiac output.

(i) *Venous tone* is diminished, thus leading to an increase in venous capacitance and an overall reduction in venous return.

(ii) *Stroke volume* may be directly reduced as a result of the depressant effect of halothane on heart muscle. However, in normal clinical dosage the heart is still capable of responding to changes in circumstances which demand an increase in cardiac output (e.g. anoxia).

(iii) *Heart rate* is often reduced by deep halothane, probably as the result of prolongation of the refractory period of the heart muscle and a slowing of conduction in the A.V. (atrio-ventricular) nodal and ventricular tissue. These effects are believed to be predominantly vagal in origin and therefore are often abolished by the administration of atropine. However, provided the level of anaesthesia is not profound and the subject is healthy, the heart rate frequently remains unchanged, and may indeed increase in response to either surgical stimulation or a fall in peripheral resistance.

(b) *Total Peripheral Resistance.*—Although there is not unanimous agreement as to the effect of halothane on the total peripheral resistance, the majority of workers have found a decrease of 15–20% with a 2% inspired concentration. This decrease is believed to be predominantly due to central vasomotor depression, although sympathetic ganglionic blockade and a direct depressant action on vascular smooth muscle have been suggested as contributory causes.

In conclusion, it may be said that halothane can have a profound effect on blood pressure by reducing both peripheral resistance and cardiac output. In practice, provided the depth of anaesthesia is not excessive and the patient's cardiovascular system is healthy, the blood pressure is maintained within normal limits.

Cerebral Blood Flow.—The cerebral vascular resistance is consistently reduced by halothane and therefore the cerebral blood flow is normally increased so long as the perfusion pressure does not fall below 65 mmHg. It should be noted that in patients suffering from severe central arterial sclerosis, the cerebral vascular resistance will not fall with halothane; therefore, any decrease in blood pressure may result in a dangerous diminution in cerebral blood flow.

Coronary Blood Flow.—Most workers have demonstrated a decrease in coronary blood flow—presumably related to a reduction in mean aortic pressure—but since this reduction is associated with a diminution in cardiac work (due to reduced peripheral resistance), the overall oxygen demands of the heart are adequately satisfied. With these considerations in mind, halothane can be considered to be a suitable agent for patients with coronary disease, but clearly it is undesirable to allow the mean aortic pressure to fall unduly.

Skin and Muscle Blood Flow.—Using forearm and finger plethysmography, a four-fold increase in peripheral blood flow has been demonstrated.

Cardiac Rhythm.—Although there exists no direct evidence that halothane produces increased cardiac irritability, dysrhythmias may arise in ventricles, atrioventricular node, or atria, and may be associated with depression of atrioventricular conduction. These dysrhythmias are likely to occur in the presence of increased catecholamine blood level. Halothane does not normally stimulate the production of catecholamines, but if their blood level is increased as a result of hypercarbia, hypoxia, surgical stimulation under light anaesthesia, or the injection of adrenaline, then severe and potentially dangerous cardiac dysrhythmias may occur (page 166), and are particularly likely to do so in the presence of halothane. The incidence of dysrhythmias associated with halothane and other anaesthetic agents is reduced by the administration of beta-adrenergic blocking agents such as practolol (page 23).

4. *Respiratory System.*—Halothane is said to produce a significant depression of minute volume even in light surgical anaesthesia, although to what extent this depression exceeds that of normal sleep does not appear to have been established. The overall reduction in minute volume is associated with a decrease in tidal exchange but an increase in respiratory rate. As anaesthesia deepens, this depression is asso-

ciated with decreased respiratory response to a rise in arterial carbon dioxide tension.

If halothane is administered with nitrous oxide (70%) and oxygen, there is evidence to suggest that the respiratory minute volume may be either increased or decreased compared with halothane and oxygen, depending upon the alveolar concentration of halothane achieved. Under the conditions prevailing in dentistry, with light surgical anaesthesia, the addition of nitrous oxide is likely to reduce the ventilatory depression produced by halothane.

Halothane is relatively non-irritant to the respiratory mucosa, there being no stimulation of salivary or bronchial secretions. Pharyngeal and laryngeal reflexes are depressed and the bronchial musculature relaxed, the drug thus being suitable for use in asthmatic and bronchitic subjects. Ciliary action is depressed.

5. *Muscular System.*—Halothane, by means of its depressant action on the central nervous system, produces moderate relaxation of voluntary (striped) muscle. If neuro-muscular blockade is achieved by a non-depolarizing muscle relaxant (e.g. curare), halothane will increase this peripheral effect.

Recovery from prolonged halothane anaesthesia is often associated with bouts of violent shivering and generalized muscular rigidity. This phenomenon is not fully understood, but is usually associated with a fall in skin temperature. The effect can be reversed by the administration of various central depressants such as pethidine and diazepam, but we believe that the correct prevention or treatment lies in the maintenance of an optimal environmental temperature of 33°C (see page 135).

Halothane relaxes smooth muscle, notably that of the uterus and the bronchial tree.

6. *Alimentary System.*—The secretion of saliva, mucous and gastric juice is not stimulated, and the incidence of post-anaesthetic nausea and vomiting is less than that associated with all inhalation agents other than nitrous oxide.

7. *Kidney Function.*—Halothane has no specific depressant effect on renal function.

8. *Liver Function.*—The effect of halothane on liver function is still controversial, but there is no evidence of direct hepatotoxicity. However, there is some evidence to suggest that halothane administration—particularly if repeated—may occasionally be associated with impaired liver function of a type difficult to distinguish both clinically and histologically from infective hepatitis. Although large-scale retrospective studies have failed to establish beyond doubt that halothane is the causative factor, it is nevertheless advisable to be cautious whenever repeated administrations are anticipated. Whilst it is not suggested that an alternative agent need necessarily be used, should there be evidence of unexplained pyrexia and/or malaise following the previous halothane administration, its further use is best avoided. Halothane is broken down in the body to a small extent, but the degradation products do not appear to be hepatotoxic.

Methoxyflurane—(Trade name—Penthrane)

Physical Properties

Methoxyflurane is a clear, colourless liquid, the vapour of which is non-inflammable and has a fruity odour. It is a stable compound, but prolonged exposure to light produces a brown discoloration said to be of no significance. It is unaffected by soda-lime, but its vapour brings about the deterioration of rubber.

Molecular weight—164; Relative density—1·43; Boiling point—104·8°C; Vapour pressure (20°C) 25 mmHg; Solubility partition coefficients—(a) Blood/gas—13; (b) Brain/blood—2·34; (c) Fat/blood—38·5; (d) Rubber/gas—7·24.

The low vapour pressure and relatively high blood solubility combine to render rapid induction of anaesthesia difficult with this agent. Likewise, recovery is slow.

Pharmacological Properties

1. *Central Nervous System.*—The pattern of depression is orthodox, overdose leading to central respiratory and vasomotor depression. Although opinions differ as to its analgesic potential, recent work carried out on obstetric patients indicates that 0·35% concentration in the inspired mixture will provide superior pain-relief to that associated with 50:50 nitrous oxide/oxygen mixtures with comparable clouding of consciousness; as an obstetric analgesic, it is thought to be as effective as trichlorethylene and less apt to produce mental confusion. In spite of these special analgesic properties, the agent has not become popular in out-patient dental anaesthesia because of the slow rate of induction and recovery associated with its effective use; future developments may indicate a sphere of usefulness in self-administered analgesia for conservative dentistry.

2. *Cardiovascular System.*—The effects on the cardiovascular system are similar to those of halothane, except that the fall in blood pressure which may be associated with the administration of methoxyflurane is due mainly to a reduction in cardiac output, whereas that associated with halothane is accompanied by a marked reduction in peripheral resistance. Thus, hypotension associated with methoxyflurane, as opposed to halothane, is characterized by pallor.

3. *Respiratory System.*—There is a moderate reduction in minute volume due to a reduction in tidal exchange, but associated with rapid breathing (tachypnoea).

4. *Muscular System.*—Voluntary muscle relaxation is moderate, and associated with central depression rather than myo-neural blockade.

5. *Alimentary System.*—There is evidence to suggest that the incidence of post-anaesthetic nausea and vomiting is considerably higher than that associated with halothane.

6.   Renal and hepatic damage have been described.

Teflurane

Teflurane is a recently introduced agent, the high volatility and low blood solubility of which indicate its potential suitability for use in out-patient anaesthesia.

However, the concentration required to produce adequate surgical anaesthesia, also produces such a high incidence of severe cardiac irregularities as to demand more extensive investigation before its ultimate safety can be assessed.

Enflurane—(Ethrane, compound 347)

This is a new fluorinated ether with similar properties to halothane, but said to be free from the latter's dysrhythmogenic properties. It may therefore prove to be of value in dental out-patient anaesthesia.

Non-Fluorinated Anaesthetic Agents

In dentistry, by far the most important agent in this group is 'Trilene', but certain other drugs will be briefly described in this section.

Trichlorethylene (B.P., U.S.P.)—(Trade name—Trilene)

$$\begin{array}{cc} Cl & Cl \\ | & | \\ H-C & = C - Cl \end{array}$$

Physical Properties

Trichlorethylene is a colourless liquid, the vapour of which is non-inflammable. It is more irritant than that of halothane. The commercial anaesthetic preparation Trilene is coloured by the addition of waxoline blue, and contains 0·01% thymol as a stabilizing agent. Decomposition into dichloracetylene, phosgene and carbon monoxide will occur on exposure to light and heat, and the agent should therefore be stored in a cool, dark environment. This decomposition is also produced by alkalis, and Trilene should not be used in association with soda-lime.

Molecular weight—131·4; Relative density—4·35; Boiling point—87·5C; Vapour pressure (20°C)—60 mmHg; Solubility partition coefficients—(a) Blood/gas—9·0; (b) Fat/blood—106·7.

The relatively low vapour pressure and high blood solubility combine to render induction and recovery from anaesthesia slow when compared with halothane. At present, Trilene is often administered from a low-efficiency vaporizer (e.g. the Goldman.—See Table XI, page 69), but there is an increasing demand for the high-efficiency temperature controlled type of apparatus. An inspired concentration of 0·5%–2% is normally used to achieve surgical anaesthesia, concentrations in excess of 2% proving difficult to breathe owing to the irritant properties of the agent.

Pharmacological Properties

1. *Central Nervous System.*—The pattern of depression is orthodox, serious respiratory and vasomotor depression only occurring with a degree of overdose unlikely to be encountered in normal clinical practice. Analgesia is the outstanding characteristic of Trilene, and the fact that effective pain-relief without loss of consciousness can be achieved by the inhalation of 0·35%–0·5% Trilene in air has led to its acceptance as a true analgesic in both obstetrics and dentistry.

2. *Cardiovascular System.*—Cardiac output and blood pressure normally remain unchanged, but dysrhythmias are not uncommon, particularly in the presence of a raised carbon dioxide tension; an excess of circulating adrenaline may produce ventricular fibrillation. Bradycardia may occur, and is thought to be due to an increase in vagal tone.

3. *Respiratory System.*—Tachypnoea is the most common respiratory disturbance; rates of up to 40 per minute may occur, particularly in children, and may lead to inefficient respiratory exchange. This characteristic is thought to be due to over-sensitization of the lung stretch-receptors (Hering-Breuer reflex). Although the drug is more irritant to the respiratory mucosa than halothane, there is no tendency to stimulate the production of excessive bronchial secretions. Ciliary action is depressed.

4. *Muscular System.*—Voluntary muscle relaxation is minimal.

5. *Alimentary System.*—The incidence of post-anaesthetic nausea and vomiting is higher than that associated with halothane, particularly when a high inspired concentration has been used.

6. *Liver Function.*—Liver damage has been reported, but is rare.

Excretion.—Trichlorethylene is broken down in the body, but it is chiefly excreted unchanged through the lungs.

Cyclopropane

$$
\begin{array}{c}
\overset{\displaystyle H_2}{\underset{}{C}} \\
H_2C\text{——}CH_2
\end{array}
$$

Cyclopropane enjoyed a brief period of popularity in an attempt to provide rapid anaesthesia in the dental out-patient without oxygen restriction. The unacceptable explosion hazard was overcome by adding nitrogen to the inhaled mixture, but the technique advocated was associated with an extremely high nausea and vomiting rate. The introduction of halothane has made the use of this costly drug unnecessary in dental practice.

Ethyl Chloride

$$
\begin{array}{c}
Cl \quad H \\
| \qquad | \\
H\text{—}C\text{—}C\text{—}H \\
| \qquad | \\
H \quad H
\end{array}
$$

For many years this inflammable agent was used for the rapid open-mask induction of anaesthesia in children, it being possible to carry out a short dental procedure after removal of the mask. It was also used to subdue the persistent mouth breathing adult, by the simple expedient of spraying it on the mouth-pack. However, its high cardiotoxic potential, and its not infrequent association with sudden cardiovascular collapse led to its abandonment in orthodox anaesthetic circles.

Divinyl Ether (Vinesthene)

$$\underset{\displaystyle H-C=C-O-C=C-H}{\overset{\displaystyle H\ \ H\quad\ \ H\ \ H}{}}$$

This inflammable and highly volatile agent was used as a safer alternative to ethyl chloride in children. In practice, its high volatility dictated that it should be used in a closed system, and the explosion hazard together with its secreto-motor stimulant effect combined to allow its replacement in anaesthetic practice by halothane—in spite of its good safety record.

From the foregoing account it would appear that halothane most nearly fulfils the criteria considered desirable in an inhalation agent for out-patient use; and therefore at the present time it must be considered the inhalational supplement of choice to nitrous oxide in both children and adult out-patients. In circumstances where cost and availability are significant factors, trichlorethylene is probably the most satisfactory alternative, but where a rapid induction and short maintenance is required, particularly in small children, the choice may lie between ethyl chloride and vinesthene. Although vinesthene is considered the safer of the two agents, induction with ethyl chloride is easier to manage, and provided hypoxia and overdose are meticulously avoided, many experienced anaesthetists would consider the drug less dangerous than is generally accepted.

Chloroform

This agent is considered too hepatotoxic and cardiotoxic for use in dental anaesthesia and therefore will not be discussed further.

Ether

This agent, in spite of its high margin of safety, is not of value in dentistry owing to its inflammability, its irritant properties, and its high blood solubility leading to slow induction and recovery. The classical Guedel description of the stages of anaesthesia originally applied to the use of open ether anaesthesia and is as follows:

First Stage or stage of analgesia. From beginning of induction to loss of consciousness.

Second Stage or stage of unconscious excitement. From loss of consciousness to onset of automatic respiration. May be characterized by struggling, breath-holding, swallowing, vomiting, coughing.

Third Stage or stage of surgical anaesthesia.

Plane 1. From onset of automatic respiration to cessation of eyeball movement.

Plane 2. From cessation of eyeball movement to commencement of intercosta
    paralysis.

Plane 3. From commencement to completion of intercostal paralysis.

Plane 4. From complete intercostal paralysis to diaphragmatic paralysis.

Fourth Stage. Overdose leading to death.

RECOMMENDED READING

1. **Uptake of Anaesthetic Gases by the Body.**
    KETY, S. S. (1950) *Anaesthesiology*, **11**, 517.
2. **Uptake and Elimination of Anaesthetics.**
    BOURNE, J. G. (1967) *Studies in Anaesthetics*. London: Lloyd-Luke. Chap. 1.
3. **Carriage of Oxygen and Carbon Dioxide in the Body.**
    KEELE, G. A. & NEIL, E. (Ed.) (1971) *Wright's Applied Physiology*, 12th Ed., Part IV.
4. **Halothane.**
    GREEN, N. M. (1968) *Clinical Anaesthesia—Halothane*.
5. **The Halothane Dilemma.**
    SIMPSON, B. R., STRUNNIN, L. & WALTON, J. G. (1971) *Br. med. J.*, iv, 96.
6. **Nitrous Oxide Impurities.**
    AUSTIN, A. T., KAIN, M. L., SMITH, W. D. A. & CLUTTON-BROCK, J. (1967) *Proc. R. Soc. Med.*, **60**, 1175.

CHAPTER FIVE

INHALATIONAL TECHNIQUES FOR EXODONTIA
IN THE OUT-PATIENT

The following account describes a simple inhalation technique which should prove satisfactory for the majority of uncomplicated adult patients.

Before allowing the patient to enter the surgery, the anaesthetist must discipline himself to adopt the following routine.

(i) Prepare all necessary drugs.

(ii) Check all cylinder contents, including spares marked 'full'.

(iii) Thoroughly familiarize himself with all the control mechanisms of the particular chair in use.

(iv) Ascertain the exact nature of the proposed dental procedure, and briefly recheck with his colleague the patient's medical history.

(v) Check the availability of routine equipment such as props, gags, packs, etc., and make sure that any additional emergency equipment is also to hand.

(vi) Know the patient's name.

It is assumed that all necessary preoperative measures as described in Chapter 1 have already been carried out, and that after exchange of the normal courtesies, the patient may be positioned in the dental chair in whatever posture is deemed appropriate to the prevailing circumstances. This controversial subject is fully debated in Chapter 8, and here we will attempt only to describe the positions in common use and the purely practical problems each may present.

1. Sitting Posture

(a) The patient's buttocks should be well back in the chair, and to ensure this, it is advisable to tilt the chair slightly backwards as shown in Fig. 48. If no backward tilt is employed, as in Fig. 46, there is a tendency for the patient to slide his buttocks forwards for comfort, thus adopting the unsatisfactory position shown in Fig. 47. Restraining straps are not necessary under the conditions obtainable with modern anaesthesia, and their use should be avoided.

(b) The position of the head should be that which offers the maximum comfort to the patient. This position can be altered if necessary as soon as the patient is asleep, in order to facilitate maintenance of the airway or surgical access (Figs. 49 and 50).

(c) The patient's hands should lie comfortably in the lap. With present day standards of anaesthesia it is unnecessary to insist that the patient puts his hands in his pockets or even clasps them in his lap. Instructions of this sort often serve only to alarm the patient, and may even add to restlessness during induction owing to a feeling of unnatural bodily restriction.

2. Supine Posture

When this position is adopted (see Figs. 20 and 51), care should be taken to ensure that the head is placed in a comfortable position and stabilized with a suitable head rest. The arms should be prevented from falling backwards between the chair and arm rest.

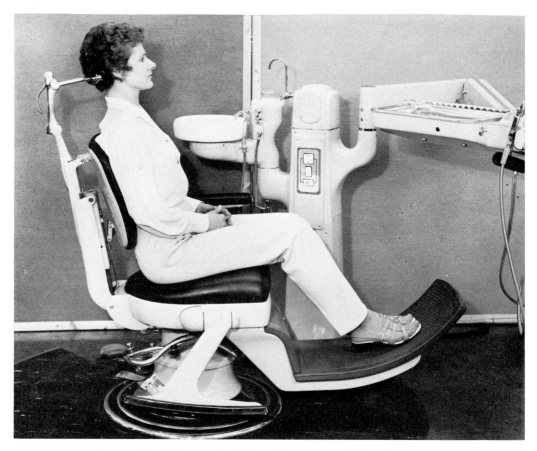

FIG. 46.—Patient sitting in fully upright posture with legs dependant

3. Reclining Posture

As seen from Fig. 52, the reclining posture represents a compromise between the sitting and supine, and it must be stressed that the prime object in this posture is to enable the legs to be raised; thus, it is essential, for the patient's comfort, to recline the back rest in relation to the seat.

The advantages and disadvantages of each of these postures are fully discussed in Chapter 8. For the majority of exodontia cases we favour the reclining posture, but the following account covers both this and the supine.

Attention will have already been paid to certain details of immediate preparation as listed in Chapter 1, but whenever possible, instructions and questioning of the patient should be carried out before finally positioning him in the chair, in order to occasion him the minimum anxiety.

INDUCTION OF ANAESTHESIA

The following account describes the use of nitrous oxide, oxygen and halothane.

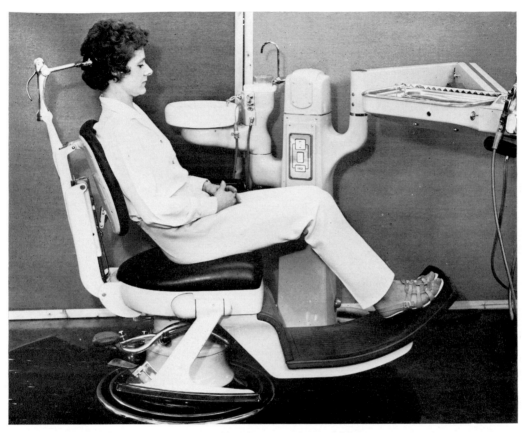

FIG. 47.—Patient sitting in upright posture
Note tendency for patient to slide buttocks forward and over-flex head

Position of Anaesthetist

The anaesthetist should either stand or sit behind the patient, depending on the posture of the latter (Figs. 53 and 54). In this position he has the maximum control of the airway and can be of greatest assistance to the dentist in supporting the head. He also has easy access to the carotid and temporal pulses, and can manipulate the chair, without moving his position, in an emergency.

Insertion of Prop

In the co-operative patient, the prop may be inserted immediately prior to the commencement of induction of anaesthesia, but it is important that no further questions should be asked of the patient following its insertion. The prop selected should be comfortable for that particular patient. If the patient proves unwilling to tolerate a prop, its insertion should be delayed until anaesthesia has been established. With modern anaesthesia this should not present any problem, since relaxation is

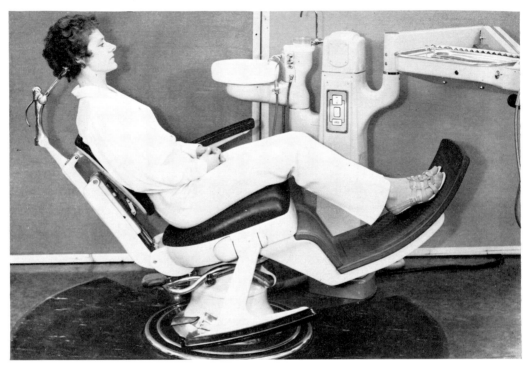

FIG. 48.—The unsatisfactory posture shown in fig. 47 has been prevented by tilting chair backwards. Note that slight flexion of the neck brings the body of the mandible into the horizontal plane

readily achieved, and any delay in commencing extraction is preferable to an induction marred by a gagging, restless patient. The prop is inserted on the opposite side of the mouth from the proposed work, unless it is desired to apply an upper forceps to an instanding lower tooth, in which case either a prop may be placed behind the instanding tooth, or alternatively a gag may be used, in order to provide unrestricted surgical access. If exodontia is to be bilateral, the side giving rise to pain should be commenced first.

Inhalation Induction

Induction of anaesthesia by the inhalation method for out-patients has been largely replaced by the intravenous route, owing to the introduction of metho-

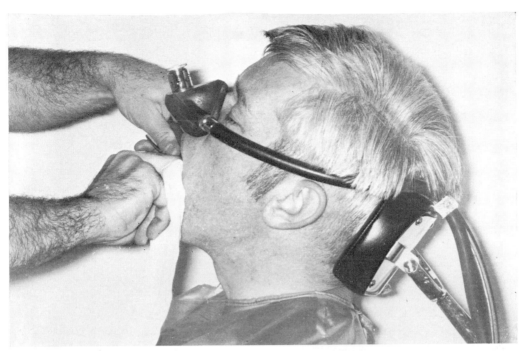

FIG. 49.—Head upright for extraction of lower tooth. Note that surgeon's right hand is pulling mandible forwards to maintain an unobstructed airway

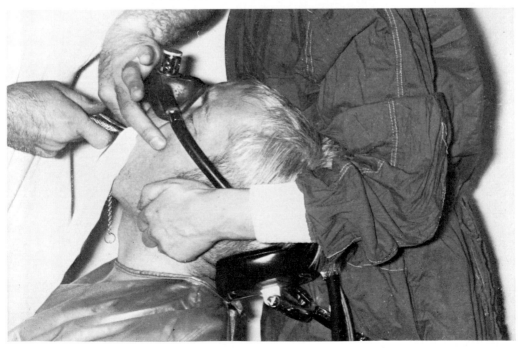

FIG. 50.—Head extended for ease of access to upper tooth. Note counter pressure applied to patient's head by anaesthetist's chest

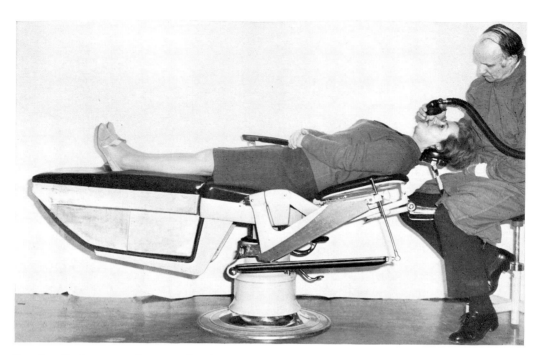

FIG. 51.—Supine posture in conventional chair (left arm rest lowered) with leg support. Compare with the more comfortable posture achieved in fig. 20 (Chap. 3) with the contoured chair

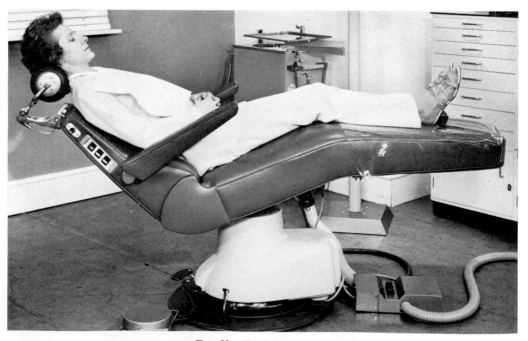

FIG. 52.—Reclining posture

hexitone and propanidid into anaesthetic practice. However, there are still many patients, particularly children, who prefer an inhalation induction and some in whom, for medical reasons, intravenous drugs are contraindicated (e.g. Ludwig's angina). In addition to this, many practitioners have little experience of venipuncture and therefore have a greater facility for the inhalation route.

Before the induction is commenced, every effort should be made to ensure a quiet environment and a relaxed patient. All instruments should be hidden from view and the only voice heard should be that of the anaesthetist.

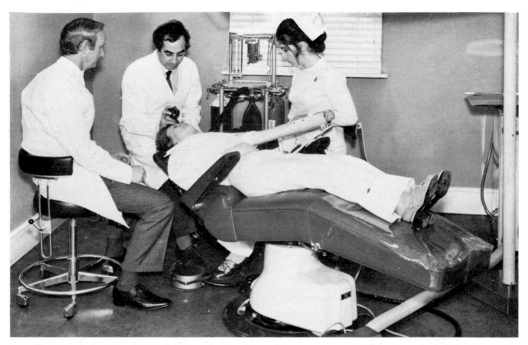

FIG. 53.—Operating team seated. Note that outlet and bag-mount on Salisbury anaesthetic machine are adapted for low-seated dentistry

The patient should be asked to close his eyes and breathe quietly through the nose, while a gaseous mixture consisting of 75% N_2O and 25% O_2 is administered through a nasal mask. If the machine is of the intermittent flow type, e.g. Walton Five, the flow-rate will be determined by the pressure control which is usually set at 5 mmHg pressure, and the gas mixture can be delivered either through a twin tube nasal inhaler, or a single wide bore tube with Goldman nose-piece. If the machine is a continuous flow type, e.g. Salisbury, the flow-rate is controlled by accurate flow-meters and for the purpose of induction a high flow-rate is advisable (9 litres/min. nitrous oxide/3 litres/min. oxygen), preferably delivered through a single wide bore tube for reasons explained on page 80.

It is not necessary, nor generally advisable, to apply the mask to the patient's face at the commencement of induction, as a state of 'amnalgesia' (page 252) can be achieved by holding the mask over the head, and allowing the gases partially to displace the air breathed. When this state has been achieved, the mask can be applied to the face and other anaesthetic vapours introduced. In the case of halothane the percentage can be increased up to 4% as quickly as is readily accepted by the patient. However, if the anaesthetist has little experience with the use of halothane in a wider context than dental anaesthesia, he should limit the concentration used to 2% owing to the increased risk of circulatory changes occurring with higher concentrations.

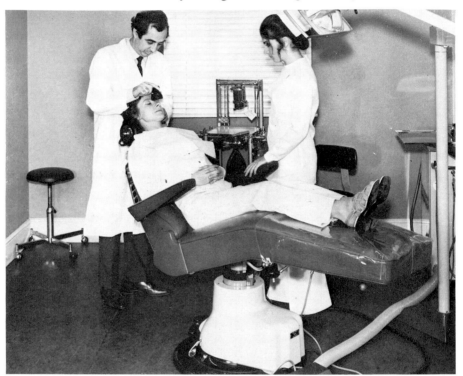

FIG. 54.—Anaesthetist standing for the induction of anaesthesia, with patient in reclining posture

Provided the mask is applied carefully and gently, the patient will retain no memory of either the odour of the anaesthetic or physical contact with the mask. It is most important that the nasal mask should completely enclose, but not obstruct the nares (Figs. 55 and 56). The simple instruction to close the eyes, relax, and breathe quietly through the nose, repeated frequently, is a valuable adjunct to the action of the anaesthetic drugs. The instruction to breathe deeply or blow the gas away is nearly always misguided, since it spoils the suggestion of sleep, and often leads to restlessness and hyperventilation, which in turn may give rise to mouth-breathing and occasionally apnoea. The commonest obstacle to smooth progress in the induction of anaesthesia is mouth-breathing, particularly in the nervous patient attempting to hyperventilate. Whilst this can usually be corrected by encouragement and persuasion, on rare occasions, when there is an anatomical cause for nasal obstruction, either a mouth cover or a full face mask should be used. If the narrow bore twin tube nasal mask is being employed in conjunction with an intermittent flow machine capable of delivering high flow-rates, a mouth cover will be effective, provided that this attachment both delivers an adequate flow of gases to the patient, and allows unimpeded expiration through an expiratory valve. Failure to satisfy these criteria may result in tumultous consequences in a patient unable to breathe through the nose. If wide

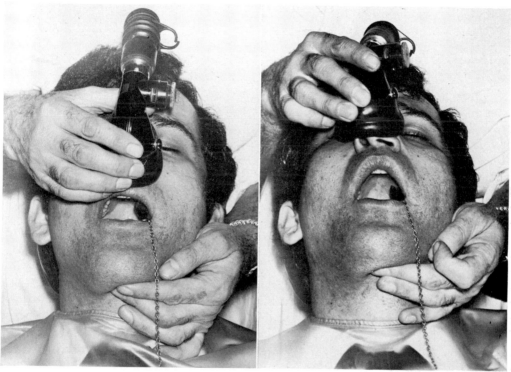

FIG. 55.—The Goldman nasal mask completely enclosing the nares. The airway is being maintained by gentle sub-mental support

FIG. 56.—The Goldman mask carelessly applied

bore tubing and Goldman nasal mask are employed—particularly with a continuous flow machine—the narrow bore mouth cover attachment will prove useless, unless the expiratory valve on the nasal mask is closed. Under these circumstances a full face mask is usually preferable.

Onset of 'Surgical Anaesthesia'

The lightest level of anaesthesia at which a surgical stimulus can be applied to an anaesthetized patient without the likelihood of a reflex response being elicited, is here described as the 'onset of surgical anaesthesia', and is conventionally accepted as coinciding with the first plane of the third stage of the Guedel classification (page 111). It is often difficult to tell exactly when this stage has been reached, as indeed this will vary considerably with the intensity of the surgical stimulus and the pain threshold of the patient. The experienced anaesthetist will know approximately how much anaesthetic is likely to have been absorbed after a given period of time. It is this knowledge, in conjunction with the onset of automatic respiration and the state of the 'eyelash reflex' which are considered by us to be the most valuable indications that the desired depth of anaesthesia has been reached. It should be stressed however, that the only ultimate indication of adequate depth of anaesthesia is the absence of an undesirable response to the particular stimulus applied.

The following features of surgical anaesthesia merit further consideration.

1. *Automatic Respiration*

During the induction of anaesthesia the respiratory pattern is variable; should this phase be characterized by striking fluctuations in rate and depth, as is common with the nervous, tense patient, then the onset of automatic respiration is easily recognized by a change in which breaths are taken at regular intervals, and inspiration and expiration bear a constant relationship to one another. This change may be almost imperceptible if it follows a smooth induction in a co-operative relaxed patient. The stertorous respiration, in which heavy forceful expiration predominates, for so long described as the prime feature of automatic respiration, is clearly associated with unsupplemented nitrous oxide and its concomitant hypoxia, and is seldom seen with the technique under discussion.

2. *Eye Signs*

(a) *Eyelash and Eyelid Reflexes.*—The reflex activity of the orbicularis muscle decreases with increasing depth of anaesthesia. During very light anaesthesia this reflex activity is brisk, i.e. the patient blinks if the eyelashes are touched, and any attempt to open the lids is actively resisted. As anaesthesia deepens, these reflexes become increasingly sluggish, and complete disappearance is often a confirmatory sign of entry into surgical anaesthesia. It should be remembered that attempts to elicit these reflexes too early, only serve to disturb the patient, and therefore should be made solely to confirm other evidence of surgical anaesthesia.

(b) *Eyeball Movement.*—Prior to surgical anaesthesia, and indeed usually until the first plane is well established, the position and movement of the eyeball is variable. It is not necessary to achieve a fixed central eyeball before commencing dental surgery; thus, the eyeball signs are of little clinical value.

(c) *Conjunctival and Corneal Reflex.*—This sign refers to the reflex closure of the eye when the conjunctiva or cornea is stimulated. It persists longer than the eyelash reflex, and since there is some danger of damaging the eye, it should not be routinely employed.

3. *Relaxation*

If a prop has not been inserted prior to induction, it is necessary to obtain sufficient jaw relaxation to enable the mouth to be opened without the use of excessive force. With halothane, such relaxation is usually present at the onset of surgical anaesthesia and the jaw may be readily opened, either by using a suitable mouth gag (page 81), or by applying downward finger pressure to the lower jaw, with counter pressure to the forehead as illustrated in Fig. 57. It is difficult to perform this manoeuvre without causing transient airway obstruction.

When, by consideration of the above signs, surgical anaesthesia appears to have been established, the mouth may be packed.

PACKING THE MOUTH

Objects

(a) *Protection of the Respiratory Tract.*—The prime object of packing is to protect the pharynx from contamination by any foreign material released by the surgical procedure. This material, if allowed to enter the pharynx, may cause protective reflex gagging, swallowing or laryngeal spasm, thus interfering with the smooth course of anaesthesia. These protective reflexes are not, however always effective in preventing contamination of the lungs. Thus, skilful packing is an important factor in achieving both safe and tranquil conditions.

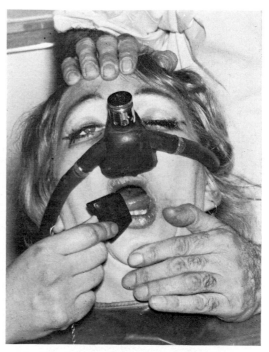

FIG. 57.—Method of inserting prop on relaxed anaesthetized patient

(b) *Prevention of Mouth breathing.*—Correct packing may be utilized to ensure the continuance of nasal breathing, which is dependent upon the close apposition of the dorsum of the tongue to the palate (Figs 58 and 59). Therefore it will be apparent that any manoeuvre which depresses the tongue will lead to mouth breathing; for the tongue is the only truly efficient central oropharyngeal partition, and therefore the keynote to successful packing is to interfere with the position of the tongue as little as possible once nasal breathing has been established. Some interference is usually inevitable but can be limited to lateral displacement; any packing material placed between the tongue and the soft palate will, by hindering the upward movement of the tongue inherent in nasal breathing, render mouth breathing likely to occur. Should such a pack be placed too far back, it may push the soft palate against the posterior pharyngeal wall, thus completely obstructing the nasopharynx (Fig. 60).

Method

(a) *Posterior Teeth.*—For the extraction of all posterior teeth it is essential that the posterior extremity of the pack makes firm contact with the mucosa overlying the ramus of the mandible, and entirely obliterates the retromolar space, thus preventing the passage of all foreign materials from the mouth to the pharynx. If the upper molar teeth only are to be extracted the pack may then be folded in layers so that it

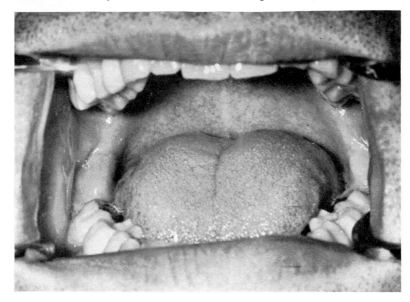

FIG. 58.—Nose-breathing, showing close apposition of dorsum of tongue to palate, thus sealing the oropharyngeal isthmus

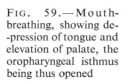
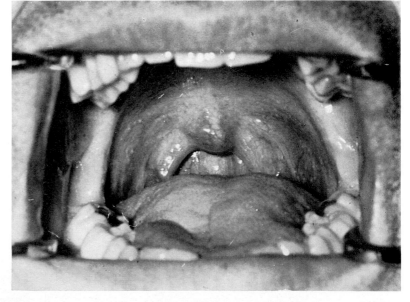

FIG. 59.—Mouth-breathing, showing de--pression of tongue and elevation of palate, the oropharyngeal isthmus being thus opened

lies across the side of the tongue and covers the lower teeth (Fig. 61), thereby isolating completely the operation area; if however, lower molar teeth are to be extracted it is essential to tuck layers of pack into the lingual sulcus (Figs. 62 and 63)—a manoeuvre which is more difficult to achieve successfully in the supine than in the upright posture. The introduction of layers of pack between the teeth and tongue in this way can also be made to displace the tongue backwards, and providing this displacement is not

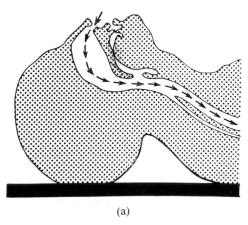

(a)   (b)

FIG. 60.—(a) Normal nasal breathing   (b) nasopharynx obstructed by pack

excessive it may aid nasal breathing by helping to keep the dorsum of the tongue in contact with the palate. Excessive backward displacement will result in respiratory obstruction and of course must be avoided. When extracting lower third molars,

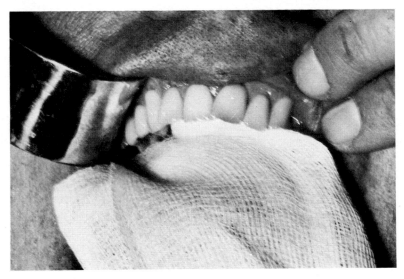

FIG. 61.—Packing upper teeth

particularly where an elevator is used and there is risk that the tooth may be displaced lingually, it is a wise precaution, in addition to this method of packing, to place thumb or finger lingually against the crown of the tooth while it is being elevated. This manoeuvre inevitably results in some displacement of the tongue, but if care is taken, this can usually be restricted to lateral compression.

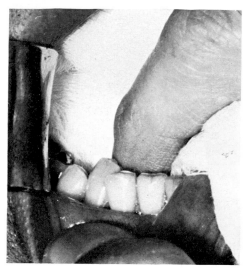

FIG. 62.—Pack being tucked deeply into lingual sulcus by index finger

(b) *Anterior Teeth.*—Isolating anteriorly placed teeth, using the same principles, presents little difficulty (Fig. 64).

(c) *Bilateral Extractions.*—When extractions are bilateral, on completion of the first side, the pack should be rearranged to cover and thus control the bleeding sockets. After insertion of prop or gag on the completed side, the second side is packed in the manner already described, with a fresh pack. Effective control of bleeding in multiple extractions will be facilitated if the first side extractions are limited to the minimum number of teeth which will enable the prop to be inserted on that side, so that the extraction of contralateral posterior, and all anterior teeth is completed under the protection of the second pack (Fig. 65).

We have found that the operator is usually in a better position to arrange the pack than the anaesthetist. Not only is he more fully aware of the exact nature of the operation to be performed and the presence of any loose teeth, but he has throughout,

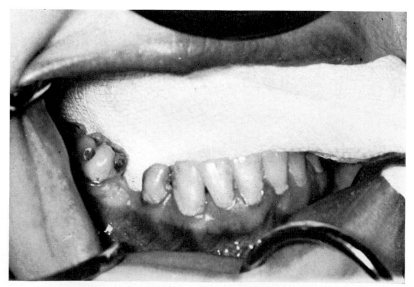

FIG. 63.—Pack in position for extraction of lower posterior teeth. Gap demonstrates that pack has been tucked deeply into lingual sulcus

a much better view of the patient's mouth. The ideal arrangement is, of course, to have a dental surgeon and anaesthetist who are used to working together as a team.

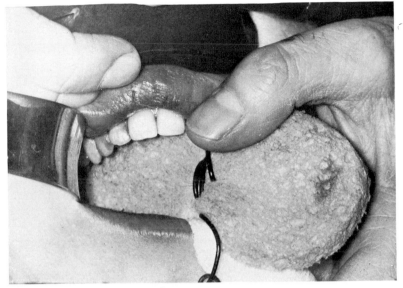

FIG. 64.—Flanged cellulose pack used in conjunction with gauze, for the extraction of upper anterior teeth

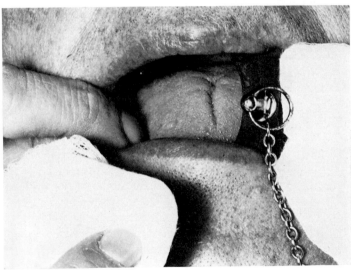

FIG. 65.—Packing for bilateral extractions. First pack covering completed area; second pack about to be inserted

Material

Whatever region is to be packed we would emphasize that flat layers of a broad pack of sufficient thickness afford much better protection than a small pack which may become rolled up into a tight bundle lying on top of the tongue.

We favour the use of gauze strips 9″ (22 cm) wide, cut into suitable lengths and folded into 3 thicknesses with the ends turned in. The texture of the gauze is of some importance, since a mesh that is too fine will reduce absorptive powers, whilst one which is too coarse is likely to fray or become caught on the cusps of teeth or in the blades of the forceps and will rapidly become sodden. An optimum gauge is about 16 ply. The lengths necessary will vary with the size of the patient and the site and nature of the procedure, but at all times no less than 4″ (10 cm) should be left hanging out of the mouth. Suitable lengths of gamgee may be used in place of the gauze, but prepared squares of gamgee and other materials supplied with tapes are not advised, owing to the danger of their slipping back into the pharynx should they become sodden with blood or saliva. This danger also applies to the flanged cellulose pack if used on its own for multiple extractions. We do, however, recommend the use of the flanged cellulose pack (page 239), in addition to the gauze pack, for all procedures which are prolonged or accompanied by considerable bleeding (Fig. 64). The cellulose pack may be changed as frequently as is necessary, without at any time disturbing the original gauze pack or allowing it to become excessively wet. Moreover, the presence of a cellulose pack will protect the gauze from becoming ensnared by a burr or needle point, should the use of either instrument prove necessary.

MAINTENANCE OF ANAESTHESIA

The induction of anaesthesia may be said to have been completed and main-tenance begun as soon as quiet, steady anaesthesia has been established, the pack inserted, and the patient rendered unresponsive to stimulation. At this stage the halothane can usually be reduced to 1% or 0·5% and the total flow to 8 l/min. (or 3 mmHg pressure on the intermittent flow machines). Provided smooth unobstructed nasal respiration can be maintained, it should be possible to keep the patient in light surgical anaesthesia for an indefinite period of time with this technique.

If it is adjudged that the surgical procedure is likely to be short (i.e. less than 2 minutes), the halothane may be turned off provided the patient does not exhibit any response to surgical stimuli. However, it must be remembered that halothane, because of its relatively low tissue solubility, is rapidly eliminated; thus, should any unforeseen surgical difficulty arise, it may be necessary to re-introduce the agent. Likewise, in procedures which are envisaged as requiring prolonged anaesthesia, it is advisable to use a maintenance dose of 0·5% halothane throughout, rather than to risk a return to reflex response and the consequent disturbance of respiratory rhythm. Where operator and anaesthetist are accustomed to working together as a team, it will usually be possible for the anaesthetist to forecast the conclusion of the opera-tion, and discontinue the halothane accordingly, thus rendering recovery as rapid as possible.

Mouth Breathing

In order to maintain stable controlled anaesthesia by the inhalation route, it is essential to prevent anaesthetic dilution by mouth breathing. The mechanism of mouth breathing, and the part played in its prevention by correct placement of the mouth pack, have already been described on page 123. Here, it must be pointed out that mouth breathing is sometimes associated with relaxation of the submandibular muscles in the upright posture, the tongue falling deeply into the floor of the mouth, thus opening up the oropharyngeal isthmus. This type of mouth breathing can be corrected by gentle external pressure in the submandibular region, the tongue being forced upwards to re-establish contact with the palate. Mouth breathing which occurs as an active response to surgical stimulation under light anaesthesia cannot be corrected by this simple manoeuvre, and indeed it is characterized by 'tightness' of the submandibular muscles; the anaesthetic must be deepened, and for this purpose a full face mask is sometimes required. It is occasionally necessary to maintain anaesthesia via a nasopharyngeal tube (page 142) in a subject in whom mouth breathing cannot be corrected by the methods described above.

Continued Airway Protection

Although the pack, if correctly placed, acts as an effective barrier from mouth to pharynx, in order to prevent it from becoming rapidly sodden, which is especially likely to occur in the supine posture, excess blood should at all times be removed by an efficient sucker. When the extractions are bilateral, on completion of the first side, the position of the pack should be arranged in such a way as to control bleeding from the extracted area. This is accomplished by using the freshly positioned prop as an additional means of applying pressure. The second side should then be packed in the manner already described.

General Supervision

During maintenance of anaesthesia, the anaesthetist has the dual task of assisting the operator and supervising the patient's general condition. When lower teeth are extracted he must support the mandible, and if the operator is unable to extract lower right teeth with his left hand, the anaesthetist will have to move to the left side of the patient in order to allow him suitable access. For upper teeth, in addition to providing counter pressure to the head (Fig. 50), the anaesthetist may improve access to the molar region by the application of firm forward pressure to the mandible on the contralateral side. For the extraction of upper anterior teeth, it may be necessary to remove a mask such as the Goldman which is characterized by a convex lower margin. These various manoeuvres must always be undertaken in such a way that the patient's airway remains unobstructed, and this task is sometimes rendered more difficult by the adoption of the supine posture, when the only effective method may lie in hyperextension of the head on the neck—a position which may increase the operator's difficulties.

The anaesthetist's attention must at all times be directed towards the patient's overall welfare, particularly as evidenced by the state of the respiratory and circulatory systems.

Respiratory System

During dental extractions, and in particular those involving difficult lower teeth, the operator frequently applies pressure on the lower jaw in such a direction as to

A.A.D.—5*

allow the tongue to obstruct the upper airway. In addition, if the supine posture is employed on a relaxed patient, the force of gravity frequently has the same effect. It is the anaesthetist's constant duty to correct even minor degrees of obstruction by correct counterpressure on the jaw. This is best achieved, as already stated, by firm pressure behind the angles of the mandible in a forward direction. When this pressure is prolonged it is advisable to cushion the pressure points with a suitable pad to avoid bruising (Figs. 66, 67, 68).

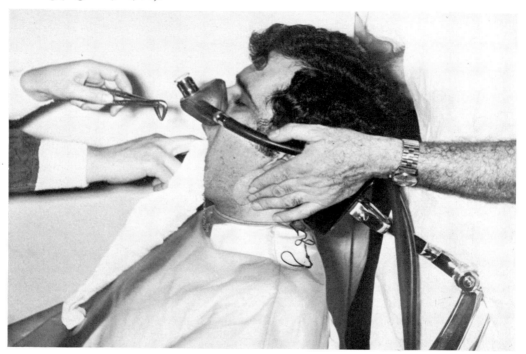

FIG. 66.—Maintenance of airway by firm pressure behind the mandible which is protected from bruising by the use of cellulose packs. Note ease of manoeuvre when self-retaining twin-tube nasal mask is used

The anaesthetist should be in a position to detect the first departure from normal respiration, by making the following observations:

(a) *Reservoir Bag.*—Provided the mask is well fitting and respiration is nasal, the movement of the reservoir bag gives an indication of the rate, depth and overall pattern of respiration. If the depth of anaesthesia is adequate, the rate will usually remain constant, irrespective of surgical stimulus. Provided the flow-rate of gases does not greatly exceed the patient's minute volume, the degree of movement of the bag will reflect the depth of respiration. At higher flow-rates, this sign is not so sensitive. The pattern of movement on the bag in unobstructed respiration is characterized by smooth excursions, in which expiration follows inspiration without a pause. Any departure from this pattern usually denotes a degree of airway obstruction, and should be immediately apparent to the anaesthetist.

FIG. 67.—Support of mandible using Goldman mask without harness. This manoeuvre is difficult for the anaesthetist with small hands

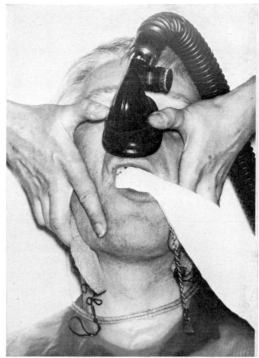

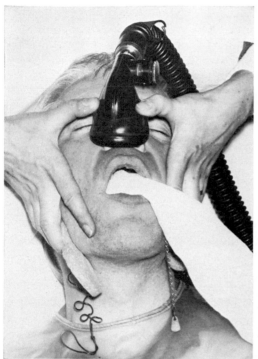

FIG. 68.—The mask has slipped out of position, obstructing the nares—a common mishap when this mask is used without a harness

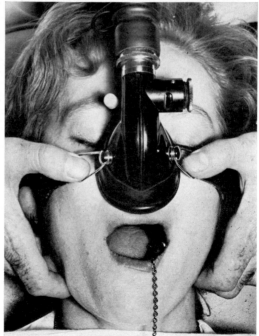

FIG. 69.—Improvement with use of harness

(b) *Chest Movement.*—In normal respiration the descent of the diaphragm, as observed by abdominal movement, slightly precedes or coincides with free expansion of the chest. Any tendency towards recession of the thoracic cage and supraclavicular fossae during inspiration, accompanied by jerky abdominal movements, suggests some degree of obstruction and is often referred to as see-saw respiration. In the fully clothed patient, this characteristic movement can be more easily felt than seen, by placing the hand over the upper part of the abdomen.

(c) *Valve Sounds.*—Under normal circumstances, the sound of gas escaping from the expiratory valve during each expiration, will serve as an audible guide to respiratory activity, and will be referred to as the 'valve sound' in subsequent description. The following alterations in the normal rhythm of the valve sound may occur:

(i) *Continuous Valve Sound.*—This may occur either in mouth breathing, or in the presence of breath holding, apnoea or complete respiratory obstruction.

In the event of mouth breathing, the additional sound of oral respiration may be heard. In breath holding, apnoea and obstruction, no oral exchange of air is heard, but the obstructed patient will usually show some abortive respiratory movement.

(ii) *Absence of Valve Sounds.*—This may occur with either the presence of a leak in the circuit, in which case the bag will also fail to fill; or with a reduction in gas flow rates due to the exhaustion of a cylinder.

(d) *Breath Sounds.*—Noisy respiration of a snoring, grunting or crowing nature almost always indicates partial respiratory obstruction, the nature of the noise depending upon the site of the obstruction.

Low pitched noise similar to that heard in snoring indicates the site of the obstruction to be supralaryngeal, the treatment of which is described on page 141. Occasionally this noise can be produced by soft palate vibration in the absence of respiratory obstruction.

High pitched inspiratory sound is invariably associated with laryngeal stridor and is described fully on page 144.

The forced expiratory wheeze associated with bronchospasm is readily recognizable, and fully discussed on page 148.

Coughing is usually due to irritation of the respiratory tract by mucus, blood or other material and, although it is a protective mechanism, its cause should be investigated and treated, should it persist. Occasionally it results from exposure to a sudden increase in halothane vapour concentration, in spite of the relative non-irritant properties of this drug.

(e) *Colour.*—The colour of the skin and mucous membranes provides a rough guide as to the state of oxygenation of the capillary blood, and should be under constant observation. It is of particular importance in the dark skinned races to observe the mucous membranes and nail beds, since overall colour changes in the skin are not apparent. It will be remembered (page 91) that cyanosis is said to be recognizable in the presence of 5 g of reduced haemoglobin per 100 ml of capillary blood. It should be stressed that the appearance of cyanosis in the anaemic patient represents a more serious degree of hypoxaemia than in the normal. For example, a patient with a haemoglobin of 70% (i.e. 10 g %) will exhibit cyanosis only when a severe degree of hypoxaemia exists, i.e. when half the total haemoglobin is in the reduced state. Finally, the prevailing lighting conditions, the visual acuity of the observer, the posture of the patient, and the state of the peripheral circulation all exert an important influence on the recognition and evaluation of cyanosis.

Circulatory System

The anaesthetist should always keep a constant watch on the condition of the patient's cardiovascular system. The use of sophisticated monitoring equipment, although desirable, is at present impracticable in the average dental surgery, and may in some instances serve only to distract the anaesthetist's attention from simpler and more important observations. We consider that the following simple observations will provide him with much important information in the majority of cases; it must be admitted, however, that recent appreciation of the high incidence of cardiac dysrhythmias in certain types of dental anaesthesia, renders a reliable and simple form of routine cardiac monitor a desirable aim for the future.

(a) *Pulse.*—It should be pointed out that, whilst simple observation of the pulse will normally reflect the heart's activity, its significance may be limited, for it is possible for a weak heart-beat (e.g. extrasystole) to fail to produce a palpable peripheral pulse. Such abnormalities are only detectable by continuous monitoring of the heart with an oscilloscope. The peripheral pulses most readily accessible to the dental anaesthetist are the carotid, superficial temporal and facial, and the sites for palpation are shown in Fig. 70. Some experience is required in order to locate and evaluate these pulses with confidence. Palpation of the carotid pulse may be difficult in the short thick-necked individual and may require firm finger pressure with the head in the mid-line. The superficial temporal and facial pulses should, however, be felt gently with the finger-tips. The anaesthetist should palpate these pulses as frequently as possible during induction, maintenance and recovery, making the following observations:

(i) *Rate.*—The normal adult resting rate is 72 beats per minute. This rate is subject to wide variation preoperatively, ranging from 50/min. in the trained athlete to 120/min in some highly nervous adults; tachycardia in the nervous patient will usually settle to a normal rate during the course of stable anaesthesia.

It is sometimes difficult to count the pulse rate accurately during dental anaesthesia and a simple pulse monitor with rate-counter may prove valuable (Fig. 39). The anaesthetist, however, is usually able to detect any significant alterations which may occur without the assistance of monitoring equipment.

Bradycardia, in which there is a reduction of more than 20 beats per minute from the patient's normal resting rate, is recognized readily and may lead to a fall in cardiac output. Such a degree of bradycardia is most commonly due to halothane overdose or vagal overactivity during induction (pages 105 and 167). It may, however, indicate severe hypoxia or hypercarbia (pages 160 and 161) or even heart block (page 170).

Tachycardia, developing during dental anaesthesia usually indicates sympathetic overactivity, which most commonly results from stimulation under light anaesthesia, mild hypoxaemia, or postural and other forms of hypotension (page 164). It may also be drug induced (page 21).

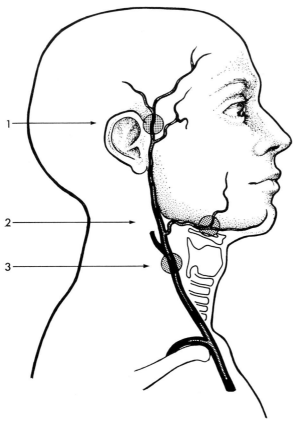

Fig. 70.—Sites for Palpation of Superficial Pulses.
1. Superficial temporal. 2. Facial. 3. Carotid

(ii) *Rhythm.*—The exact nature of any disturbance in rhythm cannot be identified with certainty by palpation alone, and therefore all abnormal rhythms should be viewed with suspicion. For example, extrasystole may sometimes be associated with the administration of halothane and trichlorethylene or, more rarely, with surgical stimulation under light anaesthesia. Withdrawal of these excitatory stimuli should result in reversion to normal rhythm. On the other hand, should the abnormality persist, more serious myocardial disturbance may be present and will require curtailment of the anaesthetic pending further investigation. For detailed discussion of this complex problem see page 171.

(iii) *Volume.*—The volume of the pulse as transmitted to the examining finger is a measure of the pulse pressure (i.e. the difference between systolic and diastolic blood pressure) and represents a useful guide to the circulatory state of the patient. Although it is impossible to assess the patient's blood pressure with any degree of accuracy from this sign, any alteration on palpation will suggest a change in the circulatory dynamics and should be further investigated.

(b) *Skin Characteristics.*—Careful observation of the skin characteristics, e.g. colour, temperature and dryness, will often serve as an invaluable guide to the state of the general circulation. Where circulatory dynamics are undisturbed, the skin will be pink, dry and normal in temperature, and in areas such as the lobes of the ears and nail beds a brisk capillary refill can be elicited. In particular, we believe that the lobes of the ears, being at the same gravity level as the brain, offer the anaesthetist a valuable and accessible site for continuous observation. If the ears appear pale or cyanosed, they should be rubbed briskly, whereupon the rapid return of pink blood will indicate an adequate tissue blood flow; if, however, they remain pale or cyanosed, this is a strong indication of serious disturbance in circulatory function which must be urgently investigated and treated. The interpretation of these signs in the manner described, assumes adequate respiratory function and normal haemoglobin, and is offered here for broad practical guidance.

Body Temperature (see page 246)

It has been established that the immobile, shocked, or anaesthetized patient should ideally be subjected to an environmental temperature of 33°C (91°F), since his own mechanisms of normal heat-production are seriously impaired. Because this temperature is uncomfortably warm for medical, dental and nursing staff, patients are usually treated in an environmental temperature of about 25°C (77°F), and unless special precautions are taken to keep them artificially warm, the fall in skin temperature will result in a response of shivering or other forms of muscle movement as anaesthesia lightens. It is therefore desirable that during both anaesthesia and recovery the patient is kept as warm as possible.

RECOVERY

Immediate Recovery

After the anaesthetic has been discontinued, direct supervision of the patient by the anaesthetist should be as carefully maintained as during the administration, and continued until the patient awakens and is able to understand and obey simple instructions.

Position

If the reclining posture has been employed, the chair may be returned to the upright position and the patient's head and neck pushed forward so that any excess blood or saliva, not controlled by the pack, will pool in the anterior portion of the mouth where it can be readily removed (Fig. 71). To allow blood or debris to enter the pharynx at any time is indicative of imperfect management. If this initial upright position is employed, it is important that the pulse is frequently palpated. When circumstances permit, we consider that the lateral horizontal position should be adopted for recovery as soon as possible (Fig. 72). This presents no problems if the

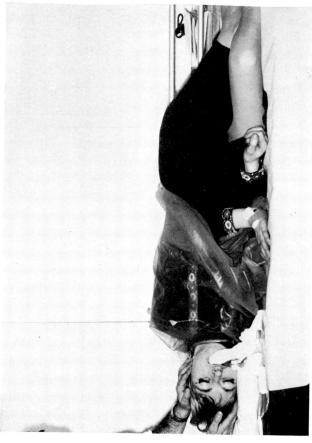

Fig. 72.—Lateral recovery position

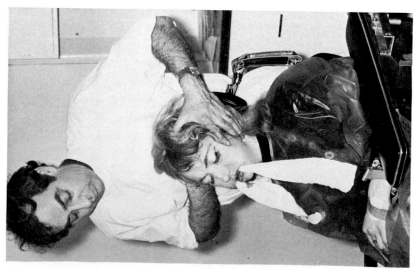

Fig. 71.—Upright recovery position

136

extractions have been carried out on a flat surface (e.g. a trolley), but in the dental surgery (office), where some form of dental chair will have been used, adoption of the true lateral position will often prove difficult or impossible. Whilst considering the lateral to be the ideal recovery position, we would nevertheless maintain that the upright—as already described—is preferable to the supine, in which the risk of airway obstruction and pharyngeal contamination with blood is considerable. Once consciousness has been fully regained, irrespective of the initial recovery position chosen, final recovery is best achieved with the patient lying down. We have found that even 5–10 minutes in this position results in a reduction in the incidence of nausea, vomiting and malaise—particularly in children.

Mouth Packs

Care should be taken to ensure that the pack or packs are positioned in such a way as to encourage maximum haemostasis. Should bleeding have been brisk, it may be necessary to insert fresh packs. These are left undisturbed until the patient regains consciousness and is able to spit out, thus avoiding postoperative nausea due to excessive swallowing of blood.

Mouth Props

If the prop is removed immediately on completion of the anaesthetic, this will enable the mouth to be closed firmly on the packs, which not only assists haemostasis but also allows accidental dislocation of the tempero-mandibular joint to be detected before consciousness is regained; this latter complication can sometimes result from vigorous attempts to maintain an unobstructed airway. Some operators, however, prefer to leave the prop in position until consciousness is regained so that they may apply finger pressure to the operation site.

It may be unwise to remove props when the patient is semiconscious as this manoeuvre may be interpreted by such a patient as part of the operation.

Oxygen

It is often recommended that oxygen be administered for one or two minutes following prolonged anaesthesia with N_2O, in order to combat diffusion hypoxia (page 91).

Ultimate Recovery

The length of time taken for the patient to be able to leave the chair for the recovery couch with assistance, after discontinuing the anaesthetic, is mainly dependent upon the duration and depth of anaesthesia and the physical and mental characteristics of the patient. Normally, it is not in excess of 3 minutes.

It is wise to keep the patient under supervision for about 30 minutes postoperatively, for it is usually within this period that postoperative sequelae may develop. These may be:

(a) *Post-Extraction Haemorrhage.*—This is a dental complication, the early recognition of which may prevent considerable inconvenience to all.

(b) *Nausea and Vomiting.*—There is a clear relationship between the incidence of nausea and the nature of the anaesthetic used. For example, cyclopropane produces a 30% nausea rate, halothane about 5%, and Trilene occupies an intermediate position. The lowest incidence of nausea is associated with the use of unsupplemented intravenous agents such as methohexitone.

Other factors, not directly related to the specific anaesthetic agent used, may influence the incidence of nausea, and in particular those patients who are prone to travel sickness are liable to experience the same symptoms during recovery from anaesthesia, and therefore should be premedicated with an antiemetic agent. It should be remembered that blood swallowed during recovery is a potent cause of post-anaesthetic vomiting.

(c) *Headache.*—Headache is not an uncommon complication of general anaesthesia. Its precise causation is not known, but it can usually be readily controlled with simple analgesics such as aspirin.

(d) *Postoperative Pain.*—It is usual for patients to experience some degree of post-extraction discomfort once the effects of the anaesthetic have fully worn off, and the early administration of an analgesic is recommended. On pages 41–48 a large range of simple analgesics is described, and any of these will usually prove suitable. However, if there is a history of sensitivity or gastric intolerance to aspirin, we have found paracetamol (Panadol) to be a satisfactory choice.

Final Instructions

It is essential that any patient who has received a general anaesthetic, however short, should be accompanied home. The patient should be made to understand, preferably in writing, that driving a vehicle is forbidden for the remainder of the day, and the consumption of alcohol is unwise. It is advisable to incorporate these instructions on the consent form (Table IV, page 17).

The foregoing account is based upon the use of nitrous oxide, oxygen, halothane sequence. We will now briefly discuss alternative techniques not involving the use of halothane.

1. 'Trilene' (page 109)

The technique of induction, maintenance and overall management with this agent is similar in all respects to that with halothane and the drug may be administered from a Goldman vaporizer (see Table X, page 67). The following differences should be noted:

Advantages of Trilene.—(a) Low cost; (b) Good analgesic properties; (c) Less tendency to produce hypotension.
Disadvantages.—(a) Slow induction and slow recovery due to the combination of low

volatility and high tissue solubility; (b) Lack of relaxation at recommended level of anaesthesia; (c) Higher incidence of postanaesthetic nausea and general malaise; (d) Increased tendency to produce tachypnoea, especially in children.

2. Cyclopropane (page 110)

Owing to its ability to produce rapid and pleasant loss of consciousness in the presence of a high oxygen concentration, cyclopropane, at one time, enjoyed a brief vogue. The explosion risk was overcome by adding nitrogen to the gaseous mixture, but the extremely high incidence of postoperative nausea and vomiting and the difficulties with continuous administration have rendered this agent unacceptable, since the introduction of halothane.

3. Methoxyflurane ('Penthrane')

Our own experience with this agent is limited, but its one advantage, namely that of analgesia, does not, in our opinion, compensate for the following disadvantages: (a) Slow induction and recovery; (b) Unpleasant odour; (c) Comparable cost to halothane.

4. Unsupplemented Nitrous Oxide

For almost a century unsupplemented N_2O was the standard anaesthetic used for dental out-patient procedures. The weak anaesthetic properties of the agent led to the use of oxygen restriction in an attempt to enhance its action. Such oxygen restriction has the following effects: (a) To allow the maximum partial pressure of nitrous oxide to be achieved in the alveolar air; (b) Possibly to expedite rapid loss of consciousness by the direct effect of oxygen restriction on the brain; (c) Initially to increase tidal volume and thus accelerate the replacement of nitrogen by nitrous oxide in the lungs; (d) To increase the cerebral blood flow and thus facilitate the uptake of nitrous oxide by the brain.

These effects increase the rate of induction of anaesthesia, but a comparable final level can be achieved without recourse to oxygen restriction, within 2 minutes rather than 30 seconds. Owing to the weakness of the agent, an adequate level of anaesthesia cannot be achieved in a proportion of patients. Moreover, even in suitable patients, either dilution of the nitrous oxide concentration in the inhaled mixture as a result of mouth breathing, or excessive surgical stimulation, can lead to emergence from an adequate depth to a state of confused excitement.

Certain workers maintained that when using nitrous oxide without oxygen restriction, the satisfactory level of anaesthesia which they achieved was lighter than the conventional excitement stage, and coined the term 'amnalgesia' to describe this state (page 252).

In spite of the advantages of rapid recovery, and the low incidence of unpleasant after-effects, we consider that unsupplemented nitrous oxide has a limited sphere of usefulness for the following reasons: (i) Unless oxygen restriction is used, the loss of consciousness is relatively slow; (ii) Inability to produce adequate anaesthesia in all circumstances, and therefore an incidence of 'awareness' during treatment; (iii)

Lack of muscle relaxation; (iv) The risk of subjecting the patient to excessive hypoxia by the use of a technique which is traditionally associated with some degree of oxygen restriction.

The introduction of halothane, methohexitone and propanidid has enabled the anaesthetist to use techniques devoid of these disadvantages. It is for this reason that unsupplemented nitrous oxide has in recent years lost favour.

RECOMMENDED READING

Body Temperature.

Climate in Theatre (1971). *Br. med. J.*, iv, 186

CHAPTER SIX

RESPIRATORY HAZARDS AND THEIR TREATMENT

Any defect in anaesthetic management which results in more than transient reduction in pulmonary gaseous exchange is potentially hazardous, and necessitates immediate diagnosis and correction. Early recognition of these defects is of paramount importance, and their causes and effects will be discussed in detail under two separate headings: A. Airway Obstruction
B. Respiratory Depression

A. AIRWAY OBSTRUCTION

In the unintubated patient, obstruction to the flow of gases in and out of the lungs may occur at three levels, namely supralaryngeal, laryngeal and infralaryngeal.

In the main, all types of airway obstruction can be recognized by certain characteristic signs. These include snoring or stridor accompanied by in-drawing of the suprasternal space, the supraclavicular fossae, and, in severe degrees, the entire thoracic cage, during attempted inspiration. These signs are often associated with over-activity of the accessory muscles of respiration.

Supralaryngeal Obstruction

1. Tongue

Supralaryngeal obstruction is most commonly caused by the approximation of the tongue to the posterior pharyngeal wall, and is frequently accompanied by a characteristic snoring sound. It may be the result of the influence of gravity in the relaxed patient in the supine position (Fig. 73); or it may be due to backward displacement of the lower jaw and tongue by the surgeon—particularly when extracting difficult lower teeth. The receding chin is frequently associated with poor mouth-opening, and indeed the very act of opening the mouth in this condition often tends to obstruct the airway. Extension of the head in relation to the neck will usually minimize this difficulty. The combination of receding chin, poor mouth-opening, large tongue and short rigid neck can render surgical access so difficult as to warrant endotracheal intubation, even in simple extraction cases. This is particularly true in children suffering from certain congenital abnormalities discussed on page 348. When obstruction is the result of surgical manipulation, it can best be corrected by the application of firm counter-pressure behind the angles of the mandible, but many experienced operators develop the technique of extracting lower teeth whilst pulling the mandible forward themselves with the steadying left hand, thus rendering the anaesthetist's task much simpler. The surgeon's fingers may also inadvertently displace either the tongue or pack backwards into an obstructing position without necessarily applying any backward pressure to the mandible itself. These mishaps have only to be recognized to be corrected, but occasionally the extraction of lower posterior teeth can present such surgical problems that some airway distortion is unavoidable; unless this is transient, the situation will demand the passage of a nasotracheal tube, in order to allow the operator unimpeded access in the absence of a partially obstructed airway. Although endotracheal intubation is the most reliable method of rectifying supralaryngeal obstruction, nasopharyngeal intubation may, at times, suffice.

Nasopharyngeal Intubation.—The most satisfactory form of nasopharyngeal airway is a soft, thin walled nasotracheal tube, cut to suitable length. The length of this tube is, in fact, critical and can sometimes only be satisfactorily determined by trial and

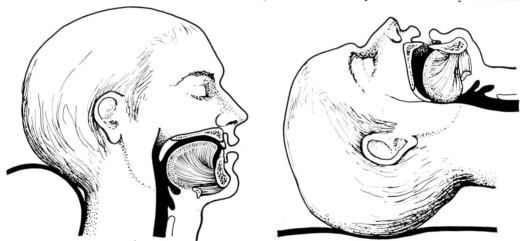

Fig. 73.—Supralaryngeal obstruction caused by the relaxed tongue in the Supine Posture

error, the uncut tube being passed until clear air sounds emerge. The tube is then cut, and a safety pin inserted through it to prevent it slipping further into the nostril. Normally the nasal mask can be reapplied, but should it be desired to connect the tube directly to the anaesthetic apparatus, the tube must be partially withdrawn after cutting, to allow the appropriate connection to be attached. We have not ourselves found flanged tubes of predetermined length (e.g. the Goldman, Fig. 37) to be consistently successful in achieving a perfect airway; nor can we recommend the traditional practice of attempting to predetermine the correct length of tube by measuring the distance between ear and nares, except as a rough guide to the probable length required.

It must be stressed that nasopharyngeal intubation should not be attempted unless first plane surgical anaesthesia has been well established, otherwise coughing, retching, excessive salivation, etc. may be provoked. In addition, a soft tube should be used, and great care exercised in its passage in order to avoid nasal bleeding which, if excessive, may necessitate endotracheal intubation or abandonment of the anaesthetic. The incidence of nasal bleeding may be reduced by the use of intranasal vasoconstrictors (e.g. ephedrine 0·5%). Finally, if the tube is to be connected directly to the anaesthetic apparatus, it is important to ensure that the connection is well seated and firmly secured within the nostril in order to avoid kinking of the tube. Occasionally a nasopharyngeal tube will enable inhalation anaesthesia to be maintained in a patient in whom mouth breathing cannot be corrected by the methods described on page 128.

2. Pack

A rare but potentially catastrophic cause of supralaryngeal obstruction, is impaction of the mouth pack in the pharynx, accompanied by tight closure of the jaws. Avoidance of this disaster depends upon the use of properly designed and positioned mouth packs as described on page 123. Although laryngotomy (page 147) is the ultimate treatment, attempts should first be made to dislodge the pack by simple methods. Even tightly clenched jaws can usually be opened with a Fergusson's gag, (preferably with Ackland blades uncovered by rubber), and it should then be possible to remove the pack either manually or with the aid of laryngoscope and Magill's forceps. Should this prove impossible and the life of the patient be in jeopardy, the anaesthetist is faced with two alternative courses of action. Either, he may administer a depolarizing muscle relaxant (e.g. suxamethonium) to facilitate removal of the pack in the manner described; or he will have to perform a laryngotomy. It must be remembered that it will take some time to draw up and administer suxamethonium, and every second counts. Moreover, since this treatment involves paralysis of the muscles of respiration, removal of the pack must be immediately followed by artificial ventilation of the lungs. Blood in the pharynx must be rapidly removed by suction, and if bleeding persists, endotracheal intubation may be necessary in order to avoid contamination of the lungs during ventilation. The experienced medical anaesthetist may be able to achieve these objects, but in inexperienced hands, laryngotomy may well prove to be both quicker and simpler.

3. Ludwig's Angina

Severe acute infections of the pharynx and floor of the mouth (i.e. Ludwig's angina) may be of dental origin, and thus be presented to the dental anaesthetist for emergency treatment as an out-patient. Such infections may lead to serious impairment of airway patency, and it cannot be emphasized too strongly that, should general anaesthesia prove unavoidable in the treatment of such a case, this should always be administered in hospital by a very experienced anaesthetist. The detailed management of these cases is described on page 282.

4. Submucosal Bleeding in a Haemophiliac

Great care must be taken to avoid any degree of trauma when intubating, packing or extubating a haemophiliac (page 286). Also, injections of local anaesthetic in the mouth are contraindicated. Severe supraglottic obstruction may result from excessive bleeding, and require endotracheal intubation or, as a last resort, laryngotomy.

Laryngeal Obstruction

1. Laryngeal Closure (Glottic Spasm)

Definition.—In normal breathing the vocal cords are relaxed during both inspiration and expiration, allowing free passage of air in and out of the lungs. Active abduction of the cords (opening of the glottic aperture) will take place when an increase in gas flow to the lungs is required, as during exercise or voluntary hyperventilation. On the other hand, varying degrees of adduction (closing of glottic aperture) may occur, either as an essential component of speech or as part of a reflex response to various internal or external stimuli. This glottic closure may be temporary, as in the reflex aspects of swallowing and retching, under which circumstances it is always accompanied by inhibition of respiration; it may, however, be prolonged, not part of a co-ordinated reflex mechanism, and associated with active respiratory effort. Under these circumstances, it is described as laryngeal spasm. It is only when this closure is incomplete that restricted airflow through a partially closed glottis gives rise to the characteristic, high pitched sound described as laryngeal stridor.

Causation.—Any violent stimulus may give rise to laryngeal spasm. Even in the conscious subject, a stimulus such as sudden immersion into cold water, can produce this response. In the unconscious subject, the same effect can be produced by a variety of surgical stimuli when the level of anaesthesia is inadequate. The level of anaesthesia required to prevent this response, will depend upon the character of the stimulus applied. For example, dilatation of the cervix or anal sphincter demands profound anaesthesia to obtund the reflex, whereas the stimulus of tooth extraction, seldom produces the response even in extremely light anaesthesia. However, by far the most common stimulus to provoke laryngeal spasm is one which can be interpreted as constituting a threat to the inviolability of the air passages. Such a stimulus may not only evoke laryngeal spasm but also other protective reflexes such as sneezing, swallowing and retching, all of which aim to divert the contaminant from the lungs. Should these reflexes prove ineffective, stimulation of the carina will evoke the final protective response, namely that of expulsive coughing, possibly assisted by an increase in ciliary action within the trachea.

Under light anaesthesia, swallowing and retching normally constitute the primary protective mechanism. Under deeper levels of anaesthesia, where these reflexes are abolished, laryngeal closure will assume this role. During very deep anaesthesia, when the laryngeal reflex is abolished, the trachea will remain unprotected and even the cough reflex will become at first ineffective and finally abolished. However, it should be stressed that it is not only in deep anaesthesia that the danger of lung contamination exists, for the chain of reflexes described is by no means perfect. This is evident from the many recorded episodes in which foreign bodies have been inhaled by the conscious subject with minimal disturbance at the time, the effects being discovered at a later date.

In the context of dental anaesthesia, the stimulus liable to provoke any of the responses described above, nearly always takes the form of mechanical irritation of the sensitive respiratory mucosa. This irritation can be caused by blood, mucus, regurgitated gastric contents, or even high concentrations of irritant anaesthetic vapours. Whilst it is widely accepted that the presence of these irritants in the vicinity of the larynx is the commonest trigger mechanism to the foregoing reflex chain, we believe that obstruction of the upper airway by pack or tongue, may sometimes be interpreted as constituting a foreign body, and thus provoke the reflex protective response of laryngeal closure. Such pharyngeal obstruction may also initiate excessive production of secretions and even predispose to 'silent regurgitation' of resting gastric juice, both of which will add to the severity of the spasm. These observations suggest that laryngeal spasm is most likely to occur at that stage of anaesthesia which is characterized by an absent swallowing but fully active glottic reflex. This proposition differs from Bourne's theory, which states that laryngeal spasm represents an inbalance between the 'protective' and the 'respiratory' functions of the larynx, and hence is likely to occur in the subject in whom depressant drugs have weakened the respiratory drive, thus allowing the protective laryngeal mechanism to predominate. The barbiturates, which are respiratory depressants, certainly have the reputation of sensitizing the larynx, although there is no factual evidence that this is so. This reputation may have been created by the practice of allowing surgery to commence at too light a level of anaesthesia when an intravenous barbiturate is used as the sole anaesthetic agent. The powerful narcotics (e.g. morphine), on the other hand, which are also respiratory depressants, are held to obtund rather than sensitize the glottic reflex. Thus, the actual mechanism of laryngeal spasm under anaesthesia would appear to be controversial, and whether it is precipitated by loss of the protective swallowing reflex or by a mechanism of inbalance as suggested by Bourne, is secondary in importance to the fact that it occurs at a particular state of central depression between very light and established surgical anaesthesia.

Treatment.—Removal of the precipitating cause is the only measure that need normally be contemplated. The most common precipitating causes are as follows.

(a) *Upper Airway Obstruction.*—The first action in treatment should always be directed towards ensuring that there is no upper respiratory obstruction.

(b) *Direct Laryngeal Irritation.*—This may result from an excess of secretions, unacceptable anaesthetic vapour concentration, or the presence of foreign material.

(i) *Excess Secretions and High Vapour Concentration.*—Excess secretions may either result from salivation, or be derived from the nasopharynx during acute infections. They are generally only evident in light levels of anaesthesia, and salivation in particular is often associated with extreme nervousness. The immediate treatment is to discontinue the anaesthetic and administer oxygen until the spasm relaxes and the pharynx is cleared of secretions by swallowing. Anaesthesia should be immediately recommenced using a high oxygen content, the anaesthetic vapour being steadily increased as quickly as the patient will tolerate without interruption of smooth respiration.

(ii) *Foreign Material.*—This may be blood, water or debris from the operation site, or regurgitated stomach or oesophageal contents—particularly if the spasm occurs during the induction of anaesthesia. Regurgitation may be suspected if the onset of spasm is unexpected and sudden, associated with hiccough, and persists in a severe form giving rise to the rapid development of cyanosis. It is more likely to occur in the supine posture, but in the presence of hiccough it is seen occasionally in the upright or reclining patient. The patient, if not already so, should be placed flat or tilted head-down and turned on to his side with the minimum delay. An attempt to suck out the mouth and pharynx may then be made, and oxygen administered until consciousness is regained. We believe that there is no place for more active treatment at the hands of any but the most experienced medical anaesthetist, who may choose to perform laryngoscopy, direct vision toilet, and endotracheal intubation with a cuffed tube. If blood or debris is the precipitating cause, it may be able to be removed by simple suction, and the position rectified by repacking. Oxygen should be administered until the spasm relaxes and anaesthesia only recommenced if the anaesthetist is certain that the pharynx is clear and the bleeding under control. If, however, the pharynx cannot be cleared or the bleeding controlled, treatment must follow the lines laid down for regurgitation. Very rarely, if all these manoeuvres fail to achieve an unobstructed airway, laryngotomy may be indicated (page 147).

(c) *Surgical Stimulation.*—Should none of the foregoing causes of spasm appear to be present, then it must be remembered that surgical stimulation under light anaesthesia can itself constitute that cause. Treatment under these circumstances consists therefore in removal of the stimulus and deepening of anaesthesia. If we accept Bourne's theory as to the essential nature of laryngeal spasm, then it would not be permissible to attempt to deepen anaesthesia with an anaesthetic agent capable of producing marked respiratory depression, that is an intravenous barbiturate. Whether or not this view is justified, we would agree with its immediate practical implication that it is dangerous to administer a central depressant in the presence of airway impairment. We therefore conclude that the correct sequence of treatment is to stop surgical stimulation, re-establish adequate ventilation and deepen anaesthesia with nitrous oxide, oxygen and halothane—nitrous oxide providing analgesia, and halothane serving both to reduce pharyngeal secretions and to provide the necessary muscle relaxation. Such muscle relaxation may also be achieved by the use of a specific muscle relaxant (e.g. Scoline), but it should be stressed that breaking the reflex spasm on the motor side in this fashion, will destroy completely the protective functions of the reflex and should only be employed when the danger of inhalation of foreign material does not exist. If a specific relaxant is used for this purpose, the anaesthetist must be capable of performing rapid intubation of the trachea, should this prove necessary.

Finally, it cannot be too strongly stressed that whatever treatment is given—and this will vary with the cause of the spasm—that treatment should be preceded, accompanied and followed by the administration of a high concentration of oxygen in the inspired mixture, and the upper airway should be unobstructed throughout.

2. Mechanical Blockage

Just as the pharynx may become blocked by a pack, so it is conceivable that impaction of a foreign body within the larynx may also produce complete respiratory obstruction. Such obstruction must be relieved as a matter of absolute urgency. This the experienced anaesthetist may be able to achieve with the aid of laryngoscope, Magill's forceps and possibly muscle relaxant drugs, but inability to rectify the situation in this manner will necessitate the performance of an immediate laryngotomy.

Laryngotomy.—Laryngotomy may be indicated for the immediate relief of obstruction at or above the level of the larynx, and the common causes of such obstruction have already been fully discussed.

In addition, postoperative obstruction may result from persistent laryngeal spasm or oedema following the treatment of fractures of the upper or lower jaws, or after an osteotomy for congenital malformation of the mandible; in either of these events, the wiring of upper to lower teeth will prevent access to the mouth and throat, and therefore may render tracheostomy or laryngotomy the only possible treatments. Ideally, the relief of these situations demands tracheostomy, but in an emergency, when an airway must be established without delay, it is quicker and safer to perform a laryngotomy, particularly as the need is most likely to arise in situations where full surgical facilities are not available.

The larynx is entered through the cricothyroid membrane (Fig. 74)

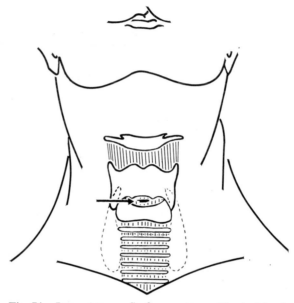

Fig. 74.—Laryngotomy: Surface anatomy. The incision is made horizontally through the cricothyroid membrane, between the thyroid and cricoid cartilages. Arrow points to incision in cricothyroid membrane

between the thyroid cartilage above and the cricoid cartilage below. The narrow space between these cartilages is readily identified by palpation in the mid-line of the neck, especially when the head is extended. There is no thyroid isthmus or large vessel in the area of the cricothyroid membrane. A small horizontal incision is made with a knife through the skin overlying the membrane, and the skin edges are separated with the fingers of the left hand. A second incision is made through the membrane itself, until a hissing sound indicates that air has entered the larynx. A laryngotomy tube should be inserted, if one is available, and an excellent instrument for this purpose is the one designed by the late Sir Terence Cawthorne (Fig. 75). If no such instrument is at hand, the opening may be made with any knife and kept patent by rotating the blade slightly in the wound.

If no knife is available, a wide-bore needle or cannula may be used.

It must be emphasized that laryngotomy is always a purely temporary procedure, since the prolonged presence of a tube in the larynx will almost inevitably lead to stenosis. Laryngotomy must always be followed by an elective tracheostomy as soon as the sudden emergency has been overcome.

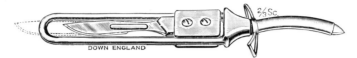

Fig. 75.—Laryngotomy: Cawthorne's instrument for emergency operation. (Reproduced by courtesy of Down Bros. and Mayer & Phelps Ltd.) The retractable blade is protruded from the handle on the instrument before the incisions are made. Thereafter the blade is withdrawn into its sheath and the laryngotomy tube is inserted

Infralaryngeal Obstruction

1. Bronchospasm

Definition.—In normal breathing, both the diameter and length of the bronchi and bronchioles increase with inspiration and decrease with expiration. This variation is slight and is thought to follow passively the normal alterations in intrathoracic pressure. However, the bronchioles in particular are capable of active alterations in their diameter, contraction of the smooth muscle within their walls serving to narrow the lumen and relaxation resulting in bronchial dilatation. When the increase in tone of the bronchiolar musculature is such as to constitute a significant increase in airway resistance, the term bronchospasm is used to describe the condition. In clinical practice, this condition is frequently exacerbated by an element of mechanical obstruction due to the presence of excessive secretions and oedema of the respiratory mucosa.

Causation.—Alterations in bronchial tone may occur under a wide variety of circumstances.

(a) *Disease.*—The two diseases commonly associated with bronchospasm are asthma and chronic bronchitis, and in both these conditions increased airway resistance is most evident during expiration. In the typical asthma of childhood, unassociated with permanent structural changes in the lungs, respiratory function may be unimpaired between attacks and the course of general anaesthesia thus remains unaffected. The aetiology of the disease is complex but it is generally accepted that emotional factors constitute the prime precipitating cause of bronchospasm, although underlying allergy may be a feature. In chronic bronchitis, there is always some element of permanent structural damage to the lungs, accompanied by excessive production of respiratory secretions. It is these secretions in association with a sensitized respiratory mucosa which may give rise to severe bronchospasm under general anaesthesia, both as a response to respiratory irritants (e.g. endotracheal intubation, irritant vapours) and to other forms of stimulation, (e.g. premature surgical intervention).

(b) *Allergy.*—The possible allergic background to asthma has already been mentioned, and acute bronchospasm (due to the liberation of histamine and other substances) may be the most dangerous feature of any allergic response. Such allergic responses represent the reaction of a previously sensitized subject to the relevant allergen which is usually foreign protein. Allergens are well known to be contained in such substances as pollens, strawberries, shellfish and animal sera. The allergic response sometimes elicited by the administration of a drug, is based upon the formation of a drug plus body-protein conjugate, which is of sufficient molecular size to develop antigenic properties.

$$\text{Drug} + \text{body protein} \rightarrow \text{Drug—body-protein conjugate}$$

Confers specificity   Confers antigenicity

The most severe form of acute allergic response is described as anaphylaxis, and in this condition, severe bronchospasm is accompanied by circulatory collapse and skin reactions of an urticarial nature (page 26).

(c) *Reflex Stimulation.*—In man, reflex bronchoconstriction most commonly results from stimulation of the respiratory mucosa in the lightly anaesthetized asthmatic or bronchitic subject. It is possible that surgical stimuli, other than those applied to the respiratory mucosa, may occasionally provoke a similar response, and indeed, there is some experimental evidence to suggest that alterations in blood pressure may also influence bronchial tone.

(d) *Chemical Stimulation.*—Any drug, which is parasympatheticomimetic in action, will tend to provoke bronchospasm. Certain anaesthetic agents, in particular the barbiturates (page 24) and cyclopropane, may act pharmacologically as bronchial constrictors, but there is no clinical evidence to suggest that their use should be avoided in the asthmatic or bronchitic subject. In addition to these drug effects, experimental work indicates that bronchoconstriction may be induced by either a rise in blood carbon dioxide or a fall in blood oxygen tension, and that these effects are due to a direct action on the brain.

Treatment.—The treatment of established bronchospasm may be difficult and protracted, and therefore every effort should be made to anticipate its likelihood and avoid its precipitation. For example, should general anaesthesia prove necessary in a bronchitic subject, special care should be taken to establish an adequate level of anaesthesia prior to the application of any surgical stimulus. In particular, all procedures likely to stimulate the respiratory mucosa should be avoided whenever possible; the most common aggravating factors are the insertion of pharyngeal or tracheal airways, and the rapid increase in inspired concentration of irritant vapours, all of which are likely, in addition to their direct irritant effect, to provoke the out-pouring of excessive respiratory secretions, which in themselves act as a further source of irritation; this latter effect may be mitigated by the administration of an anti-sialogogue.

Anaesthesia should be conducted with great care, a high oxygen concentration ensured throughout, and drugs known to produce bronchodilatation be used in pre-ference to bronchoconstrictors whenever this is possible (Table XVI). Should the patient be accustomed to taking a specific bronchodilator drug (e.g. isoprenaline spray), it may prove beneficial for him to do so immediately prior to the adminis-tration of the anaesthetic, but the risk of producing cardiac dysrhythmias with this type of therapy should be borne in mind. The recent introduction of the longer acting salbutamol is said to have diminished this risk. Premedication with a known broncho-dilator such as promethazine or aminophylline may prove helpful.

TABLE XVI

	Bronchoconstrictors	*Bronchodilators*
Premedication	Morphine	Pethidine
	Barbiturates	Atropine
		Phenothiazines
Anaesthetic	Cyclopropane	Ether
Agents	Barbiturates	Halothane

If, in spite of the above precautions, bronchospasm should occur during anaes-thesia, treatment will consist of the following measures.

(a) Removal of any precipitating factor
(b) Administration of 100% oxygen
(c) Administration of specific bronchodilator drugs. A full list of bronchodilator agents is to be found in Table XVII.The actual sequence of drugs selected in treatment will depend upon whether the bronchospasm is primarily of chemical, irritant or allergic origin.

TABLE XVII

	Bronchodilator Drugs
Long Acting	Ephedrine
	Choline theophyllinate (Coledyl)
	Methoxyphenamine (Orthoxine)
	Aminophylline
	Orciprenaline (Alupent)
	Hydrocortisone
	Salbutamol (Ventolin)
Short Acting	Adrenaline
	Isoprenaline

Aminophylline.—This drug, being a relaxant of smooth muscle, may relieve broncho-spasm of any origin. It should be administered in 2·5% solution by intravenous injection (i.e. 250 mg/10 ml). No side effects are likely to be observed if the dose is limited to 500 mg and the injection given slowly.

Hydrocortisone.—Hydrocortisone possesses anti-inflammatory and anti-allergic properties (page 290), but the onset of its beneficial effect in the treatment of bronchospasm may be considerably delayed. It should be appreciated that hydrocortisone does not prevent antigen-antibody reactions from taking place, but acts by protecting body cells from the harmful effects of such reactions. Also, the prevention of circulatory collapse which may accompany severe bronchospasm or other 'stressful' conditions is dependent upon the presence of adequate endogenous corticosteroids. It is therefore in the asthmatic, whose adrenocortical function may have been depressed by prior treatment with steroids, that the administration of hydrocortisone intravenously is likely to be of greatest value. An initial dose of 100 mg need seldom be exceeded, but may be repeated at half hourly intervals.

Isoprenaline.—Isoprenaline is a powerful bronchodilator which can be effectively administered in the form of a spray, either prophylactically to the conscious subject, or via an endotracheal tube, should one be in place.

Promethazine (*Phenergan*), *Chlorpheniramine* (*Piriton*).—If the basis of bronchospasm is clearly allergic, these drugs may be of value when administered intravenously. Promethazine should be given slowly (25 mg) owing to the risk of hypotension; chlorpheniramine should also be injected with care in a dose not exceeding 10 mg.

Adrenaline.—Adrenaline is the drug of choice in the management of bronchospasm associated with anaphylactoid reactions. It is given by intramuscular injection of 1:1000 (B.P.) solution in an initial dose of 0·5 ml followed by a further 0·5 ml at 5 minute intervals, but not exceeding a total dose of 1·5 ml. The response is rapid and may be life-saving.

In conclusion, it must be emphasized that should general anaesthesia prove necessary in the bronchitic or asthmatic patient, then stimulation of the respiratory mucosa should be avoided under light anaesthesia. The mistake most commonly made with these patients is to carry out intubation under an intravenous induction agent and suxamethonium without deepening anaesthesia before the tube is passed. Even the introduction of an oropharyngeal airway immediately after induction, can lead to severe bronchospasm. Time spent in establishing stable anaesthesia before applying any type of stimulation is time well spent.

2. Mechanical Blockage

Any foreign body which succeeds in passing through the larynx is unlikely to impact in the trachea and will therefore enter one or other main bronchus (usually the right, since in both supine and upright posture this bronchus is in more direct line with the trachea).

Contact of the foreign body with the bronchial mucosa or carina will normally initiate coughing in an effort to expel it, and this may be assisted by positioning the patient steeply head downwards on his left side, and slapping him on the back, a manoeuvre more difficult to perform efficiently in adults than in children. Should this prove ineffective, bronchial blockage will initially result in an asphyxial episode of variable severity, followed by some degree of pulmonary collapse and eventually by the development of bronchiectasis or lung abscess, particularly if the inhaled material is infected. It is, therefore, essential that any such material should be removed by bronchoscopy without delay.

In practice a tooth, rubber cover to the blade of a mouth gag, plastic suction tip, reamer or any other small object may be lost into the upper respiratory passages, such loss being accompanied by a bout of coughing and swallowing. Under these circumstances, there is always doubt as to the ultimate fate of the foreign body, and it is the anaesthetist's duty to ensure that it has not been inhaled. Full physical and radiological examination in hospital is therefore essential. We cannot stress too strongly that the loss of any foreign body during a dental procedure must be assumed to be due to its inhalation until proven otherwise. Failure to recognize and remove a bronchial foreign body may result in chronic and permanent ill health, the true cause of which may remain unappreciated. The fear of *loss of face* by the medical and dental personnel involved must never be allowed to deter them from following the correct course of action.

Occasionally the foreign body cannot be removed at bronchoscopy and a thoracotomy may prove necessary.

During transit to hospital the patient should, if possible, lie on the left side tilted head downwards.

B. RESPIRATORY DEPRESSION

In the presence of a clear airway, any reduction in minute volume below that which is required to supply the basal metabolic needs associated with the anaesthetic state, constitutes respiratory depression.

Minute volume may be decreased as the result of either a reduction in tidal volume or a fall in respiratory rate. If the tidal volume does not greatly exceed the capacity of the dead space, effective pulmonary exchange is disproportionately reduced in relation to the minute volume. Thus, for a given reduction in minute volume, a slow respiratory rate is more acceptable than a decrease in tidal exchange.

In the context of out-patient dental anaesthesia, a reduction in minute volume is most commonly associated with depression of the respiratory centre in the brain by drugs or severe hypoxia; however, a reduction in muscle power due to relaxants or disease, and also in certain circumstances, the effects of posture (page 179) may place the muscles of respiration under such mechanical disadvantage as to render the achievement of an adequate minute volume impossible.

Irrespective of the cause of respiratory depression, treatment consists primarily in the immediate establishment of adequate pulmonary exchange by artificial ventilation of the lungs. Only when this has been successfully established should specific antidotes be used.

Technique of Artificial Ventilation.—The lungs must be rhythmically inflated with a gaseous mixture containing not less than 20% oxygen. It is permissible to utilize nitrous oxide as a 'supporting' gas, owing to its lack of respiratory depressant properties; it is also permissible to utilize 100% oxygen for at least several hours, although there is evidence to suggest that a sudden change of inspired oxygen content from 20% to 100% may result in diminution in respiratory activity via the carotid body chemoreceptor reflex mechanism. Ideally, therefore, the lungs should be inflated with air or air supplemented with oxygen.

Should respiratory depression occur inadvertently during the administration of a dental anaesthetic, it will probably prove convenient to use the anaesthetic machine to inflate the lungs. Under these circumstances, all anaesthetic agents (other than

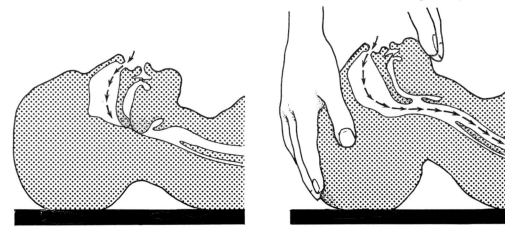

FIG. 76.—Correction of obstruction by extension of head and lifting mandible

nitrous oxide) should be discontinued. It must be stressed that in order to undertake adequate artificial ventilation the anaesthetic machine *must* possess an accessible reservoir bag of adequate capacity (1 litre), a suitable full face-mask and a fine adjustment expiratory valve. The face-mask is applied closely to the face, an air-tight fit being established so that, by adjustment of expiratory valve tension and gas flow-rate, pressure applied manually to the reservoir bag will result in adequate pulmonary inflation, as judged by the visible rise and fall of the chest and abdomen. Difficulty in achieving this is most commonly due to obstruction of the upper air passages by the tongue, and this can usually be corrected by extension of the head on the neck and forward pressure applied to the mandible (Fig. 76). Insertion of an oropharyngeal airway may prove necessary in some cases.

Insertion of Oropharyngeal Airway.—Oropharyngeal airways may be made of rubber, plastic or metal and are available in several sizes. We consider that the Guedel (Fig. 77a) pattern is the most suitable in the majority of cases, but occasionally the more tubular shape of the Phillips (Fig. 77b) is an advantage in the edentulous patient, since its wider aperture is not so likely to be occluded by the lips when the jaw is

A.A.D.—6

pulled forward; moreover, its greater bulk, by restoring the natural contour of the face, will allow airtight apposition of the face-mask to be achieved. Irrespective of design, the object is to prevent apposition of the tongue to the posterior pharyngeal wall and thus to restore the patency of the air passages. Before insertion, the airway should be well lubricated on its under surface and then carefully slid over the tongue which is pulled gently forward with a piece of gauze; the mandible is displaced anteriorly and the airway pushed into its final position, making sure that it does not trap the tongue between its under surface and the teeth. It is important to ensure that the correct length of airway is used, as if it is too long, stimulation of the epiglottis may initiate reflex laryngeal spasm, or even cause mechanical obstruction of the larynx by the epiglottis. If it is too short, it may fail to clear the maximum convexity of the tongue. For the majority of normal sized adults a No. 3 Guedel proves satisfactory.

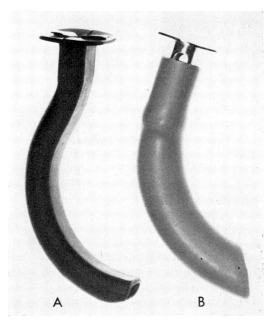

FIG. 77.—Oropharyngeal Airways

A Guedel Airway
B Phillips Airway

Note. The overlapping flange on metal insert in the Phillips airway renders it more likely to be separated from the rest of the airway when attempting to remove it with the jaws clenched

Application of Face-Mask.—Many patterns of face-mask are available. Some have been designed to follow the contours of the face, while others are unshaped and should be large enough to accommodate the chin in addition to mouth and nose. The contoured mask (Fig. 78), if fixed by a harness will tend to push the jaw backwards when the lower harness straps are tightened, and thus its application should always be under manual control. The flat pad mask (Fig. 79), if applied correctly to include the chin, will actually tend to lift the lower jaw into the unobstructed position on tightening the upper harness strap. When applied in this manner, the upper border of the mask will lie sufficiently low on the nose to avoid pressure on the eyes (Fig. 79). In any event, whatever type of mask is used for artificial ventilation, it is normally inadvisable to fix it with a harness and is best controlled by one hand, the other being used to squeeze the reservoir bag.

Inflation of the Lungs.—Having ensured that the airway is unobstructed and the mask is applied correctly, the lungs can be inflated by gentle, rhythmic manual compression of the reservoir bag. This should be undertaken at about 15 compressions per minute, each compression producing a tidal volume of about 500 ml. Care should be taken not to exceed the minimum pressure necessary to produce an adequate visible excursion, as excessive pressure may lead to oesophageal and gastric distension. Moreover, excessive pulmonary ventilation may conceivably result in prolongation of the apnoeic state due to a reduction in arterial PCO_2. The amount of pressure required will depend upon lung compliance and all the factors influencing it.

Should it prove necessary to prolong artificial ventilation for more than a few minutes in a dental surgery it is advisable to use a simple air ventilating device such as the 'Air-viva' (Fig. 81) or 'Ambu' bag rather than the anaesthetic machine, since the cylinder supply of the latter may be limited. In addition the non-return valves with which these devices are fitted prevent excessive carbon dioxide build-up. In the absence of any of the apparatus so far mentioned, the lungs may be inflated by an expired-air method. This will either be mouth-to-mouth or mouth-to-nose (Fig. 82) or via a Brook's Airway (Fig. 84). Should prolonged artificial ventilation and/or transference to hospital be necessary, endotracheal intubation may prove convenient. However, intubation is seldom essential for the purpose of adequate artificial ventilation and therefore should never be undertaken by those inexperienced in the technique. Should artificial ventilation prove necessary during the course of a surgical procedure, bleeding must be controlled by careful local pressure with a suitable pack before it can be safely

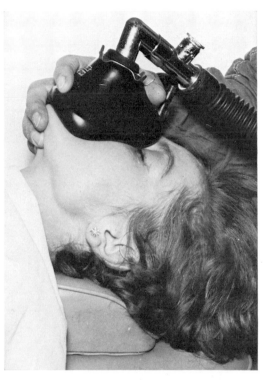

Fig. 78.—Contoured mask, hand held with jaw support

undertaken. If this is not possible, intubation with a cuffed tube will be necessary for complete protection of the lungs.

Causation and Specific Treatment of Respiratory Depression

Provided pulmonary ventilation is adequate, the anaesthetist is then, and not until then, entitled to institute specific corrective treatment. The following are the chief specific causes of respiratory depression in dental anaesthesia.

1. Barbiturate Overdose (page 27)

In dental anaesthesia, this most commonly results from faulty assessment of the correct dose of one of the intravenous agents, but can, of course, result from excessive

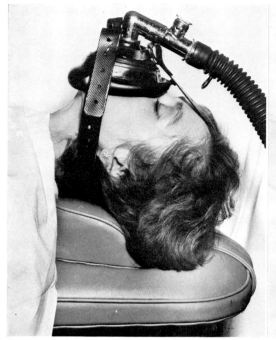 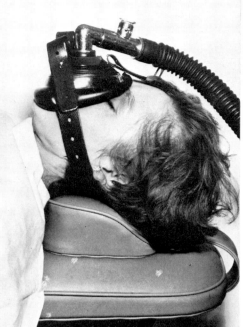

FIG. 79.— Flat pad mask correctly applied   FIG. 80. Flat pad mask incorrectly applied

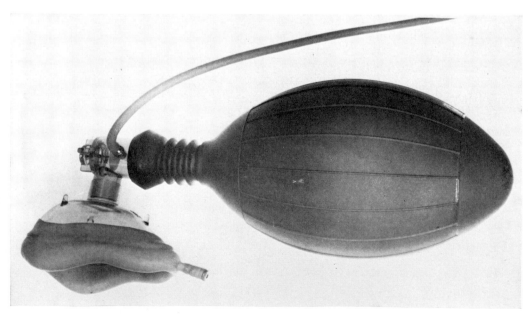

FIG. 81.—Air-Viva. Note side tube for delivery of supplementary oxygen

dosage by any route (i.e. oral, rectal or intramuscular). The unpredictable and often rapid rate of absorption from the rectum necessitates particular vigilance when this route is used. Mistakes in solution concentration are an ever present hazard.

Rapid intravenous injection of a normal induction dose may result in transient respiratory arrest, which often requires no specific treatment. However slow injection of a large dose usually produces a pattern of respiratory depression characterized by shallow breathing, which may be normal in rate. Under these circumstances, hypoxaemia may be avoided by the administration of a high oxygen concentration, provided that the reduction in tidal exchange is not excessive. It should be clearly understood, however, that the administration of oxygen can never compensate for the slow carbon dioxide build-up which is inevitably associated with all types of respiratory depression, and which will itself eventually enhance that very depression. Such a situation

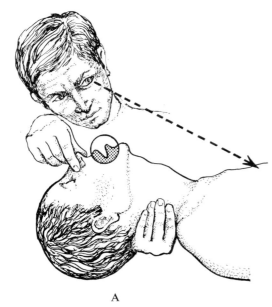
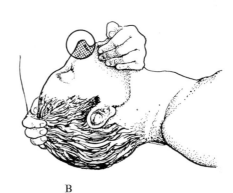

FIG. 82—A Mouth to mouth respiration
B Mouth to nose respiration

Note operator watching chest to ensure adequate expansion

A   B

may be safely tolerated for a period of up to about 5 minutes, but further prolongation must be corrected by effecting an increase in pulmonary ventilation.

Massive accidental overdose (e.g. mistaken concentration of drug) leading to prolonged apnoea will, of course, necessitate efficient artificial ventilation for as long as inadequate spontaneous respiration persists.

There is no specific antidote to the barbiturates, but the use of a non-specific central stimulant is occasionally valuable owing to its ability to break the vicious circle of barbiturate and concomitant hypercarbic depression at least temporarily, and thus initiate recovery. The most commonly used non-specific stimulants are:

Nikethamide (coramine)—2–5 ml 25% solution intravenously
Bemegride (megimide)—50 mg intravenously every 5–10 min

Vanillic Acid (Vandid, Ethamivan)—5–10 ml of 5% solution intravenously.

It is our opinion that the newer analeptics have no particular advantage over the well-tried nikethamide, which is probably the least likely to provoke convulsions, and is therefore recommended for general use.

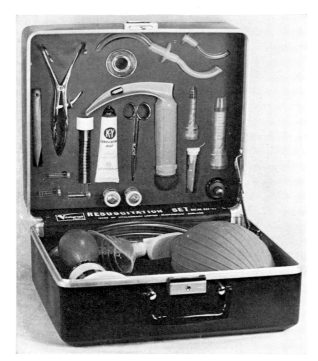

FIG. 83.—Vitalograph resuscitation set

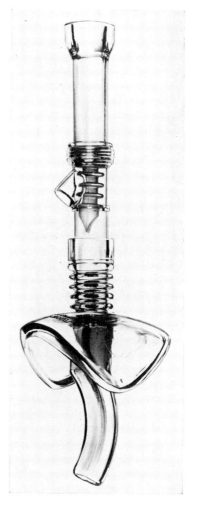

FIG. 84.—Brook's Airway

2. Opiates and Synthetic Analgesic Overdose

In dental out-patient anaesthesia, this type of depression is unlikely to be encountered other than as a result of mismanagement of the 'Jorgensen' or similar techniques. Should it occur, it is characterized by slow respiration, often of normal amplitude and can thus be distinguished from its barbiturate induced counterpart.

Should the respiratory rate fall below 10 per minute, active treatment is indicated along the general lines already described; in addition, unlike barbiturate poisoning, a specific antidote is here available and should be given.

Nalorphine (Lethidrone)—5–10 mg intravenously
Levallorphan—1–3 mg intravenously
Naloxone—0·3–0·8 mg intravenously

The first two of these drugs are themselves respiratory depressants if used on their own, but when administered in the presence of morphine or pethidine-induced respiratory depression, will reverse the depressant effects by substrate competition. Naloxone is, however, a "pure antagonist".

It should be noted that the above mentioned antidotes do not reverse any depressant effects of pentazocine.

3. Volatile Agents

All volatile anaesthetic agents will ultimately produce depression of the respiratory centre, and this is an early feature of overdose with cyclopropane but a late feature with halothane. There is no specific antidote, and treatment consists of withdrawal of the agent responsible, and artificial ventilation of the lungs which, under these circumstances, will achieve not only adequate pulmonary exchange but, by so doing, result in rapid elimination of the volatile agent concerned.

4. Drug Sensitivity and Incompatibility

Respiratory arrest may be a feature of a number of drug sensitivities and incompatibilities and should be treated along the general lines already described, and will often require hospitalization. The special relationship between the analgesics and M.A.O.I.s (page 8) and between porphyria and the barbiturates (page 26) should ever be borne in mind.

5. Muscle-Power Inadequacy

Adequate respiratory exchange is partly dependent upon the efficiency of the diaphragm and other respiratory muscles. These muscles may be weakened by disease (e.g. myasthenia gravis), or muscle relaxants, or they may be placed at a mechanical disadvantage by postural or other influences.

Treatment in all cases consists of adequate artificial ventilation as described, and specific remedies which are discussed in the appropriate chapters.

6. Oxygen Lack and Carbon Dioxide Excess

Although oxygen lack and carbon dioxide excess are initially respiratory stimulants, it must be stressed that this effect is transient, and that both disturbances progressively lead to respiratory failure. In practice, the effects of oxygen lack predominate over those of carbon dioxide excess, and constitute in dental anaesthesia the most common cause of respiratory failure. Since abandonment of the use of hypoxic techniques, prolonged airway obstruction has become the most common precipitating factor, but unrecognized failure of oxygen supply should not be forgotten as a possible cause. Although hypoxia can lead to cardiac arrest in the presence of spontaneous respiration, paralysis of the respiratory centre will inevitably follow within a few moments and may persist after successful treatment of the circulatory failure has been established. However, if respiratory depressants have been used in association with the hypoxia, respiratory failure will often precede serious circulatory depression, and thus cardiac arrest may be avoided if efficient treatment is immediately instituted.

Since hypoxia and hypercarbia can act both as cause and effect of respiratory depression, it is clear that this dangerous vicious circle must always be interrupted as soon as possible.

7. Hypocarbia

As has already been mentioned, excessive artificial ventilation may lead to lowered arterial carbon dioxide tension, which may in turn delay the return of spontaneous respiration.

In dental practice, voluntary hyperventilation during induction and recovery, which is usually hysterical, but may be the result of misguided advice, can result in sufficient lowering of PCO_2 to produce respiratory alkalosis, the chief feature of which is tetanic muscle spasm (carpopedal spasm). In addition, the cerebrovascular constriction which results from a low PCO_2 may lead to dizziness and even loss of consciousness in some subjects.

Significance and Recognition of Respiratory Insufficiency

In conclusion it must be stressed that, irrespective of the cause of respiratory insufficiency, its harmful effects are primarily due to oxygen lack and carbon dioxide excess. In addition, when associated with an obstructed airway the resultant mechanical impedance to venous return will add to the gravity of the situation by reducing the cardiac output.

It is therefore of paramount importance to be able to recognize the early signs of both oxygen lack and carbon dioxide excess.

1. Oxygen Lack (Hypoxia)

The early signs of oxygen lack are sometimes difficult to interpret as will be seen from the summary below.

(a) *Pulse Characteristics.*—There is often an initial increase in pulse rate of up to about 10 beats per minute. Clearly, such a moderate increase may be due to other factors including the anaesthetic agent in use. In addition, mild oxygen lack may sensitize the heart muscle, so that agents such as halothane which are capable of provoking dysrhythmias are more likely to do so.

Severe oxygen lack will eventually produce slowing of the pulse which is usually 'bounding' in character and associated with a rise in systolic blood pressure. If uncorrected, it will inevitably lead to cardiac arrest which may be preceded by a weak and irregular pulse.

(b) *Respiration.*—Hypoxaemia may initially result in an increase in respiratory frequency and tidal volume. Since, in the context of dental anaesthesia, there are a number of other factors which can also result in an increased minute volume, it is, in the first instance, necessary to eliminate hypoxaemia as the cause.

Ultimately, oxygen lack will lead to respiratory depression followed by arrest.

(c) *Cyanosis.*—In the subject with a normal haemoglobin content, the development of cyanosis indicates a moderately severe degree of oxygen lack. Early appreciation of the colour change will depend not only upon the lighting but also on the acuity of the observer; moreover, in certain subjects such as the dark skinned races and subjects in whom peripheral vasoconstriction is a feature, cyanosis may not be readily visible in the presence of severe oxygen restriction. Indeed, the evaluation of the significance of cyanosis must always be made in the light of all the prevailing physiological variables, and in particular those concerned with alterations in haemoglobin content and the state of the peripheral circulation. It should be noted that in the anaemic patient a minimal degree of cyanosis will indicate a serious degree of oxygen lack, whilst in the polycythaemic patient the same degree of cyanosis may be associated with an adequate blood oxygen content. For a full discussion of these problems see page 91.

(d) *Jactitation.*—Severe hypoxia may result in convulsions prior to death. Increased excitability of the motor cortex occurs when a severe degree of hypoxaemia is rapidly induced, as evidenced by the occurrence of unco-ordinated muscular twitching which is described as jactitation. This should always be considered indicative of a dangerous level of oxygen lack, and can be rapidly reversed by the administration of oxygen, provided adequate pulmonary ventilation is maintained. This phenomenon appears to be a specific feature of anaesthetic induction technique involving temporary but complete oxygen deprivation, and therefore should no longer be encountered in dental anaesthesia.

2. Carbon Dioxide Excess (Hypercarbia)

The signs of carbon dioxide excess are often modified by the presence of accompanying hypoxia, but may be seen in pure form, if carbon dioxide is administered in the inhaled mixture, or if a high concentration of oxygen is used in the presence of prolonged respiratory insufficiency.

(a) *Respiration.*—Breathing is increased in both depth and rate, and the increase in minute volume may be considerable. This initial stimulation is followed by depression and ultimately respiratory arrest. If the rise in arterial PCO_2 takes place insidiously over a number of hours, the initial stimulant effect may not be apparent. Bronchospasm, sneezing and coughing may be features of the inhalation of high concentrations (i.e. 30%) in the presence of normal oxygenation.

(b) *Pulse.*—There may be an increase in both rate and volume, the pulse being bounding in character. As the systolic blood pressure increases, reflex bradycardia may occur and dysrhythmias eventually develop, especially in a heart previously sensitized by halothane.

(c) *Bleeding*.—Owing to the increase in pulse volume, excessive bleeding may be encountered, and should this occur for no apparent reason during an operation, carbon dioxide accumulation should always be suspected as a possible cause.

(d) *Sweating*.—Sweating is a constant, early feature of carbon dioxide excess and is accompanied by peripheral vasodilatation, as evidenced by the patient's flushed appearance. Eventually, as the circulation fails and the blood pressure falls, the patient's skin will become pale and cold.

(e) *Motor Irritability*.—A minor degree of motor irritability is sometimes observed, and convulsions have been reported.

The foregoing observations should enable the anaesthetist to recognize the early signs of respiratory insufficiency. However, if proper airway supervision is meticulously exercised at all times, he should seldom encounter situations in which these signs are allowed to develop.

Whilst early recognition of respiratory insufficiency is of paramount importance, it must be remembered that it is upon the anaesthetist's ability to avoid these situations that his competence and the safety of his patient will ultimately depend.

RECOMMENDED READING

1. Laryngeal spasm
BOURNE, J. G. (1967) *Studies in Anaesthetics*. London: Lloyd-Luke. p. 66.

CHAPTER SEVEN

CARDIOVASCULAR HAZARDS

Although respiratory upsets present the anaesthetist with the majority of his problems during dental anaesthesia, circulatory disturbances—although less common—are usually more dramatic, less easy to correct, and therefore more likely to give rise to an unexpected fatal outcome.

It is necessary for the anaesthetist who is engaged in the administration of out-patient dental anaesthetics to have an approach which is both scientific and practical. Monitoring the cardiovascular system under anaesthesia can be highly sophisticated, including continuous recording of E.C.G., central venous pressure, direct arterial pressure and even cardiac output, but must always be appropriate to the prevailing circumstances and should never be dictated by hypothetical legal requirement rather than the patient's well-being. Monitoring of this type, with the exception of continuous E.C.G. recording, is only required in patients in whom the likelihood of a serious cardiovascular abnormality developing during the course of anaesthesia is so strong as to render the patient's admission to hospital obligatory. Moreover, in such cases, the anaesthetist should be fully competent to interpret any abnormality likely to be disclosed; he must form a well-balanced judgement as to the full significance of that abnormality, and be able to decide whether it merits active treatment and, if so, the form that treatment should take. As has already been pointed out on page 133 cardiac monitoring with the present range of complex and not always reliable equipment, is not yet a practical proposition in the average dental out-patient. The properly trained anaesthetist should be able to obtain adequate clinical information on the cardiovascular state of the patient from the simple clinical observations described in Chapter 5. It is the purpose of this section to describe the significance of any abnormalities disclosed by these observations, and to indicate the treatment that may be required. The majority of serious cardiovascular upsets encountered is associated with a fall in blood pressure.

LOW BLOOD-PRESSURE STATES

To clarify the following account, it is necessary to define two commonly used terms.

Fainting

Fainting is a loose lay term used to describe any unexpected loss of consciousness.

Syncope

Syncope is defined in the Oxford Dictionary as 'failure of the heart's action, resulting in loss of consciousness and sometimes death'. Within the context of this definition, such loss of consciousness is, of necessity, due to cerebral ischaemia, and is, indeed, an indication of the severity of the underlying circulatory disturbances. However, certain of these causative circulatory disturbances can occur during anaesthesia, in which case the usual presenting sign of loss of consciousness is masked.

The blood-pressure is the product of cardiac output and peripheral resistance, and it is therefore convenient to consider hypotensive states in terms of these two variables, although in reality both may contribute to the overall picture.

1. Reduction in Cardiac Output

(a) *Failure of Venous Return*

The healthy heart will pump out the quantity of blood returned to it from the venous system under all normal physiological conditions. Accordingly, if the venous return is reduced, the cardiac output will be correspondingly reduced. The following are circumstances in which such a reduction in venous return is most likely to be encountered by the dental anaesthetist.

(i) *Postural Hypotension.*—In the upright posture, venous return is influenced by the arteriovenous pressure gradient, the 'milking' action of voluntary muscle activity, the 'thoracic pump' mechanism, and the presence of venous valves; these factors tend to enhance the return of blood to the heart, and thereby compensate for the influence of gravity. Under anaesthesia, there may be impairment of muscular 'milking' action, associated with a disturbance of vasomotor tone, thus leading to the 'pooling' of blood in the venous system under the direct influence of gravity. Since the maximum circulatory capacity lies below the level of the heart, anaesthesia undertaken in the upright or sitting posture poses a special risk, which has led some authorities to advocate that all dental anaesthetics should be administered with the patient in the horizontal posture. Routine employment of the horizontal posture, however, carries with it certain disadvantages, and these are fully discussed in Chapter 8. Since it is into the dependent legs that the pooling of blood is most likely to occur in the sitting position, a reclining posture with legs horizontal seems to us to constitute the most satisfactory solution. Any benefit, resulting from the establishment of a gravity-induced pressure gradient from heart to brain by lowering the head is of doubtful significance, since it is the improvement in venous return from the lower part of the body to the heart, rather than the attempt to 'run blood through the brain by gravity' which has true physiological validity; indeed, under certain circumstances, the increased cerebral *venous* pressure which results from the head-down posture may actually predominate over the raised arterial pressure, the net result being a decrease, rather than an increase in cerebral perfusion.

The actual circumstances which may lead to postural hypotension are varied. In the conscious subject, the condition is encountered in the 'guardsman on parade' situation. Here, pooling of blood in the legs takes place when the subject stands perfectly still for a prolonged period. The absence of muscular activity largely accounts for the gradual failure of venous return, and the situation is worsened should there be accompanying peripheral vasodilatation produced for example, by a rise in body temperature. Under these circumstances, the gradual failure in venous return may lead to the subject feeling faint for some time before syncope actually occurs. In the anaesthetized subject, as already mentioned, gravity-induced pooling of blood is likely to take place as a result of the muscular flaccidity and vasomotor depression produced by deep levels of anaesthesia, and this effect is enhanced, if the anaesthetic agent in use produces either peripheral vasodilatation or central cardiac depression. The effect produced is identical to that which results from a sudden haemorrhage, and thus many of the clinical signs are similar. Reduction in venous return will inevitably result in diminished cardiac output; this, in turn, will lead to a fall in mean arterial blood pressure, and it is both the fall in arterial pressure and the concomitant decrease in central venous pressure which stimulates the baroreceptor mechanisms to produce tachycardia and peripheral vasoconstriction in an attempt to restore the blood-pressure to normal. In practice, therefore, it is the onset of tachycardia and skin pallor which should immediately draw the anaesthetist's attention to the possibility of an underlying circulatory disturbance. Owing to the serious consequences to which such a disturbance might rapidly lead if allowed to persist, and the simplicity of the initial treatment, it is essential to take immediate action before attempting to elicit confirmatory signs. The patient should be placed in the horizontal posture with the legs raised, the anaesthetic discontinued, oxygen administered, and all operative work suspended, the attention of the whole team being directed entirely towards the patient's well-being, since further resuscitative measures may prove necessary. If the underlying condition is one of uncomplicated postural hypotension, these measures will constitute the only treatment necessary to restore adequate circulatory function. However, both tachycardia and pallor may persist for a short while following the restoration of an adequate circulation. Pallor merely indicates the presence of cutaneous vasoconstriction, and it is therefore necessary to assess the capability of the circulation to provide adequate tissue perfusion. Fortunately, there is a simple clinical sign which discloses this information. If the skin of the vasoconstricted ear is vigorously rubbed, local cutaneous vasodilatation (axon reflex) will be produced, and thus the true state of the underlying circulation revealed. For, if the ear becomes flushed and pink, this will indicate that no hypoxaemia is present; furthermore, rapid capillary refill with pink blood following momentary compression of the ear will indicate an adequate capacity for tissue perfusion, and thus there exists the strong likelihood that this is taking place in those vital areas of the body which enjoy circulatory priority. We consider this simple clinical sign to be of greater value than the measurement of either pulse rate or blood-pressure. Should this sign produce a response less satisfactory than that described above, it is probable that a serious underlying cardiovascular disability exists (e.g. coronary infarction).

It should be remembered that in the dark-skinned races and patients of normally pallid complexion, postural hypotension may exist without the warning sign of pallor. In addition, in the former group of patients, capillary refill can only be observed in nail-beds and mucous membranes, in which areas its interpretation is considerably more difficult. Therefore, there is perhaps a particularly strong argument in favour of routine monitoring of pulse and blood pressure in these patients.

(ii) *Acute Hypotension of Pregnancy.*—In the supine posture, the full-term pregnant uterus— or indeed any other large abdominal tumour—may on rare occasions produce a sudden severe reduction in venous return by direct pressure on the vena cava. Because of this possibility, dental out-patient anaesthesia in the supine posture is contraindicated in these patients.

(b) *Central Cardiac Failure*

The Normal Heart.—Routine cardiac monitoring of healthy subjects undergoing general anaesthesia for dentistry discloses that a significant proportion of them develop cardiac dysrhythmias during the course of the procedure. Whilst the majority of these dysrhythmias take the form of isolated or infrequent extrasystoles and would therefore not be expected to lead to a significant fall in cardiac output, nevertheless multifocal ventricular extrasystoles sometimes leading to ventricular tachycardia, and also nodal bradycardia have been observed. One would certainly expect to find a considerable fall in cardiac output if any of these more serious dysrhythmias persisted for more than a few moments; indeed, cardiac arrest might follow either ventricular tachycardia or nodal bradycardia.

The exact mechanism responsible for the development of these dysrhythmias under general anaesthesia has not been firmly established, but the following factors have all been claimed to play a contributory role.

(i) Surgical stimulation under light general anaesthesia.
(ii) The use of halothane, particularly in children, is associated with a high incidence of dysrhythmias, whilst they are rarely seen if methohexitone is used as a sole agent.
(iii) Hypoxia and hypercarbia are both considered to be dysrhythmogenic, particularly when associated with the administration of known cardiotoxic agents such as halothane or trichlorethylene.
(iv) It has been suggested that the very anxious patient, with presumably a high catecholamine blood level, is particularly at risk, as is also the patient who has received an injection containing adrenaline.

At the present time, the true significance of these dysrhythmias is unknown, and the problem of their prevention unsolved. Intravenous premedication with atropine, whilst preventing nodal bradycardia, increases the overall dysrhythmia incidence. Selective beta blockade with, for example, practolol can be shown to be preventive, but the justification for its routine use in out-patient dentistry is doubtful. The use of unsupplemented methohexitone would clearly be helpful, but it is not possible to produce adequate, safe working conditions in a large number of the patients most at risk, i.e. children having multiple extractions. We are left with the proposition that all patients should be kept free from hypoxic and hypercarbic influences, that halothane, when indicated, should be used cautiously and that constant observation of the patient's cardiovascular state is at all times essential.

Finally, quite apart from the development of dysrhythmias, gross hypoxia or hypercarbia and massive overdose with any anaesthetic agent—inhalation or intravenous—will lead to direct myocardial depression resulting in central cardiac failure.

The Abnormal Heart.—Acute cardiac failure—often leading to syncope—may occur in the patient suffering from cardiovascular disease, whether overt or latent. This failure may be precipitated by, or fortuitously associated with, general anaesthesia; the underlying cardiac abnormalities most likely to predispose to such sudden failure are numerous, and the following are the most common: coronary occlusion, heartblock, valvular and congenital heart disease, paroxysmal tachycardia, paroxysmal fibrillation, and the rare cardiomyopathies.

A full discussion of these and other cardiac abnormalities is beyond the scope of this book, but further details can be found on pages 217 and 274.

2. Peripheral Resistance Reduction

(a) *Vasovagal Attack* (Emotional Fainting or Hypothalamic Syncope)

Fear, pain and other powerful emotions such as the sight of blood or anticipation of any unpleasant experience may be responsible for this type of syncope.

The striking anomalous feature of this reaction is the combination of signs associated with both sympathetic and vagal overactivity, i.e. pallor and sweating together with profound bradycardia. Its origin is the hypothalamus, which is that area of the brain most closely associated with the physiological response to emotion. This response is initially characterized by sympathetic activity, giving rise to cutaneous vasoconstriction, sweating and vasodilatation in voluntary muscle. This vasodilatation has been shown to be mediated in the hypothalamus through nerve tracts which are separate from those of the vasoconstrictor control pathways; thus, it is a specific characteristic of emotional sympathetic activity, and is clearly the prime response in the 'fight or flight' mechanism, which is normally followed by violent muscle activity. Should this activity not take place, and therefore the cardiac output remain constant, the reduction in peripheral resistance due to this muscle vasodilatation may lead to a fall in blood pressure.

In the particular situation of 'hypothalamic syncope', an excessive vagal activity is superimposed upon this picture, thus completing the transformation from an initial 'fight or flight' reaction to one of 'sham dead'; for the vagal response will lead, not only to bradycardia, but also to splanchnic vasodilatation which will further decrease, the peripheral resistance. It is this gross decrease in peripheral resistance, not necessarily accompanied by a significant reduction in cardiac output, which leads to the precipitous fall in blood pressure which is characteristic of this condition. Therefore under these specific circumstances, the influence of gravity on the hydrostatic pressure difference between heart and brain is the main cause of syncope. This is in contrast to the situation of postural hypotension discussed on page 164.

Treatment of the condition is simple, as alteration of the upright posture to the supine is all that is usually required to establish adequate cerebral blood-flow and thus a return to consciousness. The common practice of forcing the head between the legs will achieve this objective, but since a few minutes is often required to re-establish a return to normal peripheral resistance, the adoption of a full length horizontal posture is more satisfactory. Should consciousness not return immediately on adopting this posture, some other cause for the loss of consciousness should be sought. The administration of intravenous atropine, by reversing the intense bradycardia, may avoid the risk of dangerous cardiac dysrhythmias occurring, but it will not always influence the period of syncope by raising blood pressure.

(b) *Carotid Sinus Syncope*

A clinical picture similar to that described under 'vasovagal attack', may rarely be produced, in sensitive subjects, by the application of external pressure to the neck in the region of the carotid sinus.

(c) *Halothane*

The cardiodepressant action of halothane has been mentioned in relation to cardiac output reduction. It should here be emphasized that under light halothane anaesthesia, whilst there may be a fall in total peripheral resistance due to overall vasodilatation, nevertheless cerebral blood-flow is not reduced—and indeed may be increased (page 102). There is no reason to suppose that, in the presence of an adequate venous return, posture would greatly influence this vital cerebral blood-flow. However, in deep halothane anaesthesia (rarely required for dental purposes), the combination of loss of peripheral resistance and reduction of cardiac output may embarrass the circulatory reserves to such an extent as to render the full supine posture imperative.

(d) *Hypotensive Agents* (page 292)

Patients suffering from high blood pressure under treatment with hypotensive drugs, are liable to have a labile blood pressure which may be unduly sensitive to anaesthetic and other influences.

It is said that prolonged treatment with the M.A.O.I.s will also produce a labile blood pressure, but in this case the blood pressure is more likely to show sudden hypertensive rather than hypotensive changes (page 18).

(e) *Suprarenal Insufficiency*

Normal vasomotor response to 'stress' (e.g. shock, trauma) is dependent upon adequate suprarenal activity. Should this activity be impaired by, for example, Addison's disease or prolonged steroid therapy, the risk of vasomotor collapse should be borne in mind.

OTHER CARDIOVASCULAR HAZARDS

It is now necessary to describe certain vascular accidents which may lead to a sudden interruption of cerebral function, and which are associated with a high rather than low blood pressure.

1. Cerebral Arteriosclerosis

This condition is usually encountered in elderly hypertensive subjects who may, or may not, have a history of previous cerebrovascular accident. Whilst a reduction in blood pressure may result in cerebral thrombosis, any sudden increase can lead to cerebral haemorrhage. Under general anaesthesia, by far the most common cause of such increase is asphyxia due to obstruction of the airway; other less common causes are stormy induction, surgical stimulation under light anaesthesia, and carbon dioxide retention.

2. Cerebral Aneurysm

It is doubtful whether cerebral aneurysm itself is ever congenital, and it is thought to develop as the result of a congenital weakness in the muscular coat. These Berianeurysms may well never give rise to signs or symptoms, but under the strain of a sudden increase in blood-pressure, may rupture, thus resulting in cerebral haemorrhage which may lead to death. Once again, under general anaesthesia, the most common cause of such a rise in blood pressure is obstruction of the airway. Patients undergoing treatment with the tricyclic antidepressants carry a special risk, since a sharp rise in blood pressure may follow the injection of local anaesthetic containing adrenaline or noradrenaline. It should also be pointed out that a rise in blood-pressure, sufficient to cause rupture of such an aneurysm, may result from a convulsion following an overdose of local anaesthetic or hypoxia.

RECOGNITION AND TREATMENT OF CARDIOVASCULAR COLLAPSE

Having discussed the underlying mechanisms of acute cardiovascular collapse, it is now necessary to describe the practical details of its recognition and treatment. When the cardiovascular failure is severe and sudden in onset, cerebral circulatory inadequacy will result in loss of consciousness, which is inevitably the dominant clinical sign. However, under general anaesthesia, this will be masked, thus making it essential for the anaesthetist to be familiar with, and recognize, other less obvious signs at the earliest possible moment.

It has already been stressed on page 135 that we consider the pulse and skin characteristics to be the most important and reliable practical observations to make, particularly in relation to changes which may occur. It will be immediately appreciated that, so far as skin characteristics are concerned, changes are less readily observable in skins which are either deeply pigmented, or excessively pale, whether this pallor be normal or fear-induced. In these subjects, continuous pulse observation assumes a greater importance, and thus the use of a pulse monitor may prove particularly valuable. Some authorities would advise that the blood pressure should be frequently taken in all anaesthetized patients. We believe, however, that the value of information forthcoming in the short unintubated case is not normally commensurate with the monopoly of the anaesthetist's attention inevitably associated with the use of the ordinary sphygmomanometer or oscillotonometer.

If, in the presence of a clear airway and full oxygen delivery, obvious signs of circulatory disturbance occur, such as pallor, cyanosis, sweating, tachycardia, bradycardia, pulse irregularities or discernible changes in pulse volume, immediate action should be taken. The operation should be discontinued, the patient placed flat, with legs raised, an unobstructed airway ensured, the anaesthetic discontinued and 100% oxygen administered preferably with a face mask. This course of action, which should be the anaesthetist's immediate, automatic response, will only occupy a few seconds, provided a suitable chair is in use (page 71). At this stage a reassessment of the patient's condition should be made. Assuming that adequate, spontaneous and unobstructed respiration is present, the pulse should be carefully observed and one of the following situations may be present.

(a) *Tachycardia.*—Tachycardia is the normal, sympathetic response to postural hypotension and if the pulse is easily palpable, no further treatment is necessary and rapid recovery can be expected. Provided the rate returns to within normal limits (below 100), and capillary blood-flow improves and sweating ceases, the anaesthetic can then be continued. It is wiser under these circumstances to maintain the supine posture throughout.

Persistent tachycardia may represent either a temporary cardiac instability such as paroxysmal tachycardia, or a serious underlying cardiac catastrophe such as coronary infarction. Under these circumstances the patient's general condition, as judged by peripheral circulatory blood-flow and sweating, will probably not show a marked improvement and therefore neither the anaesthetic nor the operation should be recommenced. No further active therapeutic measures should be undertaken until an accurate diagnosis has been established. Empirical treatment with drugs such as the beta-adrenergic blocking agents, digitalis and quinidine, in the absence of an established diagnosis, may do more harm than good.

The foregoing account applies to tachycardia associated with circulatory impairment as evidenced by other clinical signs. It should be pointed out that tachycardia not uncommonly occurs as an isolated finding, and under these circumstances is often due to stimulation under light anaesthesia. It is however essential for the anaesthetist to assure himself that such tachycardia is not warning evidence of some imperfection in the anaesthetic technique, of which the most common is hypoxia. Having established this fact, he can expect the pulse rate to settle with the establishment of a stable level of anaesthesia.

(b) *Bradycardia.*—If the pulse is slow (a decrease of 30 beats per minute from normal resting level), it is likely to be due either to vagal over-activity, as in the vaso-vagal attack and halothane overdose, or to a disturbance in the cardiac conduction mechanism. This latter disturbance which gives rise to heart block is most commonly provoked either by generalized hypoxia or coronary infarction affecting the conducting tissue (page 279).

Therefore, in the presence of bradycardia it is advisable, in addition to the general therapeutic measures already recommended, to give 0·6 mg of atropine intravenously, for this will restore normal pulse rate in cases of vagal overactivity. Although it is not therapeutically effective in heart block, its administration will not prejudice either the patient's condition or the subsequent diagnosis. It has already been pointed out that the pulse does not always reflect the exact nature of the cardiac beat; for example, if a ventricular extrasystole occurs early in diastole, the strength of the contraction may not be sufficient to open the aortic valves and therefore, no beat will be transmitted to either the central or peripheral pulse. Such an extrasystole is inevitably followed by a compensatory pause and therefore, this situation will present as bradycardia if adjudged solely by palpation of the pulse. Its true nature will be recognized only by auscultation of the heart, or by electrocardiographic recording.

Bradycardia, like tachycardia, may be noted as an isolated finding, and provided there is no element of hypoxia or carbon dioxide retention, is usually due to the direct effect of halothane. Under these circumstances, the only treatment necessary is the reduction of inspired concentration or, should this prove impracticable, the intravenous administration of atropine.

(c) *Pulse Irregularities.*—Those of a temporary nature (page 134) will cease spontaneously if the emergency treatment already described is carried out. Persistent irregularities usually indicate some more serious cardiac cause, the most common being associated with coronary insufficiency. In the absence of an E.C.G. it will not be possible to arrive at an accurate diagnosis, and therefore no specific treatment other than those general measures already described should be entertained. Even should an E.C.G. record be available, it is doubtful if any specific measures undertaken under emergency circumstances are of paramount importance, as they are seldom life saving, often controversial, and may jeopardize subsequent diagnosis and treatment. We consider that it is probably unwise to administer a beta-adrenergic blocking agent or cardiac stimulant under these conditions, although in the presence of established auricular fibrillation and a progressively failing circulation, it may be justified to administer 0·5 mg of digoxin intravenously.

(d) *Alterations in Pulse Volume.*—The significance of the pulse volume as a clinical sign has already been described on page 134. A gross decrease in pulse volume, as evidenced by difficulty in feeling the pulse, is indicative of a reduction in stroke volume. In spite of compensatory tachycardia, this reduction often leads to serious impairment of cardiac output, and therefore any obvious decrease in pulse volume can be taken as confirmatory evidence of circulatory inadequacy. An increase in pulse volume is most likely to be due to carbon dioxide retention and/or hypoxia, both of which are readily corrected by simple measures.

Finally, if the emergency treatment described does not result in complete recovery, it is the anaesthetist's prime duty to supervise the smooth transference of the patient to hospital, with continuous oxygen administration, and possibly analgesic drugs should the patient regain consciousness and show evidence of cardiac pain and restlessness. If dyspnoea is present, he must ascertain the posture in which the patient finds this symptom least marked, and this may entail allowing him to sit up.

It will be seen that the signs of circulatory failure are considerably less obvious than those of respiratory failure. It is therefore obligatory that the anaesthetist should pay continual attention to both skin colour and the pulse characteristics for, in practice, it is through these observations that he will obtain the earliest possible warning of any circulatory upset. Whilst alterations in pulse rate and rhythm may provide valuable information, it is an unexpected diminution in pulse volume which constitutes the most common warning sign of serious circulatory deficiency. Should this be associated with impaired capillary blood flow, a serious circulatory state should be assumed and the possibility of impending cardiac arrest considered.

CARDIAC ARREST

Diagnosis.—Inability to palpate a central pulse (e.g. carotid or femoral, Fig. 70) necessitates an immediate diagnosis of cardiac arrest. Confirmatory evidence of this catastrophe lies in peripheral circulatory failure, dilatation of the pupils, and ultimately cessation of respiration. In the conscious subject, cardiac arrest is immediately followed by loss of consciousness.

Immediate Treatment.—Failure to palpate the central pulse demands that treatment be immediately initiated irrespective of the presence of confirmatory signs, for irreversible cerebral damage will occur within 3 minutes of arrest, unless the circulation is re-established artificially by cardiac massage. Before commencing cardiac massage, the patient should be placed in the supine posture with the legs raised, and oxygen administered after ensuring that the air passages are unobstructed. If, at this stage, the pupils react to light (or are constricted) it is justifiable to feel for the pulse again before commencing cardiac massage; for the presence of reactive pupils usually indicates either that arrest has not occurred, or that if it has, its recognition has been so immediate that the momentary delay involved in feeling for the pulse once more will not prejudice the outcome. Should this second attempt to feel the pulse prove negative, immediate cardiac massage must be undertaken irrespective of the state of the pupils. In order to do this, a decision has to be made as to whether

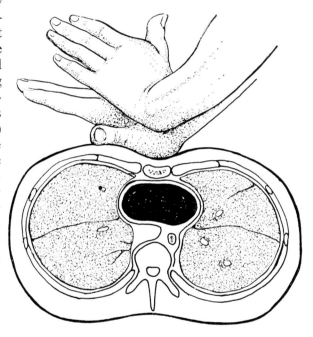

Fig. 85.—Cardiac Compression

Coronal Section through thorax showing heart being compressed between sternum and vertebral column

massage can be adequately undertaken without moving the patient on to the floor. In a well organized dental practice, this decision will have already been made by anaesthetist and dental surgeon prior to the occurrence of any catastrophe. The dental chair should allow rapid adoption of the full supine posture and should offer a rigid support to the entire thoracic region, but may require that a board (available for that purpose) is inserted between it and the patient's back. Should the chair be unsuitable in any of these respects, the patient will have to be transferred on to the floor prior to the commencement of full cardiac massage, but it is always worth thumping the sternum once or twice before transference of the patient, since this manoeuvre has been known to initiate spontaneous cardiac activity.

External Cardiac Massage.—The object is to compress the heart between the sternum and the thoracic spine, and in order to do so adequately the sternum has to be depressed about 2 inches (5 cm) with each compression (Fig. 85). This is best achieved by placing the heels of both hands over the lower third of the sternum in the manner indicated in Fig. 86 and applying, with arms straight and full body-weight, one compression per second. It is not possible to describe this procedure further, nor the variations in force and technique required in patients of varying age and physique. We cannot stress too strongly that all practitioners should ensure that they receive

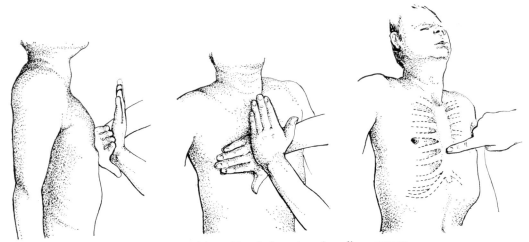

FIG. 86.—Position of hands for external cardiac massage

adequate practical instruction in this life saving procedure. If properly undertaken, a palpable carotid pulse will provide evidence of adequate cardiac output. It should also be possible to demonstrate an active capillary circulation carrying oxygenated blood, and, provided that irreversible brain damage has not already occurred, the pupils should remain or become reactive to light.

In small children, cardiac compression should be undertaken with one hand only; in infants with two fingers. In children and infants, rates of 100–120 per minute will prove necessary to maintain adequate cardiac output.

Artificial Ventilation.—True cardiac arrest is always rapidly followed by inadequate respiration (often 'gasping' in nature) or total apnoea. It is therefore imperative to institute adequate artificial ventilation of the lungs with a gaseous mixture containing at least 20% oxygen. A full account of the technique of artificial ventilation appears on page 153, to which the reader is referred. The following special considerations apply to artificial ventilation associated with cardiac arrest. It must be remembered that it is essential to clear the airway of all foreign material (e.g. vomit, blood, etc.) prior to the commencement of lung inflation. 100% oxygen should, if possible, be used at the outset, but once adequate circulatory and respiratory function has been artificially established, it is permissible to change to mixtures containing less than 100% oxygen in order to conserve what may be a limited oxygen supply. For this purpose, the

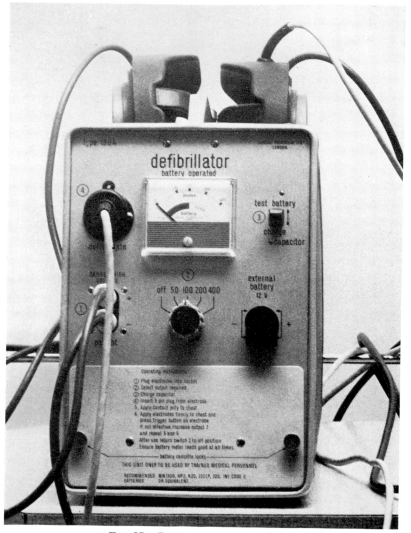

Fig. 87.—Battery operated defibrillator

air-resuscitators (page 155) are ideal, for room-air (if possible supplemented with oxygen) can be used indefinitely. In the absence of an air-resuscitator, nitrous oxide from the anaesthetic apparatus may be used as an 'oxygen-conserver', for it must be remembered that if the source of respiratory gases is artificial, a total of at least 5 litres per minute will be required in order to avoid serious carbon dioxide build-up in the absence of a suitable absorber. For convenience and efficiency, intubation of the trachea should be undertaken, provided the necessary skill and equipment are available to enable its performance without undue interruption of either cardiac massage or artificial ventilation.

One inflation of the lungs should be interposed between every group of five consecutive cardiac compressions. On the rare occasions when no assistance is available, it will prove more convenient to interpose two lung inflations between every group of fifteen cardiac compressions.

If external massage and artificial ventilation should produce early and complete recovery, the patient must nevertheless be admitted to hospital for at least twenty four hours' observation.

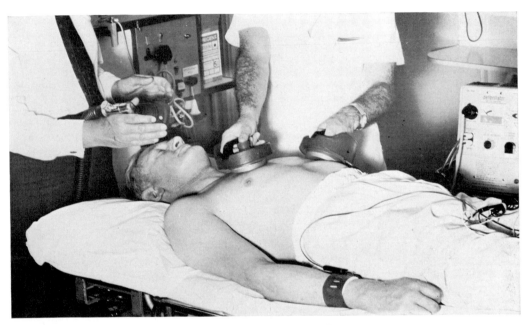

FIG. 88.—Cardiac defibrillation

NOTE 1.   Position of electrodes
       2.   Both operators cease direct contact with patient during defibrillation

Subsequent Management.—Having established an adequate supply of oxygenated blood to the vital organs by virtue of the essential resuscitative measures described, immediate arrangement should be made for transference of the patient to the nearest hospital department in which full intensive care facilities are available. However, it must now be pointed out that this transference may present certain insuperable problems which will demand that a fully equipped resuscitation team comes to the patient rather than *vice versa*. The practitioner, therefore, should have an appreciation of the possible problems involved prior to the occurrence of any emergency. The prime question is this. Can a patient, irrespective of size, be transferred into an ambulance without interrupting either cardiac massage or artificial ventilation? Massage can only be efficiently continued on a stretcher if a rigid board has been inserted beneath the patient's thoracic spine (resting on the stretcher poles), and with such a method of transport, it may prove impossible to negotiate the geography of the premises. Some ambulance services may provide special stretchers for this purpose.

If transport to hospital is feasible, it should be carried out carefully and slowly, massage and ventilation being uninterrupted. On the other hand, if the method of transference necessitates interruption of cardiac massage for more than one minute, it may be preferable not to attempt to move the patient, but such a course of action will necessitate prior liaison between practitioner and hospital authorities regarding the feasibility of bringing a team to the patient. An interchange of information regarding the adaptability of any electrical equipment involved will also be necessary. Before transference involving interruption of treatment, it may be beneficial to inflate the patient's lungs with pure oxygen for some minutes prior to the temporary discontinuation of cardiac massage, so that the maximum possible tissue oxygen concentration has already been achieved.

Whatever transport arrangement is made, the following additional therapeutic measures should be considered during the 'waiting' period.

(a) *Bicarbonate*.—Whenever circumstances permit, an intravenous drip should be set up and 150–300 ml of 8·4% bicarbonate administered over every 30 minute period, in order to counteract the inevitable metabolic acidosis accompanying tissue anoxia of any origin. The empirical quantity recommended should not be exceeded in the absence of blood pH estimation.

If the equipment for setting up a continuous drip is not available, 1 ml bicarbonate solution per kg of body-weight should be injected intravenously every 10 minutes. This means that a 10 stone (64 kg) man would need 64 ml of 8·4% bicarbonate every 10 minutes.

(b) *Other Drugs*.—In the absence of an electrocardiograph the use of drugs is empirical, since it is not possible to tell whether the heart has arrested in asystole or ventricular fibrillation, unless the chest is opened. The correct treatment for established asystole (other than cardiac massage) is the intravenous injection of adrenaline and calcium gluconate; that for established ventricular fibrillation is electrical defibrillation or, if not available, intravenous injection of procaine or lignocaine. No injections should be contemplated if their preparation and administration are likely to interfere with the uninterrupted performance of efficient cardiac massage and pulmonary ventilation. However, once these two priorities have been satisfied, the following drug therapy is recommended.

All injections should be given by the intravenous route. Intracardiac injection, once popular, may produce pneumothorax, injury to a coronary artery and interruption of cardiac compression. Intravenous injection will suffice, provided an adequate circulation is maintained by cardiac massage, and the site of the injection, wherever possible elevated and massaged towards the heart.

(i) *Adrenaline.*—0·5–1·0 ml of 1:1000 (i.e. 0·5–1 mg) solution can be injected every 10 minutes. If the heart has arrested in asystole, this injection may either initiate normal cardiac action, or it may promote ventricular fibrillation which is a legitimate step in the treatment of asystole. If, however, the heart is already fibrillating, adrenaline will often facilitate subsequent artificial defibrillation, and in any event is unlikely to worsen the situation.

It is doubtful whether any further drug therapy is indicated in the absence of electrocardiograph control.

(ii) *Calcium.*—Should the electrocardiograph show the presence of cardiac complexes, but the peripheral pulse indicate an inadequate cardiac contraction, the cardiotonic properties of calcium may be utilized.

10 ml of 10% calcium gluconate may be given at 10 minute intervals. Calcium chloride—in spite of its higher calcium content weight for weight—is better avoided, owing to its irritant properties should extravascular leakage occur.

(iii) *Procaine and Lignocaine.*—In the presence of established ventricular fibrillation, if a defibrillator is not available, or has failed to produce reversion to normal rhythm, it is worth injecting procaine or lignocaine 10 ml of 1% solution intravenously.

Defibrillation

It has been recognized recently that if arrest in ventricular fibrillation has occurred, the sooner electrical defibrillation can be achieved, the better the ultimate prognosis. The defibrillator recommended for the dental department is the portable battery model shown in Figs. 87–88.

Open-Chest Massage and Internal Defibrillation

After admission of the patient to hospital, if all other measures fail, open chest massage and internal defibrillation should be performed.

RECOMMENDED READING

1. **Cardiac Arrest.**
    GILSTON, A. A. & RESNEKOV, L. (1971) *Cardio-Respiratory Resuscitation.* London: Heinemann.
2. **The Electrocardiogram in Dental Anaesthesia.**
    RYDER, W. (1970) *Anaesthesia, 25,* 46.
3. **Cardiac Dysrhythmias in Outpatient Dental Anaesthesia in Children.**
    THURLOW, A. C. (1972) *Anaesthesia, 27,* 429.
4. **Hypotension.**
    TYRRELL, M. F. (1970) *Scientific Foundations of Anaesthesia.* Section II, Vol. 6. Ed. C. Scurr and S. Feldman. London: Heinemann. p. 117.

CHAPTER EIGHT

POSTURE

From the preceding chapters, it will have been noted that posture plays a role of some importance in both respiratory and circulatory efficiency. In recent years, the circulatory effects of posture, and particularly their influence on cerebral circulation, have monopolized the attention of many dental anaesthetists to the belittlement or even exclusion of other factors which we believe to be of equal importance. It should be appreciated that there is no posture which offers a guarantee of safety in respect of either respiratory or circulatory function. It is our intention in this chapter to present the advantages and disadvantages of those postures most commonly used for the administration of dental anaesthesia.

The choice of posture lies between the traditional upright sitting position at one extreme, and the fully supine at the other, although any intermediate position may be chosen. For the purposes of discussion, we will initially compare the salient features of the two extremes, particularly in respect of their effect on respiratory and cardio-vascular function, and their influence upon the ease with which the dental procedure may be performed.

1. Respiratory Effects

(a) *Patency of Airway.*—The upright posture facilitates airway maintenance. For even in the presence of profound relaxation, the effect of gravity will direct the relaxed tongue into the floor of the mouth rather than posteriorly into the obstructive position against the posterior pharyngeal wall, as is the case in the supine posture (page 142). In addition, when the supine posture is used, the operator will sometimes require to work at the head of the patient. In this event, the anaesthetist will be displaced from that position in which he can best maintain the patency of the difficult airway, and will therefore adopt a position at the patient's side, where his only comfortable control is by submental support, which does not always prove adequate (Fig. 89). An experienced team, comprising operator, assistant and anaesthetist, can usually overcome these difficulties, but there is sometimes a temptation to accept less than perfect permanent airway control for reasons of expediency, and indeed the less experienced team may fail to recognize such imperfection—particularly in the absence of an inhalation anaesthetic component where the reservoir bag provides visual evidence of the respiratory pattern. For these reasons, we consider that endotracheal intubation is more often indicated in the supine than in the upright posture, particularly when the dentistry is likely to be prolonged or technically difficult.

(b) *Prevention of Mouth Breathing.*—As already mentioned, in the relaxed sitting patient there is a tendency for the tongue to sink into the floor of the mouth, thus leading to mouth breathing (page 123). This may be easily rectified by gentle pressure to the submandibular soft tissues, thereby bringing the tongue and palate once more into apposition.

(c) *Airway Protection.*—It has already been pointed out in Chapter 5, that airway protection will depend primarily upon efficient packing and suction. It must now be stressed that failure to achieve this objective is probably the most common cause of difficulty and even catastrophe during dental anaesthesia. Whilst efficient packing can be achieved irrespective of posture, we nevertheless find it technically easier to accomplish and maintain in the sitting position. The probable reason for this is twofold. Firstly, there is less tendency for the pack to become sodden with blood and saliva and thus slippery, since the sitting posture encourages the pooling of fluid into the floor of the mouth where it is readily accessible to suction. Secondly, the normal position of the tongue in this posture assists the firm retention of the pack in the lingual sulcus.

There is evidence to suggest that if foreign material reaches the pharynx, some is likely to be inhaled irrespective of posture; although both the frequency of inhalation and the quantity of material inhaled are greater in the sitting posture, it must be emphasized that it is in the supine posture that the initial pharyngeal contamination is most likely to occur, with the exception of that arising from a post-nasal mucus drip (page 281). It should be clearly understood that the danger of inhalation of foreign material exists, irrespective of posture and level of anaesthesia, and therefore any breach of the pack constitutes a failure of technique which demands that the anaesthetic be discontinued and the situation rectified.

In the supine posture the danger of 'silent' regurgitation of alimentary contents is an additional hazard. This, as distinct from vomiting, is a passive process, which may occur as a result of incompetence or relaxation of the cardiac sphincter associated with relaxation of the pharyngeal musculature; gastric or oesophageal contents will flow in the direction of gravity, thus rendering regurgitation unlikely to occur in the sitting position. The medical conditions likely to be associated with regurgitation are discussed on page 5.

(d) *Respiratory Efficiency.*—Vital capacity is some 15% less in the supine than in the upright posture. This difference is due partly to alterations in lung blood-volume, and partly to the impairment of diaphragmatic movement imposed by the abdominal contents. This impairment may be of clinical significance in advanced pregnancy, obesity and in certain cardio-respiratory disorders characterized by orthopnoea, and in this type of case the upright posture should be selected.

Recently it has been shown that at low lung volume, the phenomenon of 'airway closure' may lead to some degree of hypoxaemia due to the continued perfusion with mixed venous blood of the non-ventilated areas of 'closed' lung. Low lung volume is a feature of both increasing age and the supine posture, in which it is approximately one litre less than in the upright. Thus, the upright posture may have an important overall respiratory advantage, particularly in the elderly.

2. Cardiovascular Effects

The cerebral arterial blood pressure, as compared with the conventional arm reading taken at heart level, varies with posture on the basis of ± 2 mmHg for every 2·5 cm of vertical difference between the two levels. In the upright posture, this implies a cerebral blood pressure of about 25 mmHg less than that normally recorded in the arm. It is, of course, only in severe hypotension that this gravity-induced gradient results in impairment of cerebral blood-flow, since man in his normal state is well adapted to the upright posture! The cause and effect of these hypotensive states has been fully discussed on page 164. It is generally accepted that impairment of cerebral blood-flow in the upright healthy subject is unlikely to occur unless the arm systolic blood pressure falls below 50 mmHg. It will be remembered that cerebral circulatory inadequacy can occur as a result of diminished cardiac output which may in turn be due to diminished venous return; or it may occur as a result of sudden profound hypotension associated primarily with loss of peripheral resistance (vaso-vagal attack). Maintenance of adequate venous return is of prime importance in avoiding the former, and this can usually be achieved by raising the legs without necessarily adopting the fully supine posture. In the latter condition however, the blood pressure may become so low, that the small hydrostatic difference in pressure between heart and brain in the sitting position assumes a critical importance, and under these circumstances the supine posture must be adopted. It should be remembered that whilst cerebral blood-flow is dependent upon an adequate minimum cerebral arterial pressure, the flow-rate is retarded by any increase in cerebral venous pressure, so that the *head-down* posture may prove a positive disadvantage.

3. Surgical Considerations

There is a growing tendency for conservative dentistry to be undertaken in the position shown in Figs. 20 and 53. When general anaesthesia is required, it is clearly desirable that the anaesthetist should adapt his technique to comply with the dental surgeon's preference, provided that the patient's safety is in no way jeopardized. One of the difficulties associated with the supine posture is that the conventional dental chair with adjustable head-rest is usually replaced by a contoured chair with fixed head-rest. Inability to adjust readily the position of the patient's head may add to the airway-control difficulties already inherent in this posture. Although these problems may be overcome without recourse to intubation in many patients, we nevertheless believe that the increasing popularity of 'low-seated' dentistry will result in the more frequent use of intubation if consistently safe and satisfactory operating conditions are to be provided. It is, however, often possible to maintain an unobstructed airway without intubation by placing the head in hyperextension (Fig. 89), but this requires a complete re-orientation on the part of the operator.

So far as exodontia is concerned, most dental surgeons are agreed that lower teeth are intrinsically more difficult to extract in the supine position.

Conclusions

After taking into consideration all the foregoing factors, we believe that in the unintubated patient, the reclining posture (Fig. 52) offers the most satisfactory compromise in terms of safety and convenience. This posture combines all the respiratory advantages of the upright position, together with a mitigation of the postural hypotensive disadvantages associated with dependent legs. Routine use of such a posture does, however, demand continual observation of the cardiovascular state, since it will not protect the patient from cerebral ischaemia associated with a

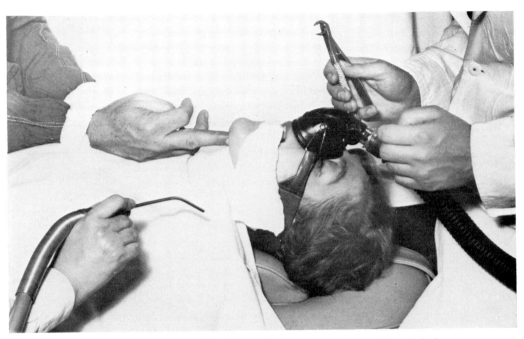

FIG. 89.—Supine posture with submental support to ensure unobstructed airway

sudden profound hypotensive episode such as occurs occasionally under prolonged deep halothane anaesthesia, or in relation to the vaso-vagal attack. But, in this event the posture is readily transformed, by lowering the back-rest, into the fully supine position with legs already raised.

The anaesthetist must appreciate that all postures have their advantages and disadvantages, and that none can be automatically considered preferable under all circumstances. For example, the pale, frightened patient with a history of fainting demands the use of the supine posture, whereas we would consider it to be contra-indicated in the unintubated obese or pregnant patient, particularly with a history of orthopnoea. Finally, there is no posture which offers the anaesthetist a guarantee against any of the hazards inherent in general anaesthesia, and to believe otherwise is to court disaster.

RECOMMENDED READING

Posture.
LOVE, S. H. S. (1970) The Complications of Dental Anaesthesia. In *General Anaesthesia for Dental Surgery*. Ed. A. R. Hunter and G. H. Bush. Altrincham: John Sherratt.

CHAPTER NINE

INTRAVENOUS AGENTS

INTRODUCTION

Since the introduction of methohexitone and propanidid—two drugs which are characterized by rapid clinical recovery—it is no longer considered unwise to use intravenous agents on dental out-patients. It is therefore generally possible to respect the patient's preference for either inhalation or intravenous methods of losing consciousness. In our experience, the majority of adults prefer the intravenous method, whilst children frequently choose to avoid an injection. However, we must stress that the competent anaesthetist should be master of all techniques and servant to none. Ideally, the choice of method should be based on a careful clinical assessment, and not dictated by deficiencies in the anaesthetist's repertoire. Should the clinical considerations demand a technique outside the scope of the anaesthetist concerned, whenever possible that patient should be referred elsewhere.

We consider that complete mastery of a simple inhalation technique, such as that described in Chapter 5 is essential before undertaking training in intravenous methods. For, whilst satisfactory anaesthetic conditions cannot be achieved by inhalational methods when airway control is inadequate, the administration of anaesthetics by the intravenous route enables anaesthesia to be induced and maintained in the presence of an obstructed airway—with possible disastrous consequences.

In this chapter we will discuss in detail only those intravenous anaesthetics in common use, i.e. thiopentone, methohexitone and propanidid. Many other intravenous agents are available, but appear to us to offer no advantages over those selected, and therefore only a brief description will be included; this reservation does not include Althesin, formerly CT 1341 (page 192), the place of which remains to be evaluated. Those techniques which entail the use of heavy sedation with intravenous drugs in combination with local, rather than general anaesthesia alone, are fully discussed in the chapter on conservation (Chapter 12). It should, however, be pointed out that these techniques have an increasing sphere of usefulness in exodontia and minor oral surgery.

Before describing the pharmacology of the intravenous anaesthetics, it is necessary to discuss in general terms the principles governing the behaviour of narcotic drugs injected directly into the blood stream.

BEHAVIOUR OF INJECTED NARCOTICS

When a drug is injected into a peripheral vein, it is carried in the blood to the right side of the heart, which then distributes it evenly throughout the pulmonary capillary circulation from which it is returned to the left side of the heart. It will thus be apparent that, provided the agent is non-volatile and therefore there is no loss to the atmosphere through the lungs, the full dose injected will ultimately be returned to the left side of the heart. Its concentration in the blood will depend not upon the concentration in the syringe, but upon the speed of injection in terms of milligrams per minute and the total venous return, which is normally equivalent to the cardiac output. The concentration in the syringe will influence only the maximum possible speed of injection able to be achieved with any given dosage. The so-called 'surge' technique (page 210) is merely a method of overcoming the inevitable delay entailed in the injection of a large bulk of fluid; a similar effect can be achieved by the use of high concentrations of drug in small bulk solution.

The drug, now evenly distributed in the blood contained in the left side of the heart, is ejected into the systemic circulation. The quantity of drug reaching the brain in one heart-beat will depend upon the proportion of the cardiac output distributed to the cerebral circulation. Under normal resting conditions this represents approximately 20% of the total output. Since the brain represents less than 5% of the total body bulk, the proportion of drug reaching it is extremely high. This proportion will be even higher in the shocked patient in whom the cerebral circulation is maintained at the expense of the remaining peripheral blood-flow; the converse may occur in the presence of cerebral arterio-sclerosis in the aged. Thus the shocked patient requires greatly reduced dosage to achieve a given cerebral effect, whilst the elderly arterio-sclerotic may sometimes require a surprisingly large dose in relation to his generally reduced metabolic and drug requirements.

It has already been pointed out that the concentration of drug in the blood, and therefore its effect on the brain, depends upon the relationship between the dose injected in a given time and the cardiac output during that time. It will thus be apparent that any significant increase in cardiac output will result in 'dilution' of the drug in the blood. Since the increase in cardiac output associated with, for example, 'anxiety' or pregnancy is not accompanied by an equivalent increase in cerebral blood-flow, it is apparent that under these circumstances, the brain will receive a relatively smaller proportion of the drug injected. This state of affairs accounts, in part at least, for the apparent 'resistance' of nervous or pregnant subjects to the effects of intravenous narcotics.

Thus far, it has been assumed that an increase in cardiac output results in an increase in non-cerebral tissue perfusion, and that therefore the blood returning to the heart from these tissues will be low in drug concentration. There is, however, one set of circumstances in which an increase in cardiac output may fail to result in increased drug 'resistance'. This situation has been described following a study of the effects of methohexitone on the human circulation; this study indicated that methohexitone may produce an increase in cardiac output associated with a degree of arterio-venous shunting rather than to an increase in tissue perfusion. This situation would of course result in a high venous concentration of the drug returning to the heart, thus minimizing the expected 'resistance', or even producing an apparent drug sensitivity.

Whilst the foregoing account is clearly an over simplification of the true state of affairs, it nevertheless serves to illustrate that many complex physiological factors influence the narcotic effect of a specific dose of drug, and that whilst a simple measurement such as body-weight may be used as an overall guide to dose range, the actual dosage indicated in a particular set of circumstances is subject to many other influences. The immediate narcotic effect of a single injection results from the achievement of a very high initial cerebral concentration. Over the succeeding minutes, this concentration falls, as the drug is given up by the brain to the blood and distributed throughout the body. The rate of this redistribution, and hence 'recovery', is dependent upon the efficiency of the peripheral circulation, the relative mass of body tissue in which the drug is soluble, and the specific solubility characteristics of the drug concerned; other biophysical features such as protein-binding and ionization may also influence the course of clinical recovery (page 188). In this context, it should be noted that any change in plasma pH resulting from over- or under-ventilation will affect protein-binding and ionization. For example, an increase in pH (i.e. low pCO_2 due to hyperventilation) will result in a reduction in protein-binding and will therefore enhance the clinical effect of a given dose of drug. The converse of this situation is also true.

Having considered in general the behaviour pattern of drugs injected intravenously, we will now consider in detail the properties of the four anaesthetic agents in common use.

Thiopentone Sodium B.P. (Thiopental Sodium U.S.P.)—Trade names—Intraval Sodium, Penthothal)

Presentation.—(a) Ampoules (0·5 g) of both 10 ml and 20 ml capacity
    (b) Ampoules (1·0 g) of 20 ml capacity
    (c) Multidose bottle (2·5 g) of 100 ml capacity
    (d) Multidose bottle (5 g) of 100 ml capacity
    (e) Suspension for rectal instillation (syringe pack) containing 200 mg per ml
    (f) Rectal suppository—250, 500 and 750 mg
    (g) Oral 'pentothal acid'
    Dosage is discussed on page 194.
Thiopentone for intravenous injection is normally dissolved in pyrogen-free 'water for injection', or 0·9% saline.

Composition.—Thiopentone is sodium ethyl (1-methyl butyl) thiobarbiturate. It is the sulphur analogue of pentobarbitone (Nembutal), and was introduced in the U.S.A. by Lundy in 1933.

Physical Characteristics.—Thiopentone is a yellow amorphous powder with an odour resembling H_2S. It is soluble in water, 2·5% or 5% solution having a pH of 10·81 (c.f. blood 7·4). A 2·8% solution is isotonic with blood. 6% sodium carbonate is added to the powder to prevent its acidification by atmospheric CO_2. The solution is relatively unstable, and should not be used after 48 hours storage or if cloudy. Both

2·5% and 5% solution are irritant to the tissues, 2·5% less so owing to its near isotonicity.

Pharmacological Actions.—In the main, thiopentone exhibits the actions common to all the barbiturates (see page 24). Its intravenous use is characterized by smooth and rapid induction of anaesthesia devoid of motor excitatory phenomena, i.e. involuntary muscle movement, hiccoughing and sneezing. Thus the drug may be considered suitable for the patient with epileptic tendencies. The resultant anaesthesia is accompanied by voluntary muscle relaxation, depression of the respiratory centre, and some degree of direct cardiac and vasomotor depression.

Whilst frank overdose will lead to marked respiratory depression or even apnoea, in normal clinical dosage the degree of depression is usually slight and transient, seldom requiring active respiratory assistance. However, it must be remembered that any anaesthetic agent which produces both respiratory depression and muscular relaxation is strictly contraindicated in the presence of upper respiratory obstruction, e.g. Ludwig's angina (page 282). Patients suffering from sublaryngeal obstruction (e.g. asthma, bronchitis) require special care in anaesthetic management, but the use of thiopentone is not specifically contraindicated. Likewise, the increased sensitivity of the ill, the shocked and the elderly to the respiratory and circulatory depressant effects of all drugs—particularly when given by the intravenous route—should ever be borne in mind. Thiopentone will, in normal dosage, produce a moderate fall in both cardiac output and blood pressure, for which the healthy cardiovascular system can adequately compensate. Whenever impairment of cardiovascular function exists, great care must be exercised in the administration of thiopentone, and two cardiac conditions demand particular caution. Firstly, constrictive pericarditis, in which the fixation of cardiac output is at a dangerously low level; secondly, aortic incompetence, in which the diastolic blood pressure is already so low that the coronary circulation may be imperilled by any further fall, however trivial. Thiopentone is regarded by some as being contraindicated in these two conditions.

Although thiopentone is in part destroyed in the liver, a single sleep-dose is not contraindicated even in cases with serious hepatic dysfunction, but repeated doses should be avoided.

Since some of the break-down products of thiopentone are said to be hypnotically active, it should be used with caution in the presence of serious impairment of renal function (page 25).

Thiopentone, in common with all barbiturates, is strictly contraindicated in porphyria (page 26).

Post-anaesthetic sequelae such as nausea, vomiting, headache and malaise are rare when thiopentone is used as the sole agent.

Summary of Main Characteristics
1. Rapid, pleasant induction free from motor excitation.
2. Risk of tissue damage with extravascular injection.
3. Moderate respiratory and circulatory depression.

A.A.D.—7

4. Absence of laryngeal depression.
5. Low analgesic potency.
6. Moderate voluntary muscular relaxation.
7. Slow final break-down and excretion.
8. Freedom from post-anaesthetic nausea and vomiting.
9. Sensitivity reactions rare.
10. Adverse relationship with porphyria.

Methohexitone Sodium B.P. (Methohexital Sodium U.S.P.)—(Trade names—Brietal Sodium (U.K.), Brevital (U.S.A.))

Presentation.—(a) Single dose bottle (100 mg) of 10 ml capacity
    (b) Multidose bottle (500 mg) of 50 ml capacity
    (c) Multidose bottle (2·5 g) of 250 ml capacity
    (d) Stock bottle (2·5 g) of approximately 17·5 ml capacity
    (e) Stock bottle (5 g) of approximately 35 ml capacity
    Dosage is discussed on page 195.

The powder is normally dissolved in pyrogen free water, 0·9% saline, or 5% dextrose. Water is the solvent of choice, but must be free from bacteriostatic agents; the resultant solution may be used so long as it remains clear and colourless (usually at least 6 weeks) but solutions prepared in saline or dextrose are not suitable for storage. Crystallization sometimes occurs and appears to be associated with exposure of the solution to the CO_2 in air. These crystals are composed of barbituric acid, and thus the supernatant solution is weaker in anaesthetic potency than that originally mixed; such solutions should be discarded.

Chemical Incompatibility.—In general, methohexitone should not be mixed with acid solutions prior to administration.

    Table XVIII provides information regarding the most commonly used combinations.

TABLE XVIII

	Immediate Precipitate	Delayed Precipitate
Atropine	Nil	Pronounced
Hyoscine	Nil	Slight
Suxamethonium	Nil	Slight
d-tubo-curarine	Nil	Slight
Gallamine	Nil	Nil
Diazepam	Heavy	
Pethidine	Heavy	
Fentanyl	Nil	Nil
Pentazocine	Heavy	
Propanidid	See under Propanidid	

Composition.—Methohexitone is sodium a-dl-l-methyl-5-allyl-5-(1-methyl-2-pentynyl) barbiturate. It is non-sulphur-containing, and was introduced into anaesthetic practice in the U.S.A. in 1956.

Physical Characteristics.—Methohexitone is a white hygroscopic powder. It is soluble in water, forming a colourless, odourless solution with an approximate pH of 11, thus rendering it bacteriostatic—a fact which is not to be interpreted as allowing relaxation of normal sterility precautions. All strengths of solution in common use are irritant to the tissues. Injection into a small or constricted vein will sometimes result in pain *proximal* to the injection. The cause of this is obscure, but admixture with lignocaine is said to reduce the incidence of this complication.

Pharmacological Actions.—Whilst the actions of methohexitone are, in the main, similar to those of other barbiturates (page 24), nevertheless induction of anaesthesia with this agent is sometimes characterized by certain excitatory phenomena such as muscle twitching, movement and hiccough. Thus, this drug is not the agent of choice for epileptic patients. Like thiopentone, methohexitone produces both respiratory and cardiovascular depression. The former is usually transient, and seldom requires special treatment. So far as the cardiovascular effects are concerned, the clinical evidence in man is inconclusive, but there appears to be general agreement that a fall in systolic blood pressure of some 20–40 mmHg is not uncommon, although a slight initial rise may also occur. Wise *et al.* found evidence suggestive of arterio-venous shunting, and observed a fall in peripheral resistance to which the heart responded by elevating its output in association with pronounced tachycardia. From the clinical point of view, a single induction dose in the healthy subject is unlikely to result in serious cardiovascular upset. The effects of prolonged administration require further investigation, but as is the case with any cumulative depressant drug, constant observation of its clinical effects in any particular set of circumstances is essential. As with thiopentone, nausea, vomiting and other post-anaesthetic sequelae are rare.

The reservations and precautions essential for the safe use of this drug in the ill, the shocked and the elderly apply with no less force to methohexitone than to thiopentone. Likewise, acute airway obstruction and porphyria constitute absolute contraindications to its use. Anaphylactoid reactions have been described, and their management is outlined on page 26.

Methohexitone is broken down, mainly by the liver, at the rate of approximately 20% per hour, and present information suggests that the overwhelming majority of break-down products are hypnotically inactive and excreted by the kidneys.

Summary of Main Characteristics

1. Rapid, pleasant induction sometimes accompanied by motor excitation.
2. Risk of extravascular injection.
3. Moderate respiratory and circulatory depression.
4. Absence of laryngeal depression.
5. Low analgesic potency.
6. Variable voluntary muscular relaxation.
7. Final break-down and excretion more rapid than thiopentone.
8. Freedom from post-anaesthetic nausea and vomiting.

9. Sensitivity reactions rare.
10. Adverse relationship with porphyria.

Recovery from Thiopentone and Methohexitone Compared

Whilst these two barbiturates share many common characteristics, it is generally accepted that clinical recovery is superior with methohexitone.

The difference in their rates of destruction within the body cannot account entirely for this superiority, and it is therefore necessary to compare certain other physico-chemical characteristics.

1. **Lipid Solubility.**—The solubility of an anaesthetic agent in fat as compared with its solubility in water is expressed as the Oil/Water Partition Ratio, and in the case of the two drugs under discussion the Peanut Oil/Water Partition is as follows:

Thiopentone 89
Methohexitone 65

This implies that if water containing 90 molecules of thiopentone per unit volume is allowed to equilibrate with peanut oil containing no thiopentone, the ultimate situation after full equilibration has taken place, will be one in which every unit volume of water will contain one molecule of thiopentone, and every unit volume of oil in contact with that water will contain 89 molecules.

This oil/water partition is represented in the body by the natural lipid/plasma partition, and the significance of this partition is that all cell membranes present a lipoid barrier to the passage of drugs from plasma into cell, thus not only influencing diffusion of drugs into the relatively avascular fatty tissues, but controlling their overall distribution throughout all the tissues of the body. Relative distribution of the two drugs between plasma and body fat has demonstrated a fat/plasma solubility ratio approximately 2–3 times as great with thiopentone as with methohexitone. For this reason, a greater quantity of thiopentone, as compared with methohexitone, will ultimately be redistributed into the fat depots, and thus relatively more thiopentone may be required to *maintain* a given blood level—and thus a given level of anaesthesia when this is required for a prolonged period. It is, perhaps, for this reason that there is a greater delay in ultimate recovery from thiopentone than from methohexitone when the drug is used to maintain prolonged anaesthesia.

2. **Protein-Binding.**—A proportion of all barbiturates introduced into the blood and tissues is bound to the plasma or tissue proteins, and thus rendered inactive. This proportion varies markedly between members of the barbiturate family, but in the case of thiopentone and methohexitone, the proportion of each drug so bound is 75% and 73% respectively, so that this characteristic is unlikely to account for any marked difference in properties.

3. **Ionization.**—The pharmacological activity of any drug depends, in part, upon that proportion of the drug which exists in un-ionized form—since it is this form which

is lipid soluble, and hence able to enter cells. The proportions in the case of thio-pentone and methohexitone under similar conditions are:

Thiopentone (un-ionized) 61%
Methohexitone (un-ionized) 76%

Thus for a given weight dosage of both drugs, a relatively greater proportion of methohexitone than thiopentone will exist in the un-ionized—and hence active—form. The proportion of any drug which exists in the un-ionized form varies according to the local tissue conditions—notably pH.

4. **Rate of Metabolism**.—Both thiopentone and methohexitone are broken down in the body, and whilst it is difficult to make a direct comparison between the relative break-down rates under controlled conditions, it is nevertheless justifiable to postulate that methohexitone must be completely eliminated more quickly than thiopentone; for thiopentone is released more slowly into the blood-stream from the fatty depots —owing to its higher fat solubility, and is thus less readily available for both break-down and excretion.

Conclusions

It will be seen from the foregoing account that the most striking physico-chemical difference between these two drugs lies in their comparative lipid solubilities.

Since thiopentone is more soluble than methohexitone in lipoid and hence nervous tissue, and yet methohexitone clinically is accepted as being $2\frac{1}{2}$ to 3 times as potent as thiopentone (i.e. to produce a given clinical effect, $2\frac{1}{2}$ times the weight of thio-pentone is required), it is necessary to offer an explanation for this apparent anomaly. It is possible that the drugs, weight for weight, have different inherent potencies, but their similarity in chemical structure would lead one to believe that this may not be the full explanation. The observed clinical potency difference is perhaps affected by a difference in redistribution characteristics. For when either drug is injected intra-venously, approximately 20% of the total quantity reaching the heart between beats is pumped into the cerebral circulation at the next heart-beat—the remaining 80% being distributed to the rest of the body. Whilst, theoretically, the first heart-beat will result in a relatively higher brain concentration of thiopentone than metho-hexitone, subsequently the blood returning to the heart from the rest of the body will contain less thiopentone than methohexitone, owing to the greater affinity of the tissues for thiopentone, so that the blood level of the drug will fall more rapidly in the case of thiopentone than methohexitone. Thus, following rapid intravenous injection under standard conditions of, say, 100 mg of either drug, the brain con-centration may be momentarily higher in the case of thiopentone, but over the clinically significant first 2 minutes will fall to subanaesthetic levels, whilst in the case of methohexitone, slower uptake by the tissues will allow the plasma, and hence brain, concentration to remain high enough to result in the production of anaesthesia over that period. Thus it is, that a higher dose of thiopentone is required to produce a comparable clinical effect, and this may account for the acceptance of the conventional concept of their relative potencies. In addition, it has already been mentioned that the relatively higher proportion of un-ionized (active) methohexitone as compared with thiopentone will contribute to the greater potency of the former in any direct weight for weight comparison.

So far as speed of recovery is concerned, it has already been pointed out that the difference in lipid solubility will account for the slower release—and therefore break-down—of thiopentone, and also that some of its break-down products are hypnotically active. It must be stressed that the complete break-down and elimination of either drug extends over a period of many hours, and from the clinical stand-point complete recovery cannot be assumed to have taken place in the absence of an intervening night of sleep.

Propanidid B.P. (A.N.)—(Trade name—Epontol (U.K.))

Presentation—10 ml ampoules containing 500 mg
i.e. 5% solution propanidid

This solution is very stable having a shelf life of 2 years at room temperature. It may be diluted further in 0·9% saline, but all such dilute solutions should be freshly prepared; under certain conditions these solutions may develop a bluish hue (Tyndall phenomenon). This is an optical effect and does not indicate any chemical change. Dosage is discussed on page 195.

Chemical Incompatibility.—Chemically propanidid is compatible with most drugs used in anaesthesia, but the manufacturers have advised against the administration of this drug mixed with methohexitone; although this advice has been challenged, we can see no valid reason for using such mixtures.

Composition.—Propanidid is propyl 4-(NN-diethylcarbamoyl-methoxy)-3-methoxy-phenylacetate) a derivative of eugenol (oil of cloves).

Physical Characteristics.—Propanidid is a pale yellow oil with a molecular weight of 337·44 and a boiling point of 210–212°C, its pH is between 4 and 5 and it is insoluble in water.

The commercial preparation Epontol is a solution of propanidid formed by the addition of Cremophor EL and 0·9% sodium chloride. The resultant solution has a pH of 4·7 and is readily diluted with normal saline. Its precursor G 9505 was characterized by a tendency to produce venous thrombosis, and although this undesirable effect appears to have been largely overcome with Epontol, it is advisable to select a large vein with a good flow. The preparation is viscous and therefore difficult to inject through a narrow bore needle. There is no pain at the site of injection even if leakage into tissues occurs, as it possesses a local anaesthetic effect.

Pharmacological Actions.—Since propanidid bears no chemical relationship to the barbiturates its pharmacological actions on all systems of the body will be described in detail.

(a) *Central Nervous System.*—There is evidence to suggest that propanidid depresses the spinal reflexes less than the baributrates, which may account for the fairly high rate of involuntary muscle movement after surgical stimulation. However, Dundee has pointed out that propanidid is not only devoid of the anti-analgesic effect seen with certain blood concentrations of the barbiturates, but itself exhibits analgesic properties.

(b) *Cardiovascular System.*—A fall in systolic blood pressure of between 25–40 mmHg is more common with propanidid than with the barbiturates, but the duration of this hypotension is shorter. The majority of patients receiving propanidid develop tachycardia. In practice, using normal clinical doses, the function of the cardio-vascular system remains satisfactory.

(c) *Respiratory System.*—Immediately following loss of consciousness, propanidid invariably leads to a short period of hyperventilation which may be followed by hypoventilation or rarely apnoea. All these effects are transient.

There is no evidence that propanidid increases the sensitivity of bronchial or laryngeal reflexes.

(d) *Side Effects*

(i) *Nausea and Vomiting.*—The incidence of nausea and vomiting when propanidid is used as the sole anaesthetic agent is minimal. However, when it is followed by the use of inhalational agents such as nitrous oxide and halothane, there would appear to be a slightly greater incidence of this complication than that associated with the barbiturates. This may be due to the fact that the rapid elimination of this drug leaves the patient unprotected from stimuli which may cause nausea and vomiting during recovery from anaesthesia.

(ii) *Hiccough.*—This complication has been observed, but is less common than with metho-hexitone.

(iii) *Allergy.*—Allergic and anaphylactoid reactions are more common than with either thiopentone or methohexitone.

One drug interaction is worthy of note. Propanidid has been shown to potentiate the action of succinylcholine chloride, whilst also reducing the incidence of afterpains normally associated with the use of this drug. This potentiation does not occur at the neuromuscular junction and is therefore probably due to alteration in enzymatic activity. In clinical practice the duration of action of a given dose of succinylcholine appears to be prolonged when used in conjunction with propanidid.

(iv) *Tissue Irritation.*—Extravenous injection results in a painless swelling, and no subsequent inflammatory changes in the tissues. Intra-arterial injection is also painless and apparently unaccompanied by serious sequelae.

Intravenous injection is followed by a higher incidence of venous thrombosis than is the case with the barbiturates.

(v) *Fate in the Body.*—Unlike the barbiturates, recovery from propanidid does not depend upon redistribution of the drug, since it is broken down rapidly in the body. Esterases in the liver, and to a lesser extent in the plasma, break down the propanidid molecule into two anaesthetically inert fractions which are non-toxic, and 90% is excreted by the kidney within 2 hours.

In clinical practice immediate recovery may not differ significantly from that seen with methohexitone, but owing to destruction rather than redistribution of the drug, prolonged drowsiness and hangover is far less common. Indeed so rapid is its destruction that it is both difficult and costly to use propanidid as the sole agent for prolonged anaesthesia.

The fate of the solubilizing agent Cremophor EL appears to be unknown. The frequency of anaphylactoid reactions is a disturbing feature of the drug.

Althesin CT 1341—Glaxo

Presentation—5 ml and 10 ml ampoules, each ml containing 12 mg of total steroid. The recommended dose is between 0·06–0·1 ml/kg intravenously,

Composition.—Althesin is a new steroidal intravenous anaesthetic agent introduced by Glaxo Laboratories in 1971 under the formulation known as CT 1341. This formulation consists of two steroids, alphaxalone and alphadolone acetate, solubilized in Cremophor EL and made isotonic using sodium chloride. Alphaxalone is the main anaesthetic ingredient and makes up 75% of the steroid content; the addition of alphadolone acetate, which has about half the anaesthetic potency of alphaxalone, is justified because it increases the solubility of the latter threefold, thus decreasing the volume of the effective dose.

Physical Characteristics.—Althesin is a slightly viscid, colourless solution, which can be readily diluted with normal saline. The solution appears non-irritant to veins and other human tissues, and can therefore be injected intramuscularly. It does not appear to deteriorate with storage.

Pharmacological Action.—The induction of anaesthesia is smooth, but in our experience is associated, in the unpremedicated patient, with minor degrees of limb movement; hiccough is less common than with methohexitone. With the recommended dose, the period of anaesthesia is longer than that seen with methohexitone, but a return of consciousness can be expected within 4–5 minutes after the standard dose of 0·6 mg/kg.

Unlike the barbiturates, redistribution to the body fat and other tissues is minimal; recovery is therefore associated with less 'hangover' than that seen with the barbiturates. Very small quantities of the drug remain in the plasma after 20 minutes, but complete excretion via gut and kidneys occupies some 48 hours.

Effects on Cardiovascular System.—The fall in blood pressure with a single induction dose of Althesin is similar to that seen with both methohexitone and thiopentone. However, the increase in pulse rate seen with all intravenous induction agents is less marked with Althesin than methohexitone; this may account for the fact that the rise in cardiac output reported with methohexitone is not apparent with Althesin or thiopentone.

Effects on Respiratory System.—The effects of Althesin on respiration are very similar to those seen with the barbiturates. There is a period of mild hyperventilation followed by a short but variable period of depression. Patients, following Althesin administration, appear to be less sensitive to the inhalation of irritant vapours than those who have received barbiturates.

Summary.—The small bulk solution, non-irritant properties, wide therapeutic index, and good recovery characteristics render it a valuable drug in out-patient anaesthesia, and of particular use in the child with small difficult veins, in whom the injection of methohexitone is often painful. Indeed, in the absence of future adverse reports, this drug may well become not only the non-barbiturate of choice, but the standard intravenous agent for many procedures*.

OTHER INTRAVENOUS AGENTS

Short Acting Barbiturates

A number of short acting intravenous anaesthetic agents has been developed over the last twenty years, but they would appear to have no clinical advantages over the four drugs mentioned above, and will only be described briefly here.

(i) **Buthalitone Sodium**—(Trade names—Transithal, Ulbreval)

This is the sodium salt of allyl-z-methyl propyl barbituric acid, and weight for weight it is about half as potent as thiopentone, over which it has no obvious advantage.

(ii) **Hexobarbitone Sodium**—(Trade names—Evipan, Cyclonal sodium)

Hexobarbitone was the first of the intravenous anaesthetics to gain popularity in 1932. Although less irritant to the tissues than thiopentone, the frequency of side effects such as muscle twitching and sneezing led to its replacement by thiopentone. Its final elimination from the body is more rapid than thiopentone.

(iii) **Thialbarbitone Sodium**—(Trade name—Kemithal)

This drug which was originally claimed to have a shorter action than thiopentone would appear to have no clinical advantage.

(iv) **Thiamylal Sodium**—(Trade name—Surital sodium)

This drug has enjoyed some popularity in the U.S.A. but is not commercially available in Great Britain. It has no clinical advantage over the other barbiturates mentioned.

Ketamine Hydrochloride B.P.—(Trade name—Ketalar)

This drug is not considered suitable for intravenous use in dentistry, but may have a limited place when used intramuscularly in children, and is therefore described in the children's section (page 222). Its use in major oral surgery is discussed in Chapter 15 (page 347).

Methods of Usage of Intravenous Agents

The following four methods satisfy all needs in dental anaesthesia.

1. **A single dose.**—This provides about 2 minutes anaesthesia for a simple procedure.
2. **A single dose plus inhalation.**—Both the inhalation component and the operation,

* Recent reports of adverse reactions suggest that Althesin should be avoided in patients with a history of asthma or other allergies.

A.A.D.—7*

in this technique, are commenced immediately following the intravenous administration, thus allowing a more prolonged operation to proceed without interruption.

3. **A sleep dose plus inhalation.**—In this technique the intravenous agent is given in
the smallest possible dose which will produce sleep, and commencement of the
operation must await the achievement of an adequate depth of anaesthesia with
the inhalation agents.

4. **Intermittent or continuous administration.**—In this technique, the object is to
achieve adequate anaesthesia for prolonged procedures without recourse to
inhalation agents.

Dosage

For the purpose of convenience, body weight and age will be used as a guide to
dosage, but it should be remembered that other factors may play an even more
important determining role (page 183).

1. Thiopentone Dosage

Table XIX summarizes the dosage pattern related to age and body weight.
Thiopentone should be prepared with sterile pyrogen-free water as a $2\frac{1}{2}\%$
solution, i.e. 0·5 g in 20 ml.

TABLE XIX.—*Thiopentone*

Method of Usage	Under 14 yrs	14–60 yrs	Over 60 yrs
Minimum sleep dose	3 mg/kg	2·5 mg/kg	2 mg/kg
Average induction or 'single shot' dose	6 mg/kg	5 mg/kg	4 mg/kg
Intermittent dose	Considered unsuitable, owing to delay in recovery		

2. Methohexitone Dosage

It is difficult to compare the relative potency of methohexitone and thiopentone,
but the results of several independent investigations lead to the acceptance of the
ratio methohexitone: thiopentone as 3:1. Thus, Table XX will act as a guide.

Methohexitone is normally prepared as a 1% solution, i.e. 100 mg/10 ml with
sterile pyrogen-free water and has a shelf life of at least 6 weeks, but may also be
used in strengths up to 5%.

3. Propanidid Dosage

Recovery from propanidid is not primarily dependent on redistribution, but
rather upon actual pharmacological break-down which is many times more rapid
than the break-down of methohexitone, thus leading to a shorter period of post-
anaesthetic central depression. This lack of cumulative effect necessitates the use
of high dosage to achieve prolonged anaesthesia by the intermittent and continuous method, thus rendering such techniques costly.

For practical purposes, propanidid can be considered to possess $\frac{1}{5}$ of the
anaesthetic potency of methohexitone, i.e. 500 mg of propanipid are equipotent

to 100 mg of methohexitone. It will be noted therefore that 10 ml of undiluted propanidid is equipotent to 10 ml of 1% methohexitone (see Table XXI).

TABLE XX.—*Methohexitone*

Method of Usage	Under 14 yrs	14–60 yrs	Over 60 yrs
Minimum sleep dose	1 mg/kg	0·8 mg/kg	0·6 mg/kg
Average induction of 'single shot' dose	2 mg/kg	1·5 mg/kg	1·0 mg/kg
Intermittent dose	Dose requirements determined by prevailing circumstances. Doses in excess of 300 mg rarely necessary or advisable		

TABLE XXI.—*Propanidid*

Method of Usage	Under 14 yrs	14–60 yrs	Over 60 yrs
Minimum sleep dose	5 mg/kg	4 mg/kg	3 mg/kg
Average induction or 'single shot' dose	10 mg/kg	8 mg/kg	5 mg/kg
Intermittent dose	Owing to rapid destruction in the body, incremental doses more closely approach induction dose, than in the case of methohexitone. Technique, therefore costly		

Owing to the absence of cumulative effects of propanidid as compared with methohexitone when the drugs are used by intermittent and continuous technique, the ratio of potency methohexitone/propanidid widens with increasing dosage.

Choice of Agent

From consideration of all the foregoing factors we believe methohexitone, and possibly Althesin, to be the most suitable intravenous agents for out-patient use. However, in epilepsy, methohexitone is best avoided. Patients suffering from porphyria must not be given any barbiturate, thus the choice lies between propanidid and Althesin.

In the diabetic, it is desirable to achieve rapid and complete recovery with minimal post-anaesthetic nausea, so that normal intake of food may be resumed as soon as possible. It would seem that propanidid has an advantage in respect of rapidity of recovery, but as it carries a higher incidence of nausea than methohexitone and Althesin, this advantage is largely nullified.

In asthma, there is a theoretical objection to the use of barbiturates owing to their parasympatheticomimetic properties, from which propanidid and Althesin are alleged to be free. However, we have ourselves frequently used the intravenous barbiturates without untoward results on asthmatic patients; we consider that the factor of paramount importance is the establishment of an adequate depth of anaesthesia with liberal oxygenation prior to surgical stimulation, for which purpose nitrous oxide, halothane sequence is eminently suitable, irrespective of the method of induction.

RECOMMENDED READING

1. **Factors Affecting the Action of Drugs.**
   LANT, A. F. (1970) *Scientific Foundations of Anaesthesia*, Sect. III, Vol. 1. Ed. C. Scurr and S. Feldman. London: Heinemann, p. 303.
2. **C.T.1341. Some Effects on Man (Althesin).**
   SAVEGE, T. M. (1971) *Anaesthesia*, **26**, 402.
3. **Steroid Anaesthesia (Althesin).**
   POSTGRADUATE MEDICAL JOURNAL (1972) Vol. 48.
4. **Anaphylactic Reaction to Propanidid.**
   THORNTON, H. L. (1971). *Anaesthesia*, **26**, 490.

CHAPTER TEN

INTRAVENOUS TECHNIQUES

Equipment

In preparation for the intravenous administration of drugs, the following equipment will be required.

1. A selection of eccentric nozzle disposable syringes.
2. A selection of suitable size disposable needles of which we recommend Nos. 12 or 17 scimitar for use with methohexitone, Althesin and thiopentone, and Nos. 1 or 12 for propanidid.
3. A tourniquet. This should provide a broad band capable of exerting even pressure, with a quick release mechanism.
4. Cleansing materials. We do not normally cleanse the skin unless there is a special indication to do so. Tincture of iodine is the most efficient agent for skin sterilization but carries the disadvantage of:
 (i) Occasional sensitivity reaction
(ii) Unsightly skin (and clothes) staining
   The gentle application of spirit, preferably by spray, has been shown to reduce significantly the bacterial flora of the skin, provided it is allowed to dry; the introduction of a needle through skin which is wet with spirit is painful. However, there is no evidence that failure to cleanse the skin results in any harmful sequelae.
5. Arm boards. For the general comfort of the patient and ease of venipuncture, a well designed arm board attached to the chair is invaluable (Figs. 23 and 24). Should such an arm board not be available, the arm must be held in the manner illustrated in Fig. 90.

Disposal of Syringes and Needles

It is important when discarding disposable syringes and needles, that a method should be employed which avoids accidental injury to those responsible for the subsequent handling of this equipment (Fig. 91). Special containers are usually provided in hospitals for the disposal of needles.

Site of Venipuncture

The following sites prove most convenient:

1. Antecubital Fossa

In this area the relationship of the brachial artery and other important structures to the superficial veins presents a constant hazard, should extravenous injection occur

(Fig. 92). It is therefore wise to select a vein on the lateral aspect of this region when-ever possible, thereby reducing the risk of arterial puncture. The superficial veins are usually large, readily visible or palpable, well fixed by supporting tissue, and relatively straight, thus rendering them particularly easy to enter, except in the obese patient where they may be obscured by excess fat. This site is not recommended for an indwelling needle unless the elbow-joint is splinted in extension, as flexion may displace or even fracture the needle.

2. Dorsum of Hand

This area has the advantage that the superficial veins are normally not in close proximity to any arteries or nerves, nor are they commonly obscured by fatty tissue.

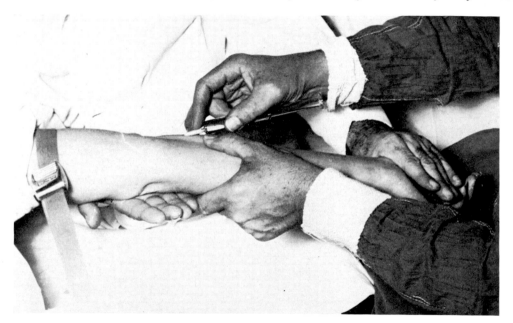

FIG. 90.—Method of holding arm for i.v. injection in veins superficial to the antecubital fossa

However, they may be tortuous and poorly supported, making them excessively mobile and consequently difficult to puncture. As the overlying skin is tough, veni-puncture tends to be more painful and bruising is especially liable to occur.

3. Flexor Aspect of Wrist and Forearm

Superficial veins may be visible in this area when they are not apparent elsewhere (e.g. small children). Attention should be paid to the possibility of superficial radial and ulnar arteries. The veins are thin walled and frail and must be punctured with care, using a small needle.

Although other sites are used occasionally, we recommend that, for the purpose

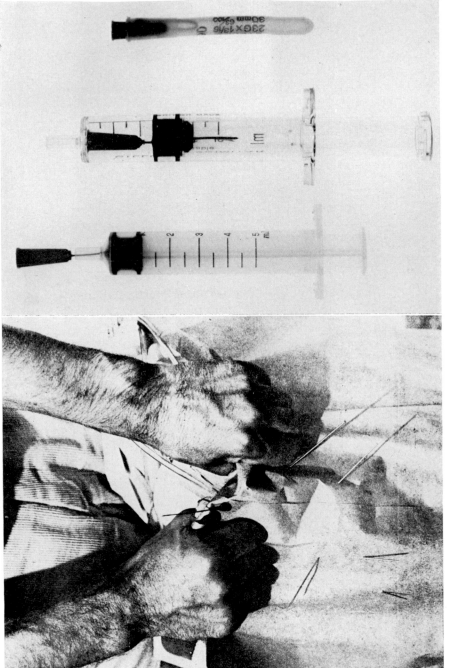

DON'T NEEDLE THE DUSTMAN   DO THIS

FIG. 91.—Disposal of needles

199

of achieving anaesthesia in the out-patient, the anaesthetist should confine himself to the areas described.

Preparation of Veins

It is time well spent to ensure a prominent vein before attempting venipuncture, and this is particularly true in children where only one attempt is usually permissible.

Most superficial veins will become readily visible if a tourniquet is tightened, just above venous pressure, proximal to the site of injection. Many superficial veins which

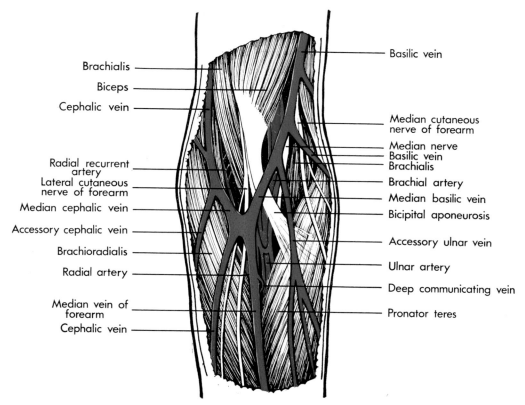

FIG. 92.—Anatomy of antecubital fossa and superficial veins

are covered by fat, may not be readily visible but can be easily palpated if the examining finger is gently drawn across the skin in a direction at right angles to the line of the vein.

If the superficial veins are constricted, they do not readily distend with blood and the following simple measures may be employed in addition to tightening the tourniquet, to produce dilatation.

(a) Active or passive movement of the limb.
(b) External friction to the covering skin.

(c) Local application of heat.

(d) Allowing the limb to be dependent for a short time before tightening the tourniquet.

Technique of Venipuncture

If venipuncture is correctly performed, the needle should ultimately lie parallel with the line of the vein. Fig. 93 shows the correct position of the needle in the vein.

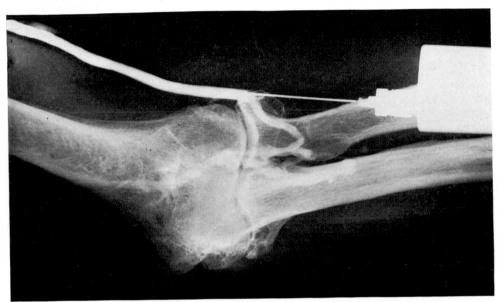

Fig. 93.—X-ray showing correct direction of needle in vein

Fig. 94 demonstrates the way in which incorrect venipuncture may lead to either superficial or deep leakage of injected fluid, in spite of the ability to aspirate blood into the syringe.

In order to achieve the parallel entry shown in Fig. 93, the following points should be noted.

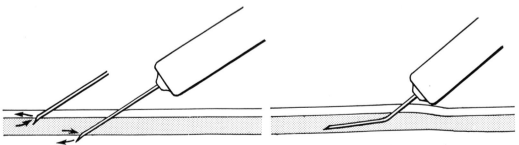

Fig. 94.—Incorrect angle of entry of needle into vein

Fig. 95.—Needle bent to enable parallel entry with central nozzle syringe

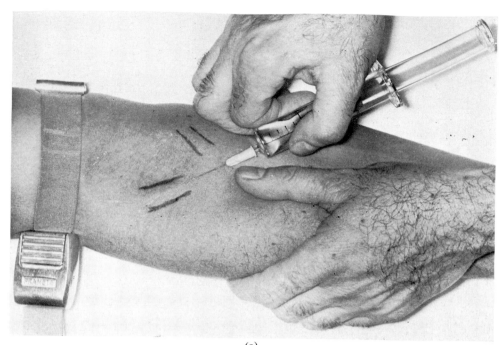

(a)

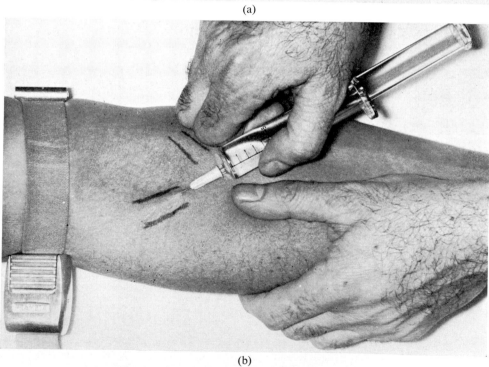

(b)

FIG. 96.—Correct method of stretching skin, holding syringe and entering vein
(a) Entering skin. (b) Entering vein

202

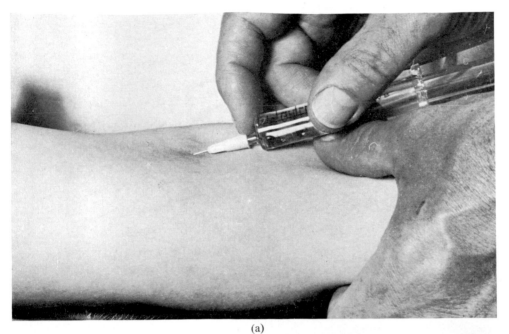

(a)

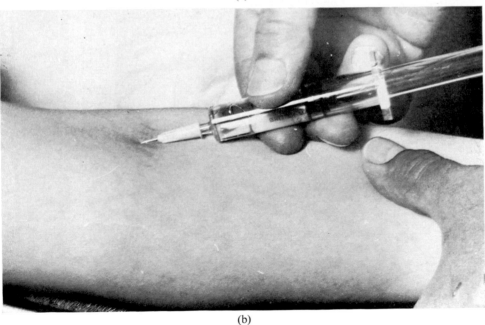

(b)

FIG. 97.—Incorrect venipuncture. (a) Left thumb stretching skin directly beneath syringe, thus preventing parallel entry. (b) Right fingers preventing parallel entry

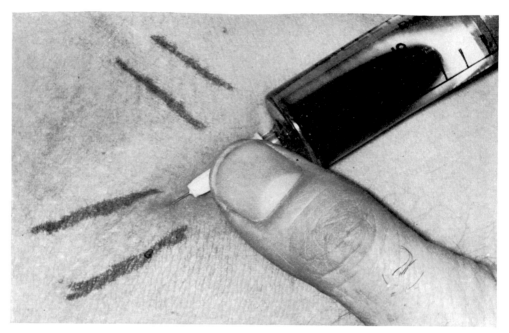

FIG. 98.—Correct method of securing syringe during injection
Note hub is steadied but not unduly depressed

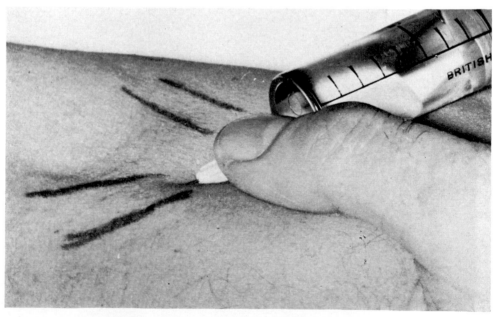

FIG. 99.—Incorrect method of securing syringe
Note depression of needle with risk of puncturing deep surface of vein

204

(a) All syringes except the 2 ml should have eccentric nozzles.

(b) It will be difficult to achieve the essential stability offered by an adequate length of needle within the vein lumen if a short needle (e.g. 20) is used. Moreover, when the anatomy is such that a flat skin surface is not available, the needle may have to be slightly bent (Fig. 95).

(c) It is important that the fingers of neither hand prevent the syringe lying flat on the skin surface (Figs. 96 and 97).

(d) The direction in which the bevel of the needle faces is not of paramount importance. However, in order to achieve parallel entry, it may be necessary to lift the vein

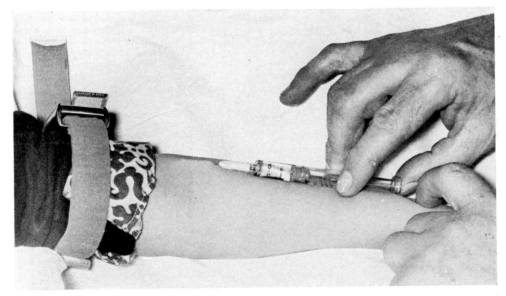

Fig. 100.—Palpation of radial artery during intravenous injection
Note superficial placement of needle

as the needle is advanced and therefore, if the bevel is directed superficially, there will be less likelihood of accidental puncture of the superficial vein wall during advancement of the needle. With bevel directed superficially, it may be necessary to depress the needle in the vein in order to prevent obstruction of the needle by the superficial vein wall during aspiration.

(e) The way in which the needle is introduced through the skin is also of importance. The skin should be gently stretched over the proposed site of injection in the manner shown in Fig. 96, since a needle cannot be introduced painlessly and rapidly through lax skin. The vein is now 'picked up' and the needle may be easily advanced along its lumen. Care should be taken to ensure that a short length of metal is always visible between the site of skin puncture and the hub of the needle, for if accidental fracture occurs, this will always take place at the junction of metal and hub. Although the moment of venipuncture is usually readily felt by the anaesthetist, it is nevertheless wise to seek confirmation by the aspiration of blood into the syringe, but inability to aspirate does not always indicate failure of entry when the vein is constricted. The tourniquet is now released and the syringe is held securely in position with the left hand while the injection is made with the right in such a manner as to ensure that any inadvertent, extravenous injection is so superficial that it is immediately visible (Fig. 98). For this reason the practice of depressing the hub of the needle is not recommended (Fig. 99). Indeed, if the needle has been correctly inserted into the vein, it will be unnecessary to steady the syringe with the left hand, which may then be used to palpate the patient's radial pulse whilst the injection is being made (Fig. 100).

On completion of the injection, the needle should be withdrawn rapidly in the precise line of introduction and the tourniquet tightened over a pad covering the site of injection to prevent bruising (Fig. 101).

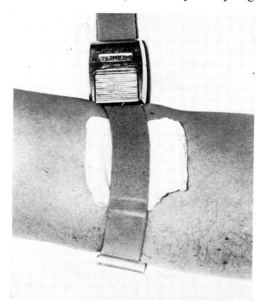

FIG. 101.—Use of tourniquet and pad to prevent haematoma

Painless Venipuncture

Attention to the following details will ensure the minimum discomfort from intravenous injections.

1. Don't use the needle intended for venipuncture to pierce the rubber cap of a stock bottle.
2. Use the smallest bore needle possible.
3. Having ensured patency of the needle, be careful to remove the drop of irritant solution from its tip before piercing the skin.
4. Do not introduce the needle through the skin wet with spirit.
5. Stretch the skin taut before puncture, which should be rapid.
6. Do not move the needle in relation to the skin, once placed correctly with adequate length within the vein.

Extravenous Injection

The following account applies primarily to thiopentone and methohexitone, but it is clearly undesirable for any intended intravenous injection to be misplaced. The irritant properties of these two drugs are generally held to be associated with their alkalinity. It should, however, be remembered that the subcutaneous injection of distilled water is extremely painful, so that the tonicity of the solution may also be an important factor.

1. **Subcutaneous Injection.**—Subcutaneous injection of the solution leads to pain, redness, swelling and possibly ulceration—severity of effect depending upon total quantity and concentration of drug injected. From this point of view it is important to avoid depressing the hub of the needle whilst injecting. Immediate treatment is directed towards aiding the dilution and absorption of the injected drug. Either 2–5 ml of 1% procaine, or 300 units of hyaluronidase dissolved in 2–5 ml of 0·9% saline, may be injected for this purpose. Subsequently local heat and rest, and analgesics may be required.

2. **Intramural Injection.**—Injection into the wall of the vein will immediately result in a characteristic swelling along the course of the vein, and it is our experience that it is this injury which most commonly leads to thrombosis; the treatment consists in resting the affected part and administering analgesics as indicated; some 'hardening' of the vein may persist for several months, but will ultimately resolve.

3. **Perineural Injection.**—Injection may occur into or around a cutaneous or even the median nerve, and this accident is particularly likely to occur if the cubital fossa is used as an injection site. The commonest injury is deposition of the drug in the vicinity of the median cutaneous nerve of the forearm, which will lead to pain in the distribution of the nerve, and subsequent anaesthesia lasting for several months. Recovery is usually complete.

4. **Intra-Arterial Injection.**—Intra-arterial injection will initially cause severe burning pain in the hand and fingers of the injected arm. Should injection persist, spasm of the end arteries will produce pallor and coldness, which will ultimately lead to thrombosis, gangrene and the possible necessity for amputation.

(a) *Prevention*
  (i) Avoidance of medial aspect of antecubital fossa.
 (ii) Palpation of intended injection site prior to tightening of tourniquet.
(iii) Pause after injection of 1 ml solution to confirm that there is no pain in hand or fingers.
 (iv) Avoid the use of solutions stronger than 2·5%.

(b) *Treatment*
  (i) Cease injecting at earliest warning sign.
 (ii) Leave needle *in situ* and inject 20 ml 0·5% procaine through it. Doubt has been expressed as to the value of this measure, but it is certainly harmless.
(iii) Continue anaesthesia using halothane to promote vasodilatation. If pallor and coldness of the fingers persist for more than a few minutes, or cyanosis, blistering, or oedema develop, the following additional measures must be considered.
 (iv) Postpone operation and admit patient to hospital.
  (v) Institute intensive heparin therapy for 4 days, using 7,500–10,000 units 8-hourly. Continue with oral anticoagulants for a further 2 weeks.
 (vi) Consider the possible merits of brachial plexus and stellate ganglion block, and even sympathetic neurectomy.

MANAGEMENT OF INTRAVENOUS ANAESTHESIA

In the management of intravenous anaesthesia, we shall describe the use of 1 %
methohexitone throughout. The preoperative assessment, preparation, and overall
supervision during and following anaesthesia, do not fundamentally differ from that
described in Chapter 5, but it should be borne in mind that all anaesthetic agents
when given intravenously are capable of producing sudden respiratory and cardiovascular depression. Moreover, whilst the anaesthetist is able to accelerate the
excretion of inhalation agents by artificial ventilation, the elimination of intravenous
drugs, once given, is outside his control.

The main methods of using intravenous anaesthetics are summarized on page 193.

1. Single Dose

Patients suitable for this technique will be those in whom no anaesthetic or operative difficulty is anticipated. A maximum of 2 minutes operating time is normally
available. The syringe should be charged with the dose of drug calculated for the
particular patient. This calculation is based on body weight and age (page 220), but
the following additional considerations will determine the final dose chosen.

(a) *Mental State*

The excitable, nervous patient frequently requires a larger than average dose,
which may justify an increase of up to 50 %. This is probably due to an increase in
cardiac output (see page 183).

(b) *Physical Condition*

(i) *Serious Illness.*—Any serious illness, particularly cardiovascular disease, demands that
intravenous drugs should be given slowly and with great care, although the total dose
need not necessarily be reduced (page 276).

(ii) *Pregnancy.*—The increased demands in pregnancy have already been discussed on
page 183.

(iii) *Obesity.*—Where there is an increase of fat in the total body mass, the dose/weight
ratio must be reduced since fat, with its poor blood supply, acts less well as an *immediate*
redistribution medium than does muscle, but ultimately recovery will be accelerated
with this reduced dose.

(iv) *Anaemia*—Caution should always be exercised when intravenous drugs are used in the
anaemic patient, and both total dosage and rate of injection reduced. The increased
sensitivity shown by these patients may in part be due to an increase in cerebral blood
flow. As a corollary to this, the patient suffering from polycythaemia may require
increased dosage.

(c) *Drug Sensitivity*

(i) *Alcohol.*—Although alcoholics are notoriously resistant to inhalation anaesthetic agents,
they do not exhibit the same degree of resistance to the barbiturates. This also applies
to opiate addiction.

(ii) *Sedatives.*—Patients who regularly take non-barbiturate sedatives and tranquillizers do not usually require any alteration in standard dosage. Dependence on the barbiturates may lead to acquired tolerance and, therefore, theoretically may require an increased dosage. However, the possibility of synergism should be borne in mind and in practice, we do not often find it necessary to adjust the standard dose, which is best determined by careful observation of the patient's individual reaction to the drug.

(iii) *Stimulants.*—Patients under treatment with stimulants such as dextroamphetamine (e.g. for slimming) are often resistant to the effects of intravenous anaesthetic agents.

(d) *Nature of Surgery*

The dosage required to produce tranquil operating conditions will depend to some extent on the severity of the stimulus.

Having determined the expected dosage by careful consideration of the foregoing factors, the injection may be commenced. The final dosage may have to be adjusted in relation to the initial response to the injection.

Practical Procedure

The patient is prepared, questioned and positioned in the manner described in Chapter 5. Venipuncture is performed and the injection commenced. After one ml has been injected, the patient is asked to confirm that there is no pain in the arm or hand. At this stage, he may be requested to open his mouth so that the prop, which has already been tested for size, can be inserted by the operator, who can then gently support the jaw during the subsequent injection. The injection is continued at a rate which is comfortable for the particular bore of needle selected. We recommend a No. 12 or 17 needle and an average rate of 10 mg per second. In the elderly, ill or shocked patient, it is necessary to inject very slowly so that any untoward effect may be noted immediately and due allowance must be made for sluggish venous return associated with poor peripheral circulation. In the healthy patient there is no advantage to be gained by slow injection. Continuous observation of the patient's pulse and appearance should be made throughout the injection, so that any circulatory change (e.g. fainting) is detected at the earliest possible moment.

On completion of the injection, the needle is withdrawn and the anaesthetist takes up the position in which he can most satisfactorily control the airway. The mouth is packed and the operation commenced.

Should the patient react excessively to surgical stimulation or the operation prove unexpectedly difficult, the anaesthetist should be prepared to add inhalation supplements. However, this is seldom necessary provided the patients are sensibly selected for this technique. Should respiratory depression or apnoea result from the injection, commencement of surgical stimulation will frequently rectify this situation, but if it does not, the operation must be discontinued and the lungs inflated with oxygen via a face mask until such time as spontaneous respiration is adequate.

Not infrequently, the patient will respond reflexly to the initial surgical stimulus by minor movement of the limbs. This response will usually subside if the surgical procedure is carried out as carefully and gently as possible. Provided such limb movement does not interfere with the operation, forcible restraint should never be applied, since it frequently potentiates unwanted motor activity.

During the extractions and the entire period of recovery, the anaesthetist must keep a constant watch on the patient's respiratory and cardiovascular function.

The patient will usually regain consciousness within 2 to 3 minutes and will be fit to walk assisted to a recovery room within 4 to 5 minutes of the initial injection. Five to 10 minutes recumbency is always beneficial. The time of final discharge will depend, not only upon the patient's own individual reaction to the procedure, but also upon the capabilities of his escort and the efficiency of the transport arrangements which have been made. The majority of patients are fit to leave accompanied within 30 minutes.

Surge Technique

This is a modification of the 'single dose' technique, in which the tourniquet is not released until completion of the injection. The total bulk of injected drug will therefore reach the heart in one or two heart-beats, thus enabling the maximum possible brain concentration to be achieved for a short time with the minimum quantity of drug. It does, however, carry the disadvantage that no adjustment to final dosage can be made in relation to the patient's initial response. On no account should the tourniquet be tightened above arterial pressure with this technique, and a test dose should be given to ensure that the needle is not in an artery.

2. Single Dose and Inhalation

Patients suitable for this technique will be:

(a) Those in whom an operating time in excess of that achieved by the single dose is required.
(b) Those who have a history of anaesthetic resistance.
(c) Those in whom it is anticipated that the operation will present specific problems requiring complete immobility and jaw relaxation.

The procedure will not differ initially from that described under single dose. The inhalation component will be added immediately following induction, so that the first minute of the operation will be carried out under the effects of methohexitone, there subsequently being a smooth take-over by the inhalation agents, so that no interruption in the surgery is necessary.

3. Sleep Dose and Inhalation

This technique is normally reserved for those patients in whom it is desirable to keep the dose of methohexitone to a minimum (e.g. fixed cardiac output disease).

It should be stressed that surgery should not be commenced until stable anaesthesia has been achieved with inhalation agents.

4. Intermittent Administration

This technique may be used as an alternative to those described under 2 or 3. It is necessary, therefore, to consider its advantages and disadvantages.

Advantages

(a) *Nausea and Vomiting.*—There is considerable evidence that the use of unsupplemented methohexitone is associated with the lowest incidence of postoperative nausea and vomiting.

(b) *Simplicity.*—The use of a single agent reduces the possible source of risk associated with 'the human error element', e.g. misidentification of drugs, failure of anaesthetic apparatus, contamination of cylinder contents, etc.

(c) *Surgical Convenience.*—Avoidance of obstruction to the operative procedure by the presence of a nasal mask. This is likely to be relevant in the following circumstances:

(i) For operative procedures on the upper anterior teeth, especially apicectomy.
(ii) For the operator who routinely performs his dentistry in the low-seated position and is unable to adjust his technique to the presence of a nasal mask. These problems can be overcome by the use of a nasopharyngeal or nasotracheal tube, if a purely intravenous technique is considered unsuitable in a particular case.

(d) *The Mouth-Breather.*—The maintenance of stable anaesthesia with this technique is not dependent upon the ability of the anaesthetist to establish free nasal respiration.

(e) *Cardiac Dysrhythmias.*—Unsupplemented methohexitone is associated with a low cardiac dysrhythmia rate.

Disadvantages

(a) *Limitations due to a Single Agent.*—There is no single intravenous agent capable of providing the full range of operating conditions which may be required in dentistry.

Methohexitone is deficient in its ability to achieve pronounced analgesia and voluntary muscle relaxation, without the production of serious respiratory and possible cardiovascular depression. These deficiencies only present as a problem in a small proportion of cases undergoing exodontia, but when the problem does arise, this technique fails to produce satisfactory operating conditions safely. In particular, excessive tongue movement may actively reject the pack from the lingual sulcus.

(b) *Control of the Airway.*—Since the only satisfactory position from which the anaesthetist can maintain a clear airway under all circumstances, is behind the head of the patient, special apparatus will be required to enable him to administer repeated injections without relinquishing control of the airway (Fig 23).

The absence of a reservoir bag removes from the anaesthetist a simple visual monitor of respiratory exchange.

(c) *Respiratory Depression.*—When the patient is limited to breathing air, and therefore a fixed oxygen percentage, there is no means of compensating for any hypoxaemia which would accompany the minor recurrent episodes of respiratory depression which may be associated with this technique.

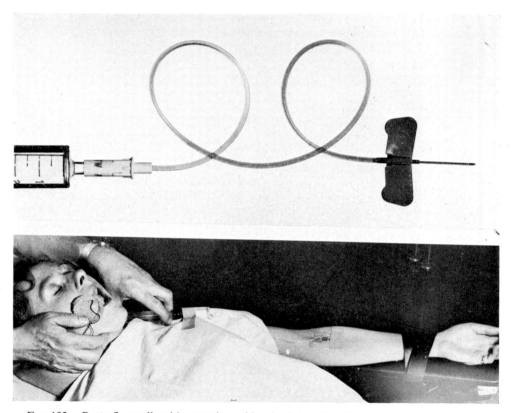

FIG. 102.—Butterfly needle with extension tubing for intermittent intravenous administration

(d) *Total Dosage.*—Avoidance of inhalation agents, will necessitate the use of a larger total dose of methohexitone than would otherwise be necessary. Immediate clinical recovery may not be delayed but total clearance will inevitably be prolonged.

From the foregoing considerations, it is apparent that the limitations of this technique will often outweigh its advantages. In practice, we find that its chief sphere of usefulness is in the patient with a difficult nasal airway, and the patient with a history of severe nausea and vomiting following inhalation anaesthesia. The special place of this technique in conservative dentistry is fully discussed in Chapter 12.

Practical Procedure

Induction.—This phase is identical to that described under Single Dose on page 208, except that special apparatus will be necessary to ensure that repeated injections can be given without recourse to more than one venipuncture. This apparatus should be as simple as possible, and we find the Butterfly needle with extension tube (Fig. 102) satisfactory. The apparatus selected should, whenever possible, enable the anaesthetist to adopt the position in which he feels he has maximum control of the airway. The use of the stock bottle with three-way tap is not recommended owing to the risk of infection.

Maintenance.—The principles of maintenance are identical to those already described under the single dose technique, except that, with this technique, incremental doses will be given as described below.

Reflex response to stimulation is the main criterion for each increment and this response may often be anticipated by the experienced anaesthetist, particularly when working with an operator whose technique is familiar to him.

The size of each increment will depend on the response to the initial dose and, if this has been correctly assessed, the first increment should be approximately half the initial dose. Subsequent increments will be progressively decreased. No dose should be given in the presence of respiratory obstruction or depression. With each increment, the anaesthetist should satisfy himself that the injection is entirely intravenous, and the peripheral pulse should, of course, be frequently checked.

It must here be emphasized that in the absence of a reservoir bag, both respiratory depression and obstruction are more difficult to recognize.

Recognition of Respiratory Obstruction

(i) *Visual.*—The rise and fall of the patient's chest and abdomen must be carefully observed. It is therefore advisable not to obscure these areas with a thick opaque plastic cover. An instrument placed on the chest and seen to be 'going up and down', indicates only that there is some respiratory effort being made; it should be confirmed that the instrument is going up on inspiration and down on expiration, and not *vice versa* as would be the case in the 'see-saw' respiration associated with partial respiratory obstruction or paralysis.

(ii) *Tactile.*—The smooth descent and ascent of the diaphragm can be felt through the abdominal wall. Any 'jerkiness' or tightening of the abdominal musculature on inspiration indicates that active attempts are being made to overcome partial respiratory obstruction.

Recovery

Although, with careful dosage, the immediate recovery is not unduly delayed, it should be remembered that where large total doses of methohexitone have been given, there is a greater likelihood of lapses of mental alertness occurring for several hours postoperatively. It is therefore important that such patients should be accompanied home by a responsible escort and that a satisfactory means of transport be arranged.

Continuous Administration

The purpose of continuous intravenous administration is to smooth out minor fluctuations in the level of anaesthesia associated with the intermittent technique, and to avoid the necessity of giving repeated increments. It carries the disadvantage that accidental overdosage is more likely to occur if careful adjustment of the 'drip' is allowed to lapse, and we consider the technique to be suitable for use only by experienced medical anaesthetists.

CHAPTER ELEVEN

CHILDREN'S ANAESTHESIA

The principles of overall safe management of anaesthesia for children do not differ essentially from those described for adults. In this chapter we will discuss those aspects of child management which require special consideration. Since the majority of children presenting for general anaesthesia for routine dental treatment are over the age of 3, the ensuing general account will cover the age-group 3–14 years. Those special problems relating to the under 3 year old age-group, will be considered separately. The final section of this chapter is devoted to the management of the abnormal child.

ROUTINE MANAGEMENT (3–14 YEARS)

The successful management of children depends upon an understanding of those features in the standard techniques described in Chapters 5 and 10 which require special attention and possibly modification. As an ever-present background to these various specific features, the entire psychological approach to the child is of fundamental importance, and will be discussed first.

1. Psychological Considerations

It is commonly accepted that the child does not usually develop a sense of reasoned responsibility before the age of 8. Thus, the psychological problems and the management of these young children differ somewhat from those of the older child and normal adult, although an immature response to stress may persist into adolescent and even adult life. For this reason, we will consider the under 8 year old age-group separately.

Under 8 year old.—Whilst many young children react favourably in their attitude to dentistry and their first dental anaesthetic as a result of successful parental handling, nevertheless many others approach what may have been presented to them as an ordeal with mistrust and insecurity. This mistrust often arises from parental anxiety and an over-protective approach to the child by the parent. Owing to emotional immaturity, the response of the child to this parental attitude, and to the unfamiliar surroundings of the dental surgery, can frequently be one of irrational fear, which is likely to be mitigated by confident and sympathetic handling. It is therefore essential for the anaesthetist to gain the child's complete trust before commencing any unfamiliar procedure. If this is not achieved, anaesthesia may be difficult and any subsequent administration a 'nightmare' for the child, anaesthetist and parent; thus,

215

time spent in establishing this trust is never wasted. It is not possible to describe in words any set method of achieving this aim, for the methods will be highly individual and only gained through a combination of humility and experience on the part of the anaesthetist. It is, however, worth mentioning certain factors which we have found to be of assistance. Any discussion with the child is best conducted from about his own level—that is to say, with the anaesthetist seated (Fig. 103). Little girls are particularly susceptible to compliments related to their dress and appearance. Toys, usually valueless in the older child, should be distractive rather than deceptive in their intent, but we personally have found distractive and hypnotic conversation to

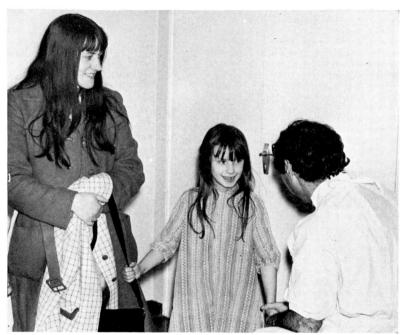

FIG. 103.—Anaesthetist seated, talking to child

be of greater value. It cannot be stressed too strongly that in this age-group, there is no place for anything but gentleness of manner and voice at all times. Having said all this, it must be admitted that in our hands there remains a small proportion of children in which our failure to establish this trust leads to a choice between postponement of treatment with subsequent premedication on the one hand, and induction without patient co-operation on the other.

Over 8 year old.—The development of a sense of reasoned responsibility in the child allows the anaesthetist to adopt a realistic adult approach, in which the child is usually open to a sensible discussion of his areas of anxiety, and can state his preferences, which should be respected wherever possible. Failure on the part of the child to co-operate with such an approach tempts one to ascribe the behaviour to 'naughtiness', and indeed firm handling often enables one to achieve a successful practical outcome with no apparent lasting psychological trauma to the child. It should, however, be remembered that 'naughtiness' is usually the manifestation of basic insecurity, and frank unkindness, as opposed to firmness, is always unjustified in handling such a child.

In consideration of the foregoing remarks, it becomes evident that the emotional state of the child, irrespective of age, is of considerable importance in successful handling, particularly so in the out-patient where there has been no opportunity for the anaesthetist to establish confidence and rapport at a preoperative visit. For this reason, it is especially important to have a close co-operation and mutual understanding between the dentist and anaesthetist, so that any explanations and promises given to the patient by the dentist at a preoperative visit are likely to be capable of fulfilment by the anaesthetist. In addition, it will commonly fall to the dentist to order, or discuss with the anaesthetist, any necessary premedication.

Role of Parent.—The attitude of the parent to dental treatment will influence considerably the child's ultimate behaviour in the dental surgery. In general, children will fall into three categories.

(a) *The Normal Co-operative Child.*—These children are usually quite happy to enter the surgery unaccompanied by their parent, but should they indicate to the contrary, the parent should be allowed to stay during the induction of anaesthesia.

(b) *The Frightened Child.*—These children should always be allowed the company of their parent during the induction of anaesthesia.

(c) *The 'Naughty' Child.*—These children nearly always become more co-operative and therefore easier to manage in the absence of the parent.

The anaesthetist's difficulty lies, of course, in distinguishing between the frightened and the naughty child. It must surely be admitted that even the most observant and experienced anaesthetist is occasionally wrong in his judgement, and if he becomes aware of his error, he will usually serve his patient best by recommending a change in the environment and person associated with any subsequent treatment, for the loss of confidence occasioned may have no other solution.

2. Medical Considerations

It is essential that a full medical history is obtained from the parent at a preoperative visit, and that a physical examination be performed by the patient's own doctor or the anaesthetist when indicated. This subject is fully discussed on pages 16 and 257, and the medical history may disclose the following conditions which are of special importance in children.

(a) *Congenital Heart Disease.*—When a history of congenital heart disease is accompanied by the signs and symptoms of decompensation, i.e. cyanosis or dyspnoea, it is essential to admit the patient to hospital for dental treatment. If there is a history of congenital disease in the absence of signs or symptoms, the anaesthetic may present no problem, but the advisability of chemotherapeutic protection against bacterial endocarditis must be considered. It is claimed by some cardiologists that in the child under ten years old, the risk of serious sensitivity reactions to penicillin exceeds the risk of the child developing bacterial endocarditis, which is comparatively uncommon in this age group. This view is not universally held, and the consensus of opinion is that penicillin coverage should be given to all congenital heart cases, with the exception of patent ductus arteriosus, and auricular septal defect.

Should penicillin have been used for infection a few days prior to extraction, then another antibiotic such as cephaloridine should be chosen for coverage. Whatever antibiotic is considered suitable, the initial loading dose should be given by intramuscular injection half to one hour preoperatively. Subsequent doses may be given orally should the risk of bacteraemia persist (page 274).

(b) *Asthma* (see page 148).—The asthma of childhood may be associated with eczema, and often has a strong psychological background. So long as the anaesthetic is not given during an attack, and is devoid of undue emotional upset, problems seldom arise. Irrespective of the method of induction, it is essential to achieve a stable level of anaesthesia, preferably with halothane, prior to the commencement of any surgical stimulation, including the insertion of mouth-prop or artificial airway. It is advisable not to interfere with any established regime of medical treatment, but it should be borne in mind that these children are occasionally taking steroids (pages 9 and 290).

(c) *Diabetes*.—A general discussion of the management of the diabetic patient is found on pages 4 and 287, and will apply in principle to children. Fortunately, the disease in childhood is rare. When it does occur it is nearly always severe and difficult to manage, and usually necessitates hospitalization. The following points deserve special mention.

  (i) It is often more difficult to avoid using general anaesthesia in the child than it is in the adult.
 (ii) The stability of the diabetic child is more difficult to achieve than that of the adult, and it is seldom possible to stabilize him on oral anti-diabetic drugs, parenteral insulin being necessary.
(iii) The presence of infection will frequently lead to ketosis in the child and unless it can be established that this is not the case, the child must be referred to hospital before treatment is undertaken.

The planned case requiring general anaesthesia can be treated as an out-patient, provided the diabetes is stable and the nature of the procedure will not interfere with the normal dietary intake. Should there be any doubt of this fact, the patient should be treated in hospital where several hours observation can be carried out postoperatively.

(d) *Upper Respiratory Obstruction*.—Nasal obstruction may occur in children with enlarged tonsils and adenoids, making uninterrupted inhalation maintenance difficult or occasionally impossible. Under these conditions it may be necessary to establish a deeper plane of anaesthesia than usual, using a full face mask, the extractions being performed after removal of the mask. Multiple extractions, if difficult, may require temporary cessation of work whilst an adequate level of anaesthesia is re-established, the mask once more being removed to enable completion of the surgery. Extreme circumstances of this sort may, in fact, justify the use of an endotracheal tube to maintain continuous smooth anaesthesia. An oral tube, whilst slightly impeding the surgeon's access, is safer for all but the highly experienced anaesthetist, whose expert sense of touch will allow him to use a nasal tube without producing nasopharyngeal trauma. Even the most experienced anaesthetist may, however, be disinclined to attempt such nasal intubation 'blind', since nasal obstruction in children is occasionally associated with the presence of a foreign body (e.g. bead or button) in the nose, and the danger exists of such a foreign body being carried blindly, partially within the lumen of the tube into the trachea, whilst direct vision laryngoscopy may reveal its presence, thus avoiding such an accident.

(e) *Idiopathic Epilepsy.*—This condition, when encountered in children, demands the same attention as described with adults (pages 5 and 290). It is particularly important to achieve a trouble-free induction, devoid of hypoxaemia and struggling. The anti-epileptic regime should not be disturbed. Should this include oral barbiturates, we do not consider that this precludes the use of thiopentone intravenously.

In spite of the large array of anti-epileptic drugs available, phenobarbitone and Epanutin are still the drugs most commonly used in children, and the development of gingival hyperplasia associated with the prolonged use of Epanutin is well recognized.

The treatment of fits, should they occur, is described on page 290.

Particular care should be taken to differentiate between true epileptic 'fits' and the 'black-outs' which may be associated with cardiomyopathy (page 5).

(f) *Travel Sickness.*—Children are prone to suffer from this complaint, the management of which is described on page 7. Recumbency during recovery is particularly desirable, and prolonged starvation should be avoided. Premedication with an anti-emetic such as Avomine may be helpful (page 39).

3. Premedication

In our opinion, there is no ideal premedicant for the out-patient child, but when the psychological approach described previously has failed to produce satisfactory results, premedication may improve the situation. The best results are often produced by either mild sedatives or full basal narcotics (page 24). Between these two extremes, moderate to heavy sedation may lead to disorientation and thus a failure to improve conditions. Table XXII serves as a non-specific guide to adult/child dose relationship.

(a) *Sedation.*—We have found the following drugs to be of some value.

(i) *Diazepam (Valium)* (page 36).—Diazepam, given by mouth in large dosage, i.e. up to 0·5 mg per kg 2 hours preoperatively, preceded by 0·1 mg per kg 3 times during the

TABLE XXII

Weight Kg	Lbs	Percentage of Adult Dose	Fraction of Adult Dose	Age of Child
15	33	33	$\frac{1}{3}$	3
18	40	40		5
23	50	50	$\frac{1}{2}$	7
30	66	60		10
36	80	70		11
40	88	75	$\frac{3}{4}$	12
45	100	80		14
54	120	90		16
65	145	100	1	

This scheme is based on the formula: $\dfrac{\text{Surface area of Child}}{\text{Surface area of Adult}} \times 100$

(Based on the original table of Butler & Richie. Reproduced from Paediatric Prescriber 2nd Ed. by Pincus Catzell. Oxford: Blackwell.)

previous day, often achieves the desired effect. If the immediate preoperative dose exceeds 0·25 mg per kg, it should not be given prior to the child's arrival at the surgery.

(ii) *Trimeprazine (Vallergan)* (page 34).—We consider that trimeprazine is the most suitable member of the phenothiazine group of drugs to use for premedication. Trimeprazine 2 mg per kg will give mild sedation within 2 hours of its oral administration, but should not be given prior to the child's arrival in the dental surgery.

(iii) *Barbiturates* (page 24).—Small doses of pentobarbitone (Nembutal) may be used orally one and half hours preoperatively, e.g. 1 mg per kg (maximum 100 mg). The pleasant elixir containing 20 mg in 5 ml will be accepted by most children; if not, the contents of a 30 mg–50 mg capsule can be mixed in a jam of the child's choice.

(b) *Basal Narcosis.*—Although it is possible always to produce a manageable child by the use of basal narcosis, this method has considerable disadvantages when used in the dental out-patient.

Firstly, the level of narcosis that may be produced demands continuous experienced nursing care from the time of administration of the drug; thus it cannot be administered in the patient's own home prior to a visit to the dental surgery.

Secondly, all present methods are associated with a recovery period of several hours.

Basal narcotic drugs can be administered by the oral, rectal and intramuscular routes. The oral route, although usually the most acceptable to the patient, achieves the least consistent results.

Oral Method

There are many drugs which can be used by the oral route for basal narcosis. We will describe two.

(i) *Pentobarbitone (Nembutal).*—In order to achieve basal narcosis, the oral dose must be heavy and given at least one and a half hours prior to anaesthesia. A dose of 6 mg per kg (2·7 mg per lb) will usually produce the desired effect, but we do not consider the method suitable for children weighing over 35 kg. The level of narcosis produced is such that the child is rousable but if handled with care, anaesthesia can be induced without interrupting sleep in the majority of cases.

It must be remembered that with barbiturate dosage of this order, both respiratory and circulatory depression may be produced—hence the necessity for constant supervision. In addition, recovery may be accompanied by considerable restlessness and disorientation.

(ii) *Trimeprazine (Vallergan)*.—A dose of 5 mg per kg (2·3 mg per lb.) will usually produce the desired effect. Compared with pentobarbitone, respiratory depression and post-operative restlessness are less commonly encountered, but the results obtained in terms of narcotic level are less reliable. Circulatory depression is occasionally a feature of these high doses, and the dose above should not be exceeded.

Rectal Method

Many soluble narcotic agents can be used by the rectal route. We will limit our description to two.

(i) *Thiopentone*.—Any preparation of thiopentone may be dissolved in tap water and given rectally in a 2% solution, but owing to the large bulk of solution required, it is more convenient to use the specially prepared rectal suspension. This contains 2 g of thiopentone in a 10 ml Abbosert syringe (i.e. 200 mg per 1 ml division on the syringe). When using this equipment, it must be remembered that, in order to obtain accurate dosage, the nozzle must be filled with suspension before adjusting the dose-marker and inserting into the rectum. The end of the syringe will have to be pierced with a pin. The basal narcotic dose is 44 mg per kg (20 mg per lb), and the onset of sleep usually occurs within 10 minutes. After administration, the child should remain on his side to minimize the chances of respiratory obstruction, and constant nursing supervision is essential. Recovery is quicker than with oral Nembutal and is usually devoid of restlessness.

(ii) *Methohexitone*.—Rectal methohexitone has been used as a basal narcotic, but not as extensively as thiopentone. Its use was described as long ago as 1960, and subsequent workers, of whom Stetson and Budd in the U.S.A. have been leading pioneers, agree that it has certain advantages over thiopentone. These are chiefly in terms of rapidity of effect and speed of recovery, with minimal 'hang-over'. A dose of 22 mg per kg (10 mg per lb) usually suffices to produce adequate narcosis. This dose may be dissolved in tap water at body temperature to make a 10% solution. The onset of sleep is usually complete within 5 minutes and the precautions advocated in relation to rectal Pentothal should be strictly observed.

Intramuscular Method

(i) *Methohexitone*.—Methohexitone may be used for basal narcosis by deep intramuscular injection. In a dose of 6 mg per kg using a 2% solution, sleep is produced within 3 minutes. The conditions produced are similar to those with rectal administration but the duration of action is considerably shorter.

(ii) *Ketamine*.—We consider that the use of this drug in out-patient dentistry should be confined to intramuscular injection in the difficult child. It will therefore be described only with this use in mind.

(iii) *Althesin*.—The small bulk of solution and non-irritant properties of the drug suggest that it may prove to be a useful intramuscular premedicant. A dose of 2 mg per kg will produce marked sedation in 15 minutes.

Ketamine Hydrochloride B.P.—(Trade name—Ketalar)

Presentation—10 and 20 ml vials containing either 10, 50 or 100 mg per ml. The 100 mg per ml is recommended for intramuscular injection.
Dose—Intramuscular route
      6·5–13 mg/kg (3–6 mg/lb)
      10 mg/kg will usually produce 12–25 minutes of surgical anaesthesia

Use for the Difficult Child.—Ketamine, unlike the barbiturates, does not have a normal sedative and hypnotic action, but is primarily a cataleptic, analgesic and anaesthetic agent. When administered intramuscularly in children in the dose recommended, it will produce an anaesthetic state characterized by profound somatic analgesia, with light anaesthesia in which skeletal muscle tone is preserved, and the pharyngeal and laryngeal reflexes are not usually abolished. In this state, minor, painful surgical procedures can be carried out.

The recovery period is prolonged, at least 2 hours being required for full ambulation. During recovery the child should remain undisturbed. The recovery in adults is frequently characterized by vivid dreaming with a certain amount of psychomotor activity and confusion, making the drug unsuitable for adult out-patient use, but this disturbance is uncommon in children.

Summary

The experienced dental anaesthetist will seldom find premedication necessary in the out-patient, since skilful and sympathetic handling of each individual child will solve the majority of problems without the disadvantage of delayed recovery associated with premedicant drugs. Whilst the methods described are not intended to be comprehensive, they could all be considered suitable for the difficult out-patient when the occasion demands. However, their chief sphere of usefulness is for the in-patient child, when premedication is more strongly indicated in view of parental separation and more complete disruption of the child's normal routine; in addition, the disadvantages of delayed recovery are less pertinent than in the out-patient.

4. Induction of Anaesthesia

Choice of Method.—In general, we find that children under the age of eight prefer an inhalation to an intravenous induction, whilst in the older age-group intravenous techniques appear to be gaining in patient acceptance. The experienced anaesthetist will appreciate those situations in which it is advisable to allow the child to make his own choice regarding the method of induction, and will also be aware of the exceptional circumstances in which it is equally advisable for the child not to be presented with the choice. These circumstances include anticipated difficulty with successful first-time venipuncture; the crying child who refuses to engage in any sensible discussion with the anaesthetist and who, in our opinion, is most easily dealt with by intravenous induction; certain rare clinical situations in which intravenous agents may be contraindicated (pages 185 and 368); and finally the child who is liable to change his mind repeatedly—whether this be 'delaying tactics' or simply due to indecisiveness.

Inhalation Induction.—There are obviously many acceptable individual variations in detailed practical management, and we will describe in detail only the particular technique which we use. Before doing so, we will list a number of points which we consider to be of special importance, irrespective of the detailed technique employed.

(i) All equipment, including the anaesthetic machine, should be as unobtrusive as possible.

(ii) If the child is to be induced seated in the chair, care should be taken to ensure a comfortable posture (Fig. 104), which may entail the use of a special children's seat. It may be considered prudent to induce the child sitting on his mother's lap, particularly when separation is likely to be difficult and convert the child's fear into panic. The mother may then be seated in the chair (Fig. 105), and the child removed from the mother's lap only when asleep.

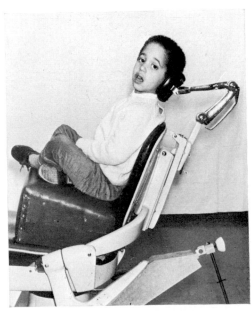

FIG. 104.—Child seated on a removable cushion

(iii) Whenever possible the child should be persuaded to close his eyes and relax prior to the commencement of induction, and this principle applies irrespective of the posture selected (Figs. 106, 107).

(iv) Since the introduction of halothane, it is no longer necessary to insert a mouth-prop prior to induction, as sufficient relaxation to obtain jaw-opening is achieved at a light level of anaesthesia.

(v) A continuous flow of quiet, hypnotic conversation *from the anaesthetist only* should commence a few seconds before the introduction of anaesthetic agents and proceed until loss of consciousness.

(vi) Until the child's senses have been to some extent obtunded by nitrous oxide (not exceeding 80%), it is inadvisable to achieve contact of mask to face, or to introduce strong concentrations of adjuvants. (Fig. 108)

(vii) The child should not be routinely restrained either manually or by a strap during induction, but it is essential that a chairside attendant is immediately available to control any unwanted movements which, if they occur, are most likely to do so between the onset of sleep and surgical anaesthesia. The child's hand may, of course, be held throughout by parent or nurse, whose own hand should not, however, be gripped by the child.

The technique which we use does not differ greatly from that for the adult described in Chapter 5. There are, however, certain points worthy of special note.

We find it both comfortable for the anaesthetist and reassuring for the child, if

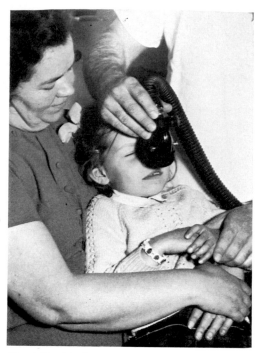
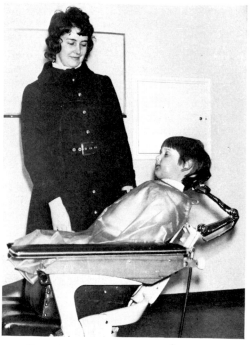

FIG. 105.—Mother seated in chair with child on lap   FIG. 106.—Child seated with eyes closed

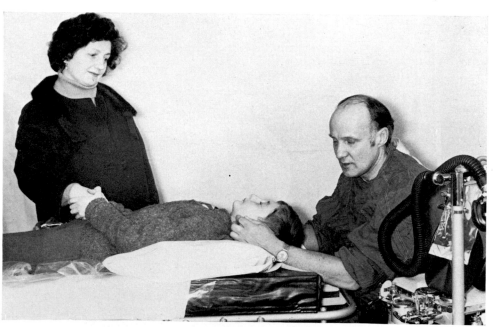

FIG. 107.—Child supine with eyes closed

the anaesthetist remains seated during induction. We usually introduce the gases from above the patient's head, using the cupped left hand to retain the gases in the vicinity of the face in the manner shown in Fig. 108. As soon as consciousness is lost, the parent is quietly led from the room, and this exit must not be delayed, since a short period of unconscious excitement, should it occur, is likely to be misinterpreted.

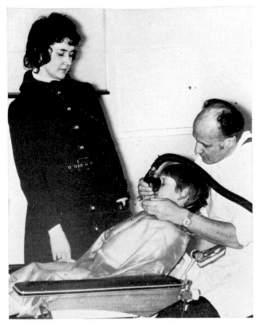

FIG. 108.—Anaesthetist seated during induction. Note mask held away from face with anaesthetist's left hand cupped to contain gases

It is advisable to use a high flow of gases, up to 15 litre per minute, until apposition of mask to face (Fig. 109), when the flow-rate can be reduced to little more than the patient's expected minute volume, which will be related to the child's size and age (Table XXIV, page 273). The percentage of oxygen and halothane necessary does not, however, differ from the adult's requirements. For convenience, this induction can be carried out with a Goldman nasal mask used to cover both nose and mouth. As soon as surgical anaesthesia has been achieved, there will be sufficient jaw relaxation for the mouth to be opened and the prop inserted. It is important to perform these manoeuvres rapidly so that the mask can be immediately re-applied to the nose for maintenance of anaesthesia, and also to reduce the period of time during which the airway may be temporarily obstructed by the manoeuvre shown in Fig. 110.

Intravenous Induction. — We cannot stress too strongly the importance of accurate first-time venipuncture in children; indeed, if there is doubt about the outcome of attempted venipuncture, it is usually preferable to use an inhalation induction.

The general principles laid down in Chapter 10 for the use of intravenous induction in adults will apply for children,

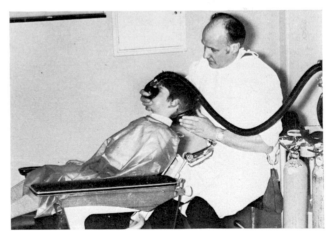

FIG. 109.—
When child is analgesic, mask may be applied to face

but specific problems exist in children which are worthy of mention, especially those relating to the unpremedicated out-patient.

(i) *The Co-operative Child* (Fig. 111).—Many of these children will elect to have an intra-venous induction. We recommend that a No. 17 or 20 rather than a No. 12 needle is routinely used; there is often nothing to be gained by using a No. 20 needle since its gauge is the same as that of a No. 17, and its very short length may prove to be a tech-nical disadvantage in its secure placement. However, in situations where the length of accessible vein is short, e.g. veins in front of the wrist, a short needle (No. 20) may be a positive advantage, and in addition its appearance will be more acceptable to the child.

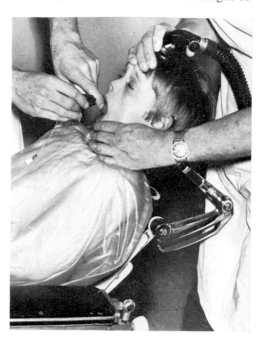

(ii) *The Crying, Frightened Child.*—The induction of anaesthesia in the child who enters the dental surgery crying is one of the most difficult problems that the dental anaesthetist has to face, and it requires a considerable amount of skill and experi-ence to achieve good results. The inhala-tion induction of these children with the child sitting on the mother's lap has been described, and may be very satisfactory if some degree of co-operation can be achieved. If the child will not listen or co-operate, then an intravenous induction is unquestionably preferable to forced application of a mask. Intravenous injection under these conditions is always difficult, and therefore experience in getting into hand veins is essential. Adequate skilled assistance in holding the child's arm must be available before any attempt is made, in order to ensure first-time veni-puncture (Figs. 112, 113, and 114).

FIG. 110.—Insertion of Prop.
Note—Pressure applied to chin with counter pressure on forehead; this may lead to transient airway obstruction

The venipuncture and injection should be completed in the shortest possible time, and we find the use of 2·5% methohexitone in a 2 ml syringe to be helpful in achieving this aim. However, pain up the arm is a frequent consequence of the injection of metho-hexitone into small veins (page 187), and a child who has been oblivious of venipuncture will frequently cry and attempt to withdraw the hand during injection. For this reason we favour the use of either thiopentone or Althesin. Thiopentone carries the disadvan-tage that, since it is unwise to exceed a concentration of 2·5%, the necessary dosage entails a slower injection than with 2·5% methohexitone. Provided Althesin proves satisfactory in other respects, it will, in our opinion become the agent of choice for this technique. Whichever agent is used it is advisable to penetrate both skin and vein in one movement as, however firmly the arm is held, it is not always possible to prevent a minor degree of pronation or supination, either of which alter the relationship between the selected point of cutaneous puncture and the underlying vein. The injection should

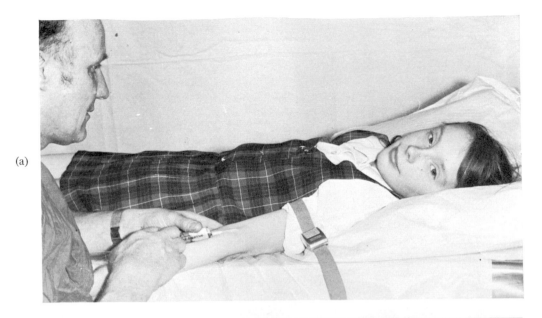

(a)

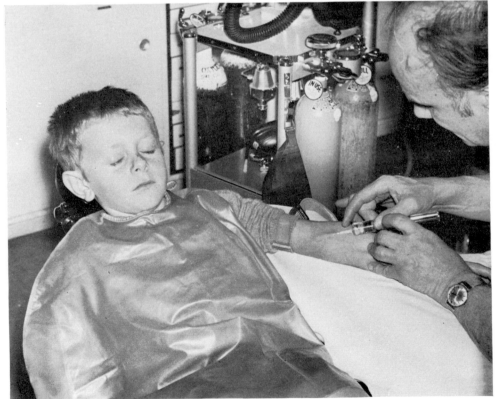

(b)

FIG. 111.—Intravenous induction in the co-operative child. (a) Supine. (b) Sitting

be commenced without delay, and with experience this is made possible by dispensing with confirmatory blood aspiration. We consider it essential to follow carefully the painless venipuncture technique described on page 206. It is also important to palpate carefully the selected site of venipuncture since accidental arterial injection is an obvious additional risk under these difficult circumstances, as is extravascular leakage.

(iii) *The Unco-operative Child.*—The unco-operative child is usually ill-disciplined and insecure, and benefits greatly from very firm but kind handling, preferably in the parent's absence. These children may be exasperating in the extreme, but under no circumstances

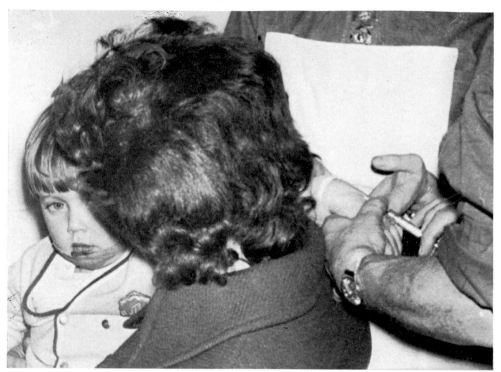

FIG. 112.—Method of I.V. induction for the difficult child. The child sees nothing of the injection and is frequently unaware of it. Note 2 ml syringe

must any professional attendant show a loss of temper. With firm and determined handling, it is almost always possible to obtain the minimum degree of co-operation necessary to perform successful venipuncture, the technique used being that described in the previous section.

5. Maintenance of Anaesthesia

The period of maintenance of anaesthesia for routine exodontia is not as a rule unusually prolonged in children. The anaesthetist should be able to predict with some accuracy the expected length and necessary depth of anaesthesia in any particular case. It should be remembered that the extraction of deciduous teeth becomes progressively easier as root-resorption progresses. The extraction of permanent teeth

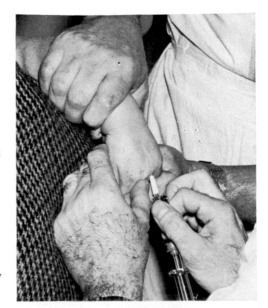

FIG 113.—Method of holding child's hand

FIG. 114.—Venipuncture on flexor aspect of wrist in small child. Note bent needle, method of holding hand securely, and assistant releasing tourniquet

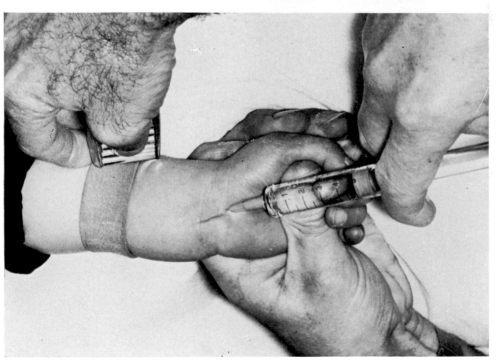

whether for orthodontic deformity or caries, presents the same technical problems as are encountered in the adult.

The principles governing safe maintenance do not materially differ from those appropriate to the adult. Tissue saturation with anaesthetic agents occurs relatively rapidly, so that whilst it is permissible to use a normal induction concentration of halothane, it must not be forgotten that the required level of anaesthesia is achieved rapidly, and that therefore the reduction in halothane concentration to the main-tenance level of 0·5% will prove necessary sooner than in the adult, if dangerously deep anaesthesia is to be avoided.

Airway control may present its own particular problems in children, and these are commonly related to the presence of large tonsils and adenoids, and also to the

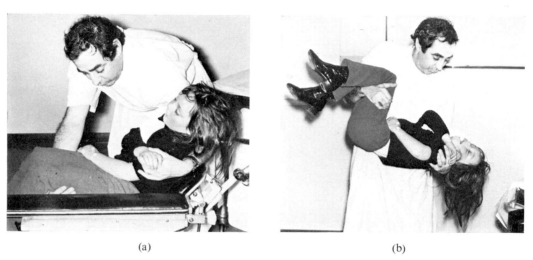

(a)   (b)

FIG. 115.—Transport of child. (a) Note control of arms. (b) Head-down posture

general limitation of working space in the small mouth. In addition, certain con-genital abnormalities, which will be described later, pose their own particular problems.

The incidence of cardiac irregularities associated with dental anaesthesia is greater in children than in adults. These irregularities usually take the form of ventricular extrasystoles, and rarely ventricular tachycardia, but their significance in terms of cardiac function remains to be elucidated.

6. Recovery

It is generally more convenient for recovery to take place other than in the dental chair, and the transport of the child from chair to recovery couch is important. The child should be lifted in the manner shown in Fig. 115 so that the arms are well secured, and should always be carried slightly head down—still securing the arms firmly as shown.

Whenever possible the child should be allowed to recover undisturbed whilst lying on his side (Fig. 116). If, for any reason, immediate recovery has to take place in the sitting position, the posture illustrated in Fig. 117 should be adopted, but even if the child walks from the dental chair to the recovery area, we believe that it is beneficial for full recovery to be allowed to take place with the child lying down, for this practice appears to reduce the incidence of post-anaesthetic malaise.

'Inexplicable delayed recovery' is not encountered in children, provided anaesthesia has been properly managed, and conditions such as diabetic coma eliminated. It is probable that most of the reported cases have followed either a period of cerebral hypoxia or frank overdose—whether or not these causes have been recognized at the time by the

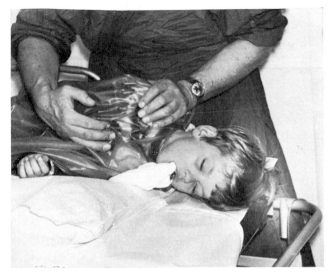

FIG. 116.—Recovery position.
Note position of pillow

administrator. However, delay in full awakening may be encountered in the child who has lost his normal sleep as a result of dental pain, or for any other reason.

There is one post-anaesthetic syndrome characteristically seen in children which merits special mention. Following what may have been a simple, satisfactory and completely trouble-free anaesthetic, the child develops one or more of the following signs and symptoms: pallor, sweating, change of mood to one characterized by silence or whimpering, nausea and 'tummy-ache', finally culminating in vomiting, after which there is usually rapid improvement. We find that this syndrome is frequently associated with a history of travel-sickness, and symptoms can be eliminated or minimized by the prophylactic pre-anaesthetic administration of an

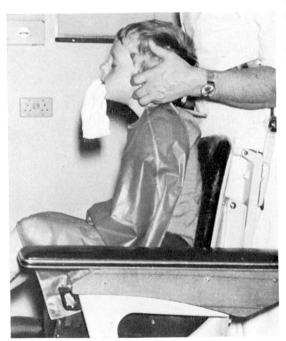

FIG. 117.—Recovery sitting

anti-emetic drug (page 39), and undisturbed recovery lying down. Prolonged pre-anaesthetic starvation may be a contributory factor, and for this reason we consider it advisable that all children should have some form of light nourishment within 6 hours of the intended anaesthetic (see page 15).

Management of the Under 3 Age Group

Occasionally these small children require general anaesthesia for dental treatment. Usually this treatment follows trauma to the upper incisor teeth, but sometimes multiple extractions may be required for rampant caries.

1. Trauma

The majority of these injuries result from a fall, and may be sustained as early as the first year of life. Usually only a short anaesthetic is required for the extraction of one or two teeth which have already been loosened. The child may be induced either lying on his side on a trolley, or in the mother's arms, and the method of induction may be by either inhalation or intravenous route, both halothane and methohexitone being well tolerated. A full face-mask may be used for induction, and removed completely for the extractions, but it is essential that adequate packing and suction are employed. The child should be placed in the lateral position as soon as treatment is completed. Should the injury require more prolonged treatment, it is advisable to use endotracheal anaesthesia.

It should be pointed out that if the injury occurred shortly after a meal, food may be retained in the stomach for many hours after the accident and, together with swallowed blood, may constitute a serious vomiting hazard.

2. Multiple Extractions

These cases may prove difficult owing to limited access to the mouth and the brisk haemorrhage from which the air passages must be protected. It is therefore recommended that only an experienced team should attempt to treat them. Although meticulous packing and efficient suction enable anaesthesia in the majority of cases to be maintained with a small nasal mask, intubation may sometimes be considered the safer course.

If intubation is not employed, extraction should be carried out with the child, either sitting upright with the head well forward, or lying tilted head downwards.

Endotracheal Anaesthesia

Intubation in children presents special problems which are discussed on page 272.

Congenital Abnormalities

There are a number of congenital abnormalities which may be present in children, which will effect the management of dental anaesthesia. The most relevant of these conditions will be discussed below.

1. **Down's Syndrome** (Mongolism).—The mongol child is usually co-operative and easy to manage, but the following common abnormalities may require special care.

(a) Congenital cardiac defects are not uncommon in these children and may require antibiotic cover before dental treatment.

(b) The tongue is frequently large which will often make adequate packing, without producing respiratory obstruction, difficult to achieve.

(c) Persistent nasal catarrh is a frequent feature of this condition which, when accompanied by an underdeveloped nasal bone, may render nose-breathing impossible. Under these circumstances, either a full face mask, which can be removed for work of short duration, or an orotracheal tube, will have to be used. If a nasotracheal tube is used the nasopharynx should be well sucked out before insertion.

(d) The presence of much subcutaneous fat frequently makes venipuncture difficult. The anterior aspect of the wrist often has to be used (Fig. 114).

2. **Congenital Spastic Tetraplegia.**—There is a large variety of spastic disorders seen in children, the aetiology of which is often difficult to determine. Dental problems are common among these children due to defective chewing, tooth grinding and malocclusion, the treatment of which frequently requires sedation or general anaesthesia.

When approaching these children, it should be remembered that, although the majority of them will be severely mentally handicapped, and 50% have an I.Q. below 70, nevertheless about 25% have an I.Q. above 90. Very careful handling is particularly important in this latter group as their main problem is one of communication rather than understanding. The anaesthetist must therefore exercise patience in establishing some means of communication, as failure to do so may lead to considerable frustration; it is always wise to have the parent or guardian present during the induction of anaesthesia and recovery, as he is the most likely person to be able to understand what the child is trying to communicate.

Many of these children are highly emotional and are readily upset by a change in environment or doctor. In consequence, some 'pre-visit' sedation may be desirable. Diazepam has proved to be a useful drug for this purpose; barbiturates are often not suitable as the disorientation produced may make the child even less co-operative.

Frequently these children are adequately co-operative, but dental treatment is made impossible because of athetoid movements; under these circumstances intravenous diazepam is usually all that is required to obtain satisfactory conditions for dentistry. If general anaesthesia is considered necessary, then an intravenous induction is preferred, as uncontrolled movements make inhalation induction difficult. Owing to the tendency to convulsions, methohexitone should be avoided.

3. **Epidermolysis Bullosa Dystrophia.**—This rare and interesting disease, affecting structures of epidermal origin, is of particular relevance to the dental anaesthetist

as these children are very susceptible to dental caries. The following features should be noted and the necessary precautions taken.

(a) *The Effects of Trauma.*—The main feature of the disease is the formation of vesicles and bullae on the skin following trauma. The degree of trauma needed to produce these changes may be slight, but friction rather than pressure is more likely to produce damage. In the least severe form of the disease, epidermolysis bullosa simplex, the lesions are usually confined to the hands and feet and are superficial to the basal membrane, so that healing usually occurs without scarring. In the most severe form, epidermolysis bullosa dystrophia, all the epidermal structures including nails, teeth and mouth are affected, so that infection and severe scarring frequently result. Death usually occurs before puberty.

(b) *The Association with Porphyria.*—Many authorities claim that there is a close association between this disease and haematoporphyrinuria and therefore care must be taken to ensure there is no evidence of porphyria before giving barbiturates (page 26.)

(c) *Steroid Therapy* (page 9).—These patients are commonly on long term steroid therapy and therefore careful enquiries should always be made concerning the patient's current treatment.

General Management

Epidermolysis Bullosa Simplex.—This mild form of the disease seldom presents many difficulties for the anaesthetist, as the lesions are usually restricted to the hands and feet.

Induction of anaesthesia should be by an inhalation method or intravenous, using Althesin or propanidid. The use of barbiturates intravenously or in premedication is best avoided unless very careful screening for porphyria has been carried out. The limbs should be carefully protected throughout the anaesthetic. This is best achieved by ensuring that limb movements do not occur at any time during induction and maintenance. If steroid therapy is being used, it may be considered necessary to take special precautions (page 291).

Epidermolysis Bullosa Dystrophia.—Owing to the widespread nature of this form of the disease, which may involve face, mucous membranes and occasionally larynx, many problems arise. The actual method of anaesthesia used will depend upon the individual circumstances, and we can only make a few suggestions for guidance.

For simple dental procedures these patients can be treated as out-patients, but if any difficulties are anticipated, either surgically or as the result of the particular form of the disease, they should be admitted to hospital. If a few simple extractions only are to be performed, the authors have found that a single dose of intravenous agent is all that may be required, thus avoiding any further traumatic contact with the patient. Great care must be exercised with the application of a tourniquet. If an inhalation induction is employed the nasal mask should not be applied to the face before the skin and lips have been protected with wool or gauze soaked in hydrocortisone. As the mucous membranes are frequently affected, intubation and packing must be avoided whenever possible. The need for these procedures can be reduced by operating in the lateral or the tonsillar position, keeping the mouth open with a suitable gag and insufflating the anaesthetic gases through a small tube placed in the side of the mouth. It is suggested that, if multiquadrant extractions are needed, then each side should be done on a separate occasion, so as to avoid the trauma which would inevitably be involved in the changeover.

4. **Myasthenia Gravis.**—This is a disease of unknown aetiology characterized by impairment of transmission at the motor nerve junctions in skeletal muscle. The dental anaesthetist is most likely to be faced with its problems in children who require some sedation or general anaesthesia for dental treatment.

The treatment, which depends upon the use of anticholinesterase drugs, is often difficult and complex and lies beyond the scope of this book, but a few observations concerning the management of sedation and anaesthesia for dental treatment may be helpful.

(i) If sedation is required for these patients, this should be carried out in hospital, where all emergency facilities are available.
(ii) All sedative drugs which have an effect on muscle tone, such as chlorpromazine and the diazepines should be avoided.
(iii) If general anaesthesia is unavoidable, we recommend the use of an inhalation technique using N_2O, O_2, halothane. Muscle relaxants are strictly contraindicated.

5. **Hurler's Syndrome** (Gargoylism, Dysostosis Multiplex).—This genetically determined condition is due to a metabolic disturbance involving an abnormal storage of mucopolysaccharides. It is characterized clinically by a large skull with prominent supra-orbital ridges and depressed nasal bridge, a typical claw-like hand, large tongue and short neck. Mental retardation is common.

The diagnosis is likely to have been established before the patient is seen by the dental anaesthetist and he may be presented with one or more of the following problems.

(a) Nasal breathing is often difficult or impossible due to a profuse nasal discharge and large adenoids in association with the depressed nasal bridge.

(b) Airway maintenance is made difficult, particularly in the presence of a mouth-pack, owing to the large tongue. Intubation is usually necessary and should present no difficulty.

(c) Cardiac insufficiency is common in these children, and considerable care has to be taken to preserve normal oxygenation. This cardiac insufficiency is due to the deposition of mucopolysaccharides in the valves and coronary vessels, as in connective tissue elsewhere in the body. Cardiac murmurs, ventricular hypertrophy and angina are not uncommon features.

6. **The First Arch Syndrome.**—This syndrome includes a number of conditions such as, Treacher Collins, Pierre Roben, cleft palate and microstoma, all of which present problems to the anaesthetist. These conditions are described and their management discussed in Chapter 16.

CHAPTER TWELVE

GENERAL ANAESTHESIA AND SEDATION FOR CONSERVATIVE DENTISTRY

THE DEMAND

Despite the availability of dental treatment under the National Health Service in the United Kingdom, some 60% of the population do not avail themselves of this facility. Many factors may contribute towards this overall dental apathy, but any technique which might lead to the abolition or reduction of fear and discomfort would contribute to a small extent towards a wider acceptance of regular dental care. It should not, however, be forgotten that all methods of general anaesthesia carry with them an inherent risk; this risk, in ideal circumstances, is very small, and may be justifiable in terms of the overall benefits conferred, but the decision to utilize powerful central nervous system depressants should never be taken lightly. Local anaesthesia has many obvious advantages in out-patient work, particularly in the realm of dental surgery where the regional techniques are usually both simple and satisfactory. Used alone, or in conjunction with sedation, local anaesthesia should remain the dental practitioner's first method of pain relief, and the more complex techniques of general anaesthesia should be reserved for those cases in which there is a clear indication for their use. This indication should not be influenced by the practitioner's convenience, or indeed by his special interest in a particular technique. Although it is neither desirable nor possible to dogmatize regarding what constitutes a 'clear indication', it is nevertheless necessary to offer some broad guidance, and for this purpose we may classify patients requiring conservative dental treatment into the following four categories.

Category I

Patients who are unable to receive treatment under unsupplemented local anaesthesia for any of the following reasons:

(a) Repeated failure to achieve local anaesthesia.
(b) Repeated adverse reactions (e.g. fainting) to local anaesthesia in spite of preventive measures.
(c) Unco-operative children.
(d) Patients suffering from neurological disorders in which involuntary motor activity is a dominant feature.
(e) Psychological influences.
  (i) Extreme fear in an otherwise normal subject
  (ii) Mental retardation and other psychological disabilities.
(f) Special conditions such as haemophilia, or patients requiring multiquadrant dentistry with chemotherapy coverage.

Category II

Patients who would prefer to be unconscious during treatment, but who could be persuaded to accept local anaesthesia.

Category III

Patients who have no personal preference, but elect to leave the choice of method of pain relief to the practitioner in charge.

Category IV

Patients who express a preference for unsupplemented local anaesthesia.

Patients in categories I and IV present no problem. In the absence of clinical considerations to the contrary, general anaesthesia or heavy sedation should be available to those in category I, just as it should not be employed on those in category IV. The justification for using general anaesthesia on patients in categories II and III will depend entirely upon the prevailing circumstances. Under ideal conditions, general anaesthesia could be considered justifiable; the more slender the clinical indications, the closer to 'ideal' should these conditions be. Fortunately, recent developments in pharmacology have so widened the sphere of usefulness of heavy sedation in combination with local anaesthesia, that full general anaesthesia for conservative dentistry is seldom necessary. It is nevertheless advisable to enumerate the conditions which we would consider to be ideal, should such an anaesthetic be contemplated.

1. Presence of an anaesthetist, skilled in dental anaesthesia, who has received a wide anaesthetic training, and who, in particular, is thoroughly familiar with all modern resuscitation techniques—including endotracheal intubation under difficult circumstances.
2. Presence of a skilled operator (other than the anaesthetist), who has considerable experience in performing conservation under general anaesthesia.
3. Presence of adequate, trained ancillary staff to assist.
4. Presence of all facilities and equipment as detailed on page 13.

TECHNIQUES IN COMMON USE

Broadly speaking the following four general anaesthetic techniques are of value in conservative dentistry.

1. General anaesthesia with endotracheal intubation.
2. General anaesthesia with nasopharyngeal intubation.
3. General anaesthesia without intubation.
4. Post-anaesthetic methohexitone amnesia (commonly called 'ultra-light').

In the last of these techniques, true anaesthesia, in the commonly accepted sense of the term, is not maintained continuously, but is nearly always produced at some stage or stages of the procedure. We consider it necessary, therefore, to classify technique 4 as belonging to general anaesthesia, for many of the dangers and management problems inherent in continuous general anaesthesia are equally, if not so obviously, relevant to this intermittent anaesthetic technique. Only by treating it with the care and respect normally accorded to full orthodox general anaesthesia, can it be employed safely and efficiently.

We will now consider these four techniques in some detail.

1.   Endotracheal Anaesthesia

The presence of a nasotracheal tube and pharyngeal pack affords the operator unrestricted access to the entire mouth. The removal of water and debris by suction becomes a convenience rather than an urgent necessity, and the operator's technique is entirely unhampered by considerations relating to the patency of the airway.

The actual anaesthetic technique, its justification, contraindications and possible sequelae are discussed in full in Chapter 13, and the same considerations apply, irrespective of the nature of the dental procedure.

2.   Nasopharyngeal Intubation

The insertion of a nasopharyngeal tube rather than an endotracheal tube will provide many of the advantages of the latter, without the need for relaxants and laryngoscopy. As with an endotracheal tube it can be attached directly to the anaesthetic apparatus thus avoiding the inconvenience sometimes caused to the dentist by a bulky nasal mask. However, it must be remembered that the nasopharyngeal tube will not give the same security of airway control as the endotracheal tube, and that its insertion may present serious difficulties by initiating nasal bleeding behind the mouth pack. Careful insertion and the use of properly designed tubes will minimize these difficulties (page 142). The use of ephedrine nasal drops prior to intubation may also be helpful in this respect. When inserting these tubes, care must be taken to ensure that an adequate depth of anaesthesia has been reached. If anaesthesia is too light, gagging and excessive salivation are likely to result, and may lead eventually to severe laryngeal spasm. A mouth pack is essential with this technique.

3.   General Anaesthesia without Intubation

General anaesthesia, using any of the techniques described in Chapters 5 and 10 can readily be adapted to fulfil the conditions necessary for the performance of conservative dentistry. Although the basic principles underlying these techniques remain unaltered, the following modifications of practical procedure are necessary.

(a) *Mouth Packs.*—The tendency for gauze or gamgee to become entangled with the burr renders it necessary to use packing material of a more compact nature. A suitable pack is that described by Drummond-Jackson, and illustrated in Fig. 118. This pack should be placed in such a manner as to form an effective seal between operating area and pharynx, and this object is usually achieved by tucking the pack into the lingual sulcus, and ensuring that its posterior border makes firm contact with the mucosa covering the lingual aspect of the ramus of the mandible (Fig. 65). Arrangement of these packs for conservation on anterior teeth is shown in Fig. 119. It may be necessary to change such a pack frequently—the frequency depending upon the quantity of water in use and the efficacy of suction; the pack should not be allowed to become sodden, and before use should be moistened with tap water and firmly wrung out. It is often advisable to use this pack in conjunction with an underlying gauze pack which remains undisturbed throughout the procedure. They should be sterilized by soaking in antiseptic solution (e.g. 1 % cetrimide) or by boiling.

(b) *Suction.*—The control of water (from the cooling system of the high speed drill) and dust, is best achieved by the use of high velocity suction. This type of suction presents the advantage over conventional high vacuum suction in that efficient removal of foreign matter can be effected over an air-gap of half an inch (13 mm). Moreover, the suction ends are specifically designed to solve the problems peculiar to dentistry (Fig. 28). Whenever possible, the wide-bore tip should be operated by the dental assistant posterior to the site of cavity preparation, so that the main water spray is prevented from saturating the pack (Fig. 119). It is clearly more difficult to achieve this aim when work of a complex nature is undertaken in the lower molar region, than it is when work in the upper anterior, and therefore more accessible, portion of the mouth is in progress. A safe and successful outcome to conservative procedures performed under general anaesthesia will largely depend upon the absolute efficiency with which the pharynx is protected against the encroachment of any foreign material.

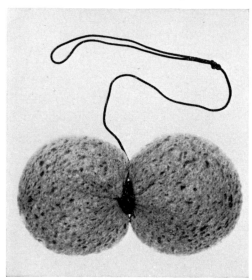

FIG. 118.—Flanged cellulose pack (Drummond-Jackson)

(c) *Posture.*—We have already, on page 181, expressed a preference for the reclining posture, which the majority of dental surgeons find satisfactory for exodontia. For conservation, however, where the 'low-seated' position is rapidly gaining favour, the anaesthetist is expected to administer the anaesthetic to a fully supine patient without disturbing the normal 'four-handed' routine. This he may find difficult to achieve, since his access to the patient's airway is extremely limited (Fig. 89). He will, therefore, be forced to depend upon either the dental nurse or himself maintaining a clear airway by submental support with the patient's head fully extended. This manoeuvre is often successful in simple cases, but cannot be guaranteed when access to the operation area, or the patient's anatomical configuration, presents difficulties. Under these

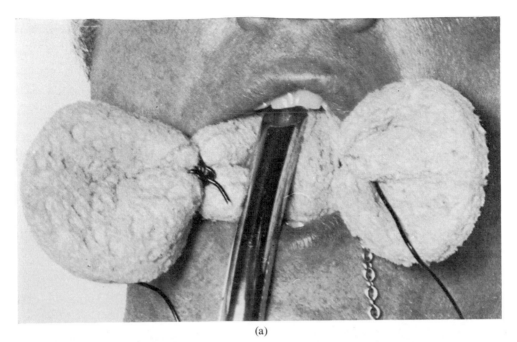

(a)

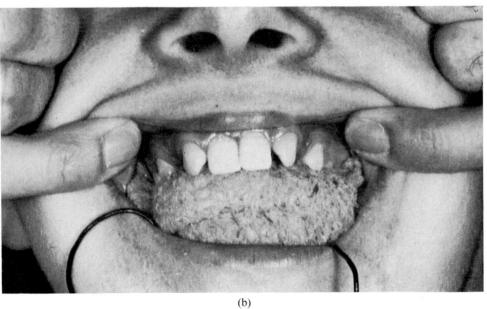

(b)

FIG. 119—A Two flanged packs and large-bore aspirator in position for conserbation on upper
anterior central incisors.

  B   Flanged packs tucked into Sulcus to expose lateral incisers.

241

circumstances, either endotracheal intubation, or an alteration in position of the whole team in order to allow the anaesthetist to support the mandible from the head of the chair, will be the only alternatives, if an unobstructed airway is to be maintained.

Certain advantages accruing from the use of purely intravenous methods of anaesthesia in dentistry have already been described on page 211. These advantages are particularly valuable in conservative work, owing to the increase in accessibility which the avoidance of a nose-piece affords the operator, enabling him to undertake work of a prolonged and complex nature more efficiently. The superiority of intermittent methohexitone over other intravenous agents has already been stressed in relation to exodontia (Chapter 10), and the same criteria of preference apply to conservative dentistry. The equipment most suitable for the administration of these drugs intermittently is the butterfly needle with extension tube (Fig. 102). The advantage of this equipment is that it is all disposable, and is therefore devoid of the risk of virus transmission, which is inherent in the use of three-way taps used in conjunction with a stock-bottle.

The technique of maintaining satisfactory anaesthesia and operating conditions, with short acting intravenous drugs only, is not an easy one. All the safeguards (packing, suction, etc.) already described apply with equal force whether or not an inhalation agent is used. In the absence of an inhalation supplement, with its wide range of anaesthetic and analgesic potential, certain motor excitatory phenomena (e.g. hiccoughs, spontaneous head and limb movements) are more likely to occur. Moreover, painful stimulation, particularly when applied to a nervous or 'pain-sensitive' patient, often evokes a reflex motor response (e.g. movement, laryngeal stridor). These motor responses, whether spontaneous or pain induced, may interfere greatly with both the smoothness and the safety of the whole procedure, and can be abolished by the use of an inhalation supplement. If, however, an entirely intravenous technique is considered desirable, the incidence of these motor responses may be reduced by the use of intravenous premedicants of the following two types.

(i) *Analgesics.*—The lack of analgesic properties associated with the barbiturates may be responsible, in part at least, for many of the motor responses described above. Prior administration of any powerful recognized analgesic drug will serve to diminish reflex response to painful stimulation both in frequency and degree. The most widely used intravenous analgesic for this purpose is pethidine 25 mg (average healthy adult), but the authors have found both fentanyl 0·05 mg and pentazocine 30 mg to be satisfactory, and relatively free from unpleasant after-effects. Whatever analgesic drug is favoured, it should never be forgotten that all powerful analgesics are depressants of the respiratory centre, and marked variations in individual susceptibility are sometimes exhibited. Great caution in their administration should be exercised, particularly when the intravenous route is employed and an additional respiratory depressant (e.g. methohexitone) is to be used. It is also absolutely essential to establish that the patient is not taking M.A.O.I. drugs (page 7), and if the drug selected is subject to the restrictions of the Dangerous Drugs Act, all necessary legal requirements must be fulfilled.

(ii) *Antisialogogues.*—The presence of excess secretions in mouth, pharynx or trachea, will frequently result in coughing or bouts of laryngeal stridor. When the level of anaesthesia is readily able to be deepened by inhalation agents, secretory activity is depressed, and the administration of antisialogogues is usually unnecessary; when, however, a purely intravenous technique is employed for prolonged procedures, excessive secretion may become troublesome, and it is therefore wise to precede the induction of anaesthesia by the administration of an antisialogogue, e.g. atropine (0·6 mg) or hyoscine (0·2 mg). This may be premixed with the analgesic agent, if used. Although the use of this type of intravenous premedication is not essential, we have found it of value in obtaining smooth operating conditions in the case where difficulty is anticipated.

Anaesthesia is induced with a normal dose of methohexitone (page 194) e.g. 80 mg, a prop of comfortable size and design being placed between the teeth just prior to loss of consciousness. If the methohexitone has been preceded by an intravenous analgesic, as described, it will be necessary to wash through the needle with saline or aspirated blood before proceeding with the methohexitone administration. It is essential that the airway should be maintained by gentle jaw-support from the very first moment of unconsciousness; any excess saliva or mucus should be carefully removed from the mouth and pharynx by suction, and the flanged cellulose pack already described gently inserted. The appropriate suction ends should now be positioned, and the first increment of methohexitone (20 mg–40 mg) given, just prior to the commencement of work. Further increments (not exceeding 40 mg) are administered as required, their actual amount and frequency being a matter for individual assessment. Excessive movement in response to stimulation, or attempts to push the pack out with the tongue, usually constitute an indication for a further increment, but the vigilance and experience of the anaesthetist, the dexterity and gentleness of the operator, and the efficiency of the assistant operating the suction, will determine successful outcome, rather than adherence to a strict dosage or timing regime.

At no time should obstructed breathing, laryngeal stridor or excessive movement be allowed to continue uninvestigated. It is also vital that the anaesthetist should carry out frequent checks on the circulatory system, and he must in particular assure himself that the peripheral pulse is at all times satisfactory. Nor, of course, should any increment of methohexitone be given unless he is certain that respiration is unobstructed, and normal in both rate and depth. Here, it must be stressed that in the absence of inhalation anaesthesia, the normal assistance afforded the anaesthetist by the movement of the reservoir bag, and the rhythmic sound of the expiratory valve, will no longer be available. Breathing will usually be quiet, and the noise of the air-rotor and the suction apparatus will render it impossible to monitor breathing by ear. The only guides which the anaesthetist has to the patient's respiratory efficiency are visual and tactile (page 213); at all times the rhythmic rise and fall of the patient's chest and abdomen must be carefully observed. This movement should be adequate in degree and quite 'smooth'. Any suggestion of 'jerkiness' or undue tightening of abdominal musculature indicates some degree of respiratory obstruction. Unless the anaesthetist is completely satisfied that respiratory and circulatory activity is normal, all dental treatment must be suspended until the cause of the suspected abnormality has been investigated and brought fully under control. During anaesthesia with intravenous agents only, although the laryngeal reflexes usually remain brisk, the danger of inhalation of foreign material is ever present; thus, those precautions designed to protect the pharynx should never be relaxed.

If, despite the administration of premedicant drugs, excessive movement on the part of the patient creates unsatisfactory operating conditions, the anaesthetist has three courses of action open to him.

Firstly, in cases where local anaesthesia is not contraindicated, the relevant area may be blocked or infiltrated. It must be remembered that a solid prop on the opposite side will impede the angulation of syringe necessary to accomplish inferior dental block, and a mouth-gag should therefore be used. If effective, such local supplementation will greatly diminish the tendency of the patient to exhibit reflex response to surgical stimulation during the subsequent light general anaesthesia.

Secondly, the anaesthetist can deepen anaesthesia with inhalation agents such as nitrous oxide and halothane, and having established a stable, controlled level of anaesthesia, maintain it by using a combination of intermittent intravenous and inhalation techniques. If, in spite of these measures, operative access and airway control continue to present difficulties, then endotracheal intubation may constitute the only means of obtaining satisfactory conditions in safety. From this procedure, the experienced anaesthetist should not shrink, but the inexperienced anaesthetist who is not prepared to intubate in the dental chair, would be well advised to abandon the case rather than allow work to continue whilst the airway is in jeopardy.

Thirdly, instead of deepening the anaesthetic, the anaesthetist may achieve improved operating conditions by allowing the patient to become conscious but heavily sedated. This technique is described in full under 4 below.

4. Post-Anaesthetic Methohexitone Amnesia

When cavity preparation has been successfully completed under intermittent methohexitone anaesthesia, as described above, it is often possible to allow the patient to regain consciousness whilst lining and filling of the cavities is being performed. During this phase of the procedure, most patients will obey simple verbal instructions, generally co-operate, and yet retain no memory of having been awake, even though some of the manipulations may have been painful. This striking phase of co-operative amnesia can be utilized, not only to complete, but also on occasions to prepare cavities; if, however, cavity-preparation requires more than a few minutes, it will prove necessary to administer further increments of methohexitone (e.g. 10–20 mg), and this will usually result in a short period of anaesthesia during which the risk of airway obstruction will exist; conservation is thus largely carried out on a patient who is co-operative but often completely amnesic. Such a patient is spared many of the hazards inherent in continuous anaesthesia, whilst enjoying the benefit of oblivion. For most of the procedure he is able to 'maintain his own airway', and thus continuous jaw-support is unnecessary; on the other hand, the pharynx should still be protected against the entry of foreign material by packing and suction; for although the 'protective' reflexes are active, and the patient is only unconscious for very short periods, it must ever be borne in mind that completely conscious subjects who have received no depressant drugs whatsoever, do occasionally inhale foreign material. Patients in the state of post methohexitone amnesia are clearly less able to protect themselves than fully conscious patients, and thus it is strongly advised that none of the usual protective precautions are relaxed, particularly if much water is in use or the patient is tilted backwards towards the supine position. In addition, the normal rules relating to food, drink and journey home should be strictly observed.

Results with this technique are unfortunately variable and often impossible to assess in advance, but the following considerations have a direct bearing upon the chances of success.

(a) *Nature of Dentistry.*—The less severe the stimuli, the greater the chance of quiet toleration by the patient.

(b) *Skill of Operator.*—The greater the degree of overall gentleness on the part of the operator, the greater the chance of success. This applies not only to painful stimuli but to any manoeuvre tending to distort the airway or to provoke the gagging reflex.

(c) *Handling by Anaesthetist.*—It is very important that during the phase of initial unconsciousness the airway should not be allowed to become obstructed even momentarily, and that the whole short anaesthetic phase should be completely smooth. In particular, the pharynx must be absolutely protected against the encroachment of foreign material, and any initial saliva or mucus must be carefully removed by suction.

The authors are of the opinion that the administration of premedication intravenously as described on page 242 serves to increase the chances of success, as does also the use of local infiltration, where this is not contraindicated.

(d) *Rapport.*—The more nervous and pain-sensitive the patient, the more difficult it becomes to achieve success with the amnesic technique. Very nervous or hysterical patients will sometimes start to phonate and move excessively as soon as anaesthesia lightens to a degree approaching 'accessibility', and all efforts on the part of the anaesthetist may fail to produce satisfactory operating conditions. These cases often require anaesthesia to be deepened with inhalation agents, and occasionally endotracheal intubation may prove necessary in order to be able to carry out satisfactory dentistry under safe conditions. Should the operator attempt to continue his work on such a patient in the amnesic state, he may well be able to perform dentistry to the patient's temporary satisfaction, for the patient—although wildly unco-operative—will usually retain no memory of the procedure. Such dentistry is likely to be of inferior quality, and where it represents the only alternative to no dentistry at all, it might be considered justifiable. But where it would be possible to perform better dentistry by using either a more sophisticated and demanding anaesthetic technique, or by using local anaesthesia, it is clearly quite unjustifiable to accept poor operating conditions simply because the anaesthetic technique used is both easy for the anaesthetist to administer and attractive for the patient to receive.

There is no doubt that the patient's disposition cannot be considered in isolation, and that the relationship between patient and anaesthetist is of considerable importance. The provision of satisfactory, tranquil operating conditions in the amnesic state, depends to some extent upon the utilization of simple hypnotic techniques. Frequently, movement and other reflex reactions to painful stimulation can be controlled by confident reassurance; but there are also many occasions when it cannot, and a more reliable method of providing good operating conditions must then be sought.

(e) *Maintenance of Body Temperature*.—In lengthy procedures carried out under methohexitone, a fall in the patient's body temperature is not unusual, and this may lead to shivering which seriously disrupts the smooth progress of treatment. The ideal skin—and thus environmental—temperature is 33°C, and since this is too warm to provide comfortable operating conditions, some separate means of maintaining the patient's body temperature should be employed.

When attention is paid to the foregoing considerations, post-anaesthetic methohexitone amnesia can provide excellent operating conditions—in which the patient's co-operation is retained—under circumstances of maximum safety and comfort. Unfortunately, the patient whose need for general anaesthesia is greatest, is often the least likely to be successfully controlled in the amnesic or 'ultra-light' state, and on these occasions a more complex anaesthetic technique will have to be used.

Summary

Whilst we have attempted to describe separately full anaesthesia produced by intermittent methohexitone, and conscious amnesia associated with the true 'ultra-light' state, it must be acknowledged that in practice, whenever painful conservation is to be performed, success is difficult to achieve unless periods of full anaesthesia are incorporated in the technique. Indeed, a recent investigation into the efficacy and safety of 'ultra-light' methohexitone anaesthesia revealed that in spite of every attempt being made to maintain 'verbal contact' with the patient, periods of full anaesthesia were inevitable; that these were often associated with bouts of airway obstruction which sometimes went unrecognized by experienced clinical observers, and that this frequently resulted in hypoxaemia; that the aspiration of radio-opaque material placed behind the pack occurred, in spite of the presence of 'the protective' reflexes; that the eyelash and swallowing reflexes were unreliable as guides to the level of consciousness; that all in all, the 'ultra-light' technique was a difficult one to practise in the pure form in which it is claimed to be safe for use by the single-handed dentist, and that it has few advantages and many disadvantages when compared with routine local anaesthesia.

From this work coupled with our own experience, we must conclude that pure conscious amnesia is seldom practised by the advocates of 'ultra-light' anaesthesia, and we believe that the majority of nervous patients are more safely and efficiently served by the use of local anaesthesia in conjunction with intravenous sedation. For those patients in whom either local anaesthesia is contraindicated, or the degree of fear demands periods of complete unconsciousness during treatment, one of the methods of anaesthesia described in this chapter will prove suitable. The choice of technique will depend largely upon the complexity of dentistry to be undertaken, and indeed it is our experience that only the simplest and most basic forms of conservative dentistry can be successfully carried out under non-intubated general anaesthesia. All the more advanced restorative procedures appear to us to require either full endotracheal anaesthesia or local anaesthesia, if necessary supplemented by sedation.

Heavy Sedation and Local Anaesthesia

The combination of local anaesthesia and heavy sedation has for years been utilized to ameliorate the discomfort and anxiety entailed in many surgical and diagnostic procedures. Historically, these techniques range from the traditional 'Twilight Sleep' to modern neuroleptanalgesia. In dentistry, however, it is only comparatively recently that widespread interest in the use of these combination techniques has been aroused. In particular, the 'Jorgensen' has probably been chiefly responsible for stimulating and spreading an awareness amongst dentists and doctors alike of the need for methods which lie between full general anaesthesia on the one hand, and unsupplemented local anaesthesia on the other. The Jorgensen technique has been used in the U.K. primarily for restorative dentistry, but its suitability in the realms of minor oral surgery and exodontia is also recognized. As the ranks of the tranquillizing drugs have continued to swell, so have dental anaesthetists searched for a drug, or combination of drugs, more suitable for the dental out-patient than those utilized in the 'Jorgensen'. In recent years much interest has centred around the use of intravenous diazepam for this purpose. In the succeeding paragraphs we will describe both Jorgensen's technique, and the various ways in which diazepam is currently employed in dentistry to eliminate fear and discomfort. It is possible, perhaps even probable, that superior techniques and drugs will emerge in the near future, but it seems to us at the time of writing that diazepam, in terms of safety, simplicity and efficacy, constitutes a most significant advance towards this final objective. It should, at this point, be stressed that the success of any deep sedation technique is dependent upon the skill of the dental surgeon in patient management, operative manipulation and, in particular, in his ability to achieve painless but totally effective local anaesthesia.

The 'Jorgensen'

The technique entails the administration of three drugs by the intravenous route, namely pentobarbitone (Nembutal), pethidine (Demerol) and hyoscine (Scopolamine).

The patient is reclined or placed supine, and pentobarbitone is administered intravenously at the rate of 10 mg every 30 seconds. For this purpose a 250 mg ampoule may be dissolved in 10 ml of pyrogen-free distilled water. The total dose of pentobarbitone used varies widely from patient to patient, and may lie anywhere in the full range between 10 and 250 mg, it being generally considered wise never to exceed the latter dose in a healthy young adult. The factors which determine the end point of the injection are not easy to state in scientific or precise terms. Any strong subjective or objective symptom or sign such as pronounced drowsiness, dizziness, blurred or double vision, ptosis, may be taken to signify that a further 10–15% of the quantity of pentobarbitone already administered is said to bring the total dose up to its optimal level. The syringe is now detached from the needle (after first withdrawing blood in order to wash the needle through), and a mixture containing pethidine 25 mg and hyoscine 0·4 mg is administered. If, as is occasionally the case, the quantity of pentobarbitone injected has been less than 100 mg the subsequent mixture of pethidine and hyoscine should be correspondingly reduced. For example, if 50 mg pentobarbitone has produced the desired effect, then pethidine 12·5 mg and hyoscine 0·2 mg should be used. All that now remains is for the relevant working areas to be covered by local anaesthesia. We have found that, in strict contrast to the diazepam techniques, it is usually beneficial to wait some 5 to 10 minutes before administering the local anaesthetic, since it appears to take this time for the Jorgensen drugs to achieve their optimum effect; indeed there is occasionally an over-reaction to any attempted interference immediately following the administration of these drugs. Needless to say, it is imperative that local anaesthesia should be achieved with the greatest possible gentleness. The use of surface analgesia, blood-heat solution, and slow injection are technical refinements too often neglected but of paramount importance. If four-quadrant dentistry entailing bilateral inferior dental block is undertaken, then the first lower quadrant should be completed at the outset, preferably covered by a short acting local anaesthetic solution, followed by both upper quadrants, so that the second inferior dental block is not administered until the first has worn off. Many operators would, however, consider the use of bilateral inferior block unjustifiable under all circumstances. The level of sedation achieved is usually satisfactory from both the patient's and the operator's point of view. Patients may sleep, but remain co-operative throughout. They should always be escorted home, and the time taken for complete recovery to occur is, unfortunately, variable. 'Hangover' effects are usually experienced for some hours, occasionally for days.

The technique has the great advantage that it has been used safely and successfully for many years on thousands of cases. This sphere of usefulness covers not only the nervous patient, but also the normal patient for whom it is essential to complete what would otherwise be an intolerably great amount of dentistry at one sitting; and, finally, the spastic patient in whom it is impossible to achieve the necessary degree of muscular relaxation without the use of drugs. There are, however, certain inherent disadvantages which have led us to abandon the technique in favour of diazepam. The use of pethidine, an addictive Dangerous Drug in circumstances where pain-relief is dependent upon local anaesthesia, is difficult to justify, particularly in an environment where the employment of mono-amine oxidase inhibitors is widespread. The recommended full dose of hyoscine seems unnecessarily large. The combination of three powerful central depressant drugs is not ideal when simpler alternatives are available. The long period of heavy sedation produced, renders the technique unjustifiable in situations where less than 2 hours dentistry is required, and thus limits

its sphere of usefulness. The long and variable 'hang-over' period sometimes results in an unwarranted and unexpected degree of incapacity on the part of the patient.

Finally, the reader should be reminded that the use of methohexitone or any other intravenous anaesthetic agent to replace or supplement pentobarbitone renders the technique no longer one of pure sedation, and should, therefore, not be described as a 'Modified Jorgensen'. There have already been two fatalities in the U.K. associated with the use of methohexitone in this context, and in one of these cases the dentist claimed that he was unaware that he was giving a general anaesthetic.

Diazepam (Valium)

The use of diazepam as an oral tranquillizer is well recognized, and as such it is effective in dentistry. In the past few years, it has also been used by the intravenous route to produce a much deeper level of sedation, and it has been shown to be remarkably free from potentially dangerous side effects. The sphere of usefulness of the drug covers both restorative and operative dentistry. Whilst its main use lies in the fact that its employment will enable the very nervous patient to accept conservative dentistry under local anaesthesia, we have also found the technique of particular value in the patient with a history of either persistent retching or fainting. We will now attempt to give some broad guidance as to the practical management of a nervous patient about to undergo conservative dentistry under intravenous Valium.

Provided Valium only is to be used, the patient may be instructed to eat a snack or light meal some 2 to 3 hours prior to the dental appointment. The usual careful medical history will have been taken, any medication being, of course, especially noted, and after the customary immediate preoperative preparations regarding clothing, toilet, etc. the patient is comfortably positioned in the chair. The reclining posture is the one most readily accepted by the majority of patients, and even if the fully supine position is ultimately intended to enable low-seated dentistry to be performed, sedation should be initially induced in the position of maximum comfort for the patient. We reject the suggestion that fainting is more likely to occur in the reclining than the horizontal posture, but we do believe that the frequency with which this complication is encountered varies inversely with the abilities of the practitioner both in terms of patient management and practical skill (page 336). A faint occurring during the induction of sedation, or subsequently, should be readily recognized by any moderately observant practitioner, and the patient's posture may be altered accordingly. We recommend that venipuncture is performed, whenever possible, in a large cubital vein since postinjection thrombosis is much less likely to occur than if a small vein with sluggish flow is used. We do not dilute the Valium, but elevate the limb and gently massage the vein centrally following injection, during which we use barbotage; barbotage involves diluting the solution in the syringe with blood after each small increment. Dosage in any particular case is a matter of direct observation and personal judgement, and whilst the appearance of pronounced ptosis has been claimed as the most reliable guide, we are much more inclined to accept the patient's own change in attitude and overall behaviour, which is often quite striking. The usual dose required for an adult is 10–15 mg, our general working limits being

A.A.D.—9

5–20 mg. The injection is made slowly, taking perhaps 1 to 2 minutes, a gentle flow of confident, quiet, reassuring conversation being always helpful. The maximum phase of sedation commences immediately following completion of the injection, and lasts for about 10 minutes; it is during this 10-minute period that the necessary injections of local anaesthetic are made, and we cannot stress too strongly that overall success is almost entirely dependent upon the gentleness and skill with which this is conducted, and the perfection of clinical anaesthesia which results. A failed block is much more likely to be a genuine failure on the part of the administrator than a pretence on the part of the patient, and a final satisfactory outcome is more likely if this simple truth is squarely faced, and remedied. Sedation is very deep during this first 10 minutes, and amnesia, which is entirely antegrade from the time of the Valium injection, is likely to be complete, so that even though the patient may have grimaced during the local injections, any discomfort is not remembered. It is also during this 10-minute period that the efficacy of the so-called 'protective reflexes' appears to be blunted, so that it would appear wise to treat the patient as though anaesthetized from the point of view of lung protection. Time must be allowed for complete local anaesthesia to be achieved, and work may then be commenced. The level of sedation appears to lighten rapidly, but the degree of tranquillity fortunately appears to remain unchanged for about one hour, and sometimes for much longer. From the practical point of view, cavity preparation of a fairly extensive nature may usually be completed during a 30-minute period characterized by moderate sedation, variable but sometimes complete amnesia, and excellent tranquillity. Lining and filling are then undertaken while the patient, recovering from sedation, remains highly co-operative and composed. After one hour, most patients appear normal, but some postural unsteadiness and hypotension may actually be demonstrable. Patients should, if possible, rest reclining for half to one hour following treatment, and should always be accompanied home and subjected to the same postoperative restrictions as those applicable to full general anaesthesia (page 17). Delayed 'hangover' effects are not nearly so common as with the 'Jorgensen', but have been observed.

Restorative dentistry of an advanced or complex nature presents management problems which are often in excess of those associated with simple fillings. Whilst anterior crown preparation generally lends itself to the type of management technique described above, the more complex posterior reconstruction procedures sometimes demand incremental doses of Valium or even short periods of analgesic intensification, in which nitrous oxide or intravenous analgesics may have to be employed. These 'composite' techniques border on general anaesthesia, and it must be admitted that full mouth reconstruction for a nervous patient often requires full intubated general anaesthesia.

Special Circumstances

So far, our account has been largely confined to dealing with the nervous patient to whom the advantages of intravenous sedation have been explained, and who has elected to try the technique. With these patients, success with unsupplemented Valium is of a very high order. However, many patients referred for special treatment have been led to believe that they will be unconscious, and such patients will often demand reassurance that they 'will know nothing whatever about the treatment'. We believe that it is never justifiable to be untruthful, but find it often possible to avoid giving a direct answer until the injection of Valium is taking effect, when, with tactful handling, the patient will often agree to allow treatment to commence without being fully unconscious. Under these circumstances, it is our custom to assure them that, should they wish it, they can always be fully anaesthetized at any time. Having got thus far, it is very rare indeed to encounter anything short of full success with unsupplemented Valium. On the other hand, some of these very nervous patients will still express a strong preference for complete unconsciousness after receiving the full dose of Valium, and under these circumstances we proceed with a small anaesthetizing dose of Brietal. Before doing so, the patient is told 'you are now going to go to sleep completely, and when you wake up, all the painful work will be done, and we will just be finishing off—trimming and polishing the fillings; you will still be very drowsy, but your co-operation at this stage enables us to do our best work'. Usually 20–30 mg Brietal suffices, and indeed we have found that there is seldom any reflex reaction to the injection of local anaesthetic with this small dose, whereas a larger dose is often accompanied by undesirable reflex response to stimulation. The Brietal may be given through the Valium needle provided this has been washed through by withdrawal of blood before changing syringes. If the upper jaw only is to be infiltrated a small prop may be placed in the mouth before loss of consciousness, but if inferior dental block is required, a prop placed on the opposite side of the mouth interferes with the usual angulation of the local syringe, and we recommend the use of a Doyen gag, for the syringe may be introduced between its open jaws. Any trickle of blood from the local injection site must be controlled by suction and, if necessary, a flanged pack. Once the intraoral injections have been made, it is advisable to await the return of 'verbal contact' before commencing dentistry. The patient should be immediately reassured that 'everything has gone satisfactorily and the final stages of polishing etcetera are now in progress'. It is, in our experience, almost invariable that treatment can now be successfully commenced and blissfully completed. The employment of this technique does, of course, demand that the patient should be fully prepared (e.g. food and drink) for a general anaesthetic.

Our ultimate objective in the use of these techniques is to wean the patient back to the acceptance of normal dentistry under local anaesthesia—perhaps with the assistance of oral Valium. Whilst we have enjoyed a good measure of success, the patients do tend, unfortunately, to become 'operator-dependent', and when such work is undertaken at a clinic, it is seldom possible to persuade the patient to return to his own dentist; but we consider it preferable for the patient to become 'operator dependent' than to become 'drug-dependent'.

Finally, when unsupplemented Valium is to be used, we consider that the presence of a second medical or dental practitioner is entirely optional. When, however, there is any likelihood that Brietal or other anaesthetic agents may be required, the presence of a second practitioner is desirable. For not only may the airway require maintenance during the local injections, but on the rare occasions when emergence from anaesthesia is not associated with peaceful co-operation, the presence of an anaesthetist will enable the dentistry to be completed under full general anaesthesia, including endotracheal intubation should this prove necessary.

'Relative Analgesia'

Recently there has been a revival of interest in the use of nitrous oxide—oxygen mixtures to provide analgesia in the conscious dental patient. Langa, in the U.S.A., has evolved an elaborate technique of patient-management which stresses the importance of ascertaining the precise proportions of the two gases necessary for any particular patient. He believes that these proportions are critical if good results are to be achieved, and claims that he is able to carry out the vast majority of restorative dental procedures without recourse to local anaesthesia.

Some twenty years ago Klock, in the U.S.A., and Tom, in the U.K., advocated the use of nitrous oxide—oxygen mixtures designed to produce a level of anaesthesia between the conventional 1st. and 2nd. stages, a level for which they coined the term 'amnalgesia', and which they claimed gave good conditions for the extraction of teeth.

These techniques have never achieved widespread popularity, and the authors have limited personal experience of their use in dentistry. It would appear, however, that the value of nitrous oxide-oxygen analgesic mixtures in the control of postoperative and labour pains is gaining increased recognition. The theoretical background to this interesting subject has recently been comprehensively reviewed by Parbrook.

RECOMMENDED READING

1. **Diazepam in Out-patient Dentistry.**
   HEALY et al, (1970) Br. med. J. iii, **13**.
2. **Sedation for Conservative Dentistry.**
   BRITISH DENTAL JOURNAL (1970) Vol. 128 No. 1. Multiple papers.
3. **Methohexitone in Conservative Dentistry.**
   MANN, P. E. et al (1971) Anaesthesia **26**, 3.
4. **Nitrous Oxide Analgesia.**
   PARBROOK, G. D. (1971). In General Anaesthesia in Dental Surgery. Ed. A. R. Hunter and G. H. Bush. Altrinciham: Sherratt. p. 33.
5. **Nitrous Oxide Analgesia.**
   LANGA, H. (1968). Relative Analgesia in Dental Practice. Philadelphia: Saunders.
6. **Intravenous Anaesthesia.**
   DRUMMOND-JACKSON S. L. (1971). Intravenous Anaesthesia. S.A.A.D.
7. **Biochemical Evidence of Anxiety in Dental Practice.**
   EDMOMDSON, H. D. et al. (1972) Br. med. J., iv, **7**.

CHAPTER THIRTEEN

GENERAL ANAESTHESIA FOR THE DIFFICULT CASE
(including minor oral surgery)

Introduction

The detailed anaesthetic management described in Chapters 5 and 10 in the main refers to patients undergoing simple dental treatment in the average dental surgery. In this chapter we propose to discuss those types of treatment which are suitable only to be undertaken when more elaborate facilities are available (page 13). These facilities cover anaesthetic requirements for both out-patient and in-patient treatment, and in the following paragraphs we will attempt to indicate which of these two modes of treatment is appropriate in any particular set of circumstances. The decision is based on the following considerations:—

A. SURGICAL CONSIDERATIONS

The type of case which demands these more elaborate facilities is that generally classified as minor oral surgery (M.O.S.), and is likely to require endotracheal intubation in order to provide safe and satisfactory operating conditions. The indications for intubation in dentistry are almost invariably surgical, and are applicable when the interests of the operator, in terms of surgical access, clash with the interests of the anaesthetist, in terms of airway control and protection. Thus, operations in the lower molar region, by encroaching upon the airway, are more likely to require intubation than are operations of similar duration upon the anterior teeth. Likewise, operations in which bleeding is likely to be profuse, and particularly when this bleeding is not localized (e.g. in multi-quadrant extractions), may necessitate intubation, even though the surgical procedure itself is simple. Operations in which the nasal mask obstructs surgical access (e.g. apicectomy on upper incisors), may well justify nasopharyngeal or endotracheal intubation, unless a solely intravenous technique is considered satisfactory.

The anaesthetist will learn to recognize the case which is likely, irrespective of the nature of the operation, to present the maximum technical difficulty in relation to the composite problem of airway control and surgical access. Thus, the patient with poor mouth-opening, receding jaw, large tongue, and tight cheeks is likely to require endotracheal intubation for a surgical procedure which, in an average patient, would not warrant it. It must be remembered, however, that it is this very type of patient who is the most likely to present technical intubation problems, so that the pros and cons of intubation must be carefully assessed. Finally, the experienced surgeon and anaesthetist, by virtue of their close co-operation, will be able to avoid recourse to intubation more frequently than will their less experienced colleagues.

It was, and still is, often taught that the surgical indications for intubation in dentistry are synonymous with the indications for in-patient hospital treatment. We, however, consider that in the healthy subject many operations requiring intubation can be safely and successfully carried out on an out-patient ('day-stay') basis, provided certain safeguards are observed.

1. No special surgical difficulty involving excessive tissue trauma should be anticipated. This, of course, is difficult to guarantee, but as a general guide any impacted wisdom tooth, the removal of which is likely to occupy an experienced surgeon longer than 30 minutes, is probably better removed as an in-patient. This view is based on the assumption that the longer and therefore more difficult cases are also more likely to give rise to severe postoperative swelling and discomfort, which can be more satisfactorily treated on an in-patient basis.

2. Operative bleeding is seldom severe in M.O.S. and in the intubated patient there is no risk of inhaled blood, provided adequate pharyngeal packing and suction are employed. However, bleeding may exceptionally be unexpectedly difficult to control, and it is essential that facilities for the admission of such cases are readily available, whether this be from a hospital out-patient department, or a private dental surgery. Should excessive bleeding be anticipated, either from a past history of such experience or from a proven bleeding diathesis, this will constitute an absolute contraindication to out-patient surgery.

Occasionally, in spite of normal history and adequate operative haemostasis, reactionary dental haemorrhage may occur unexpectedly several hours postoperatively, and thus after the patient's discharge. It is therefore essential that the out patient and his escort be given explicit instructions, both verbal and written, as to the proper course of action should this complication occur. These instructions should include both technical advice as to the simple emergency control of haemorrhage, and also, a clear statement regarding whom to contact. If this type of work is to be undertaken in a dental surgery, either the dental surgeon concerned or his deputy should be readily available for 24 hours postoperatively.

B. ANAESTHETIC CONSIDERATIONS

With adequate facilities available, there is no contraindication to the administration of a general anaesthetic to the healthy patient for the performance of minor oral surgery on an out-patient basis. In particular, provided no gross technical difficulty is anticipated, endotracheal intubation can be safely undertaken, and we find that undesirable postintubation sequelae are no more likely to occur in the out-patient than the in-patient, and should they do so, can be managed satisfactorily. The relevant sequelae are as follows:

1. 'Scoline' After-Pains (see page 260)

This unpleasant symptom occurs in some 30% of adult patients, usually on the day following the administration of Scoline. It is, however, extremely uncommon in children. We consider that this complication is unpleasant enough to warrant avoidance of the use of this drug on most occasions, and it is nearly always possible to perform intubation without it (see page 261). Should its use prove desirable, it is always necessary to warn the out-patient of the possible development of muscle pains on the following day, and to reassure him that these pains are not of serious consequence.

2. 'Sore Throat'

This symptom may indicate the presence of pharyngitis, laryngitis or tracheitis.

Pharyngitis may be caused by over-drying of secretions with an antisialogogue, associated with tight packing and traumatic instrumentation. Laryngitis and tracheitis are most commonly caused by allowing the patient to cough on the tube under light anaesthesia, but may follow the use of an unsterile tube.

Severe laryngitis may theoretically result in laryngeal oedema of sufficient degree to threaten the airway. In practice, this serious complication is confined to infants, and is thus not relevant to dentistry. Should hoarseness associated with difficulty in breathing or swallowing develop following extubation, the patient must be admitted to hospital for continued and continuous observation, but we have never encountered this problem in practice.

3. Severe Post-Anaesthetic Nausea, Vomiting and Malaise

With the anaesthetic techniques recommended in this chapter the above symptoms do occasionally occur, but rarely persist long enough in their severe form to warrant admission to hospital. Should they persist, however, the anaesthetist will have to decide whether admission has become unavoidable, since there comes a time when further improvement in the 'recovery environment' is unlikely to occur. Fortunately, admission is seldom indicated since the journey home may be rendered tolerable by the administration of an anti-emetic drug, and the anaesthetist should make an attempt to pay a postoperative visit to the patient's home. We have formed the opinion that there is a maximum time period suitable for general anaesthesia in the out-patient which, if exceeded, may lead to general malaise and other complications which can only be satisfactorily supervised on an in-patient basis. Whilst it is not possible to dogmatize, we consider that operations in excess of $1\frac{1}{2}$ hours (e.g. extensive periodontal surgery or restorative procedures) are not, on the whole, suitable to be undertaken on the out-patient, since anaesthesia of this length often warrants undisturbed rest for some 24 hours postoperatively. Probably, the most suitable technique for such prolonged cases involves the use of muscle relaxants, controlled respiration and minimal (if any) halothane, followed by reversal of the relaxant. Many anaesthetists would consider that such a technique is only justifiable in the most sophisticated out-patient environment, where overnight stay is available if necessary, i.e. the day-stay clinic rather than the dental surgery.

Thus we may conclude that intubation *per se* is not likely to be a valid indication for the routine admission of patients undergoing minor oral surgery, provided that adequate out-patient facilities are available. In general terms, any surgical procedure which in itself requires endotracheal intubation, should only be undertaken on the out-patient in the absence of any illness characterized by cardiorespiratory, meta-bolic or other serious bodily dysfunction. On the other hand, if the surgery is short and uncomplicated, requiring simple, non-intubated anaesthesia, the patient suffering from such dysfunction does not necessarily require in-patient admission. Each case must be considered on its merits, but irrespective of whether the patient is admitted or treated as an out-patient, the anaesthetic should always be administered by an experienced specialist anaesthetist.

The in-patient management of medically unfit patients is discussed in Chapter 14.

C. SOCIAL CONSIDERATIONS

It will now be apparent that both the nature of the surgery and the medical con-dition of the patient exert an important influence on the choice between in-patient and out-patient treatment. However, by far the most common deciding factor is the social background of the patient, particularly where the performance of minor oral surgery under endotracheal anaesthesia is concerned. It is essential that comfortable private transport to the patient's home, and a responsible escort have been arranged. In addition, an assurance must be obtained that immediate bed-rest and unskilled nurs-ing attention are available for at least 24 hours. The patient's regular medical and dental attendants should be kept informed of the entire procedure, and, in addition, the patient himself should know whom to contact in case of difficulty. Inability to comply with these simple rules dictates that the relevant treatment is better under-taken as an in-patient.

To summarize, the availability of out-patient facilities as described in Chapter 1, page 13, will carry the following advantages:

(a) Saving hospital beds.
(b) Allowing certain patients to avoid hospitalization, if it is their wish.
(c) Increasing the availability of general anaesthesia in those cases in whom it is preferable but who, without these facilities, would have to be treated under local anaesthesia.

TECHNIQUE OF ANAESTHESIA FOR MINOR ORAL SURGERY IN THE OUT-PATIENT

The technique of induction and maintenance of anaesthesia for minor oral surgery only differs from that described under exodontia if the patient is to be intubated. The following account describes the management of a typical minor oral surgical case requiring intubation as an out-patient, and it is our opinion that this should be undertaken only by a specialist anaesthetist, whose experience is not confined to dentistry.

Preoperative Assessment

The importance of preoperative assessment, particularly from the point of view of 'home conditions', has already been stressed. If the cases are carefully selected by an experienced practitioner, the overall results of out-patient treatment are likely to be both satisfactory, and appreciated by the patient.

We consider it essential that a full medical history be obtained, and it is generally held to be desirable that the following investigations be routinely performed; urine testing, haemoglobin estimation, blood grouping with serum retention for possible cross matching, and sickle-cell testing in the appropriate patients (page 284).

So far as physical examination of the patient is concerned, it is usually assumed that this is advantageous, although the examination traditionally performed is quite arbitrarily limited to the use of the ceremonial stethoscope. Such a procedure bears no resemblance to a full physical examination, and will rarely reveal any relevant abnormality which is not suggested by a carefully conducted medical history. Indeed, it is our contention that the justification for not performing a 'traditional' physical examination lies in the superior value of a history taken by an experienced anaesthetist with a wide background of general medical knowledge. In addition to the examination described in Chapter 1, there are certain other observations which we consider of particular relevance in these more complicated cases. The patency of the nasal airway in relation to the intended passage of a tube should be carefully established. If the use of a laryngoscope is anticipated, the presence of crowns, bridgework, loose teeth etc. must be noted, and all necessary precautions taken. The blood pressure and pulse characteristics form a useful basis for the assessment of subsequent circulatory change during anaesthesia. It will be noted that an examination incorporating these points does not require the patient to undress. Fuller examination will, of course, be undertaken if the history warrants it.

The one relevant finding unaccompanied by symptoms, which is likely to be revealed by routine auscultation of the chest is a heart murmur. This murmur may result from unrecognized fully compensated valvular disease, or be purely functional, and therefore of no significance. Such a random finding unaccompanied by any symptoms or other signs does not influence the selection or conduct of an anaesthetic, but may demand penicillin cover for dental treatment (page 274), irrespective of whether that treatment is undertaken under local or general anaesthesia. The ideal, therefore, is that all patients about to commence a course of dental treatment, who have not been clinically examined by a medical practitioner within recent years, should be advised to obtain such a check-up before the proposed dental treatment is commenced, and this examination is best carried out in the medical rather than the dental consulting room.

Premedication

Traditional premedication with an opiate or pethidine is the most potent single cause of prolonged recovery and post-anaesthetic nausea; also the use of anti-sialogogues by intramuscular injection may, by excessive drying of secretions, increase both the incidence and severity of postoperative sore throat.

With careful, sympathetic handling, the vast majority of out-patients do not require any sedative premedication, but if they do, a simple oral tranquillizer will suffice. The advisability of administering atropine will depend upon the anaesthetic

A.A.D.—9*

to be employed. With most modern techniques which do not entail the use of respiratory tract irritants such as ether, the antisialogogue effect of atropine is not usually necessary, but where intubation is carried out under light anaesthesia with the help of Scoline, excessive secretions may prove troublesome without it. In addition, intubation under light anaesthesia, the use of Scoline, and high halothane concentrations all may produce bradycardia due to vagal stimulation. This effect is prevented by the prior administration of atropine, preferably intravenously, and 0·6 mg will normally provide adequate protection against vagal cardiac stimulation, and prevent excessive respiratory secretions without producing the 'over-drying' effect often associated with the intramuscular use of antisialogogues. It should be noted that atropine is unstable in the presence of a barbiturate if the mixture is not used immediately.

INDUCTION AND MAINTENANCE OF ANAESTHESIA

The object of the induction phase in these patients is to produce conditions suitable for endotracheal intubation. As these conditions usually require good relaxation of voluntary muscles, it is necessary to describe briefly those drugs which are known as the muscle relaxants before discussing induction techniques.

The Muscle Relaxants

Relaxation, and finally paralysis, of the voluntary muscles can be achieved by two groups of drugs.

The first acts by blocking the nicotine-like action of acetyl choline, and in so doing prevents electrical depolarization at the neuromuscular junction, which normally accompanies muscular contraction. This group of relaxants includes d-tubo-curarine (Curare), gallamine (Flaxedil), pancuronium (Pavulon) and alcuronium chloride (Alloferin), all of which are normally administered by intravenous injection, and which differ from each other mainly in speed of onset and duration of action. Below are listed for each, the approximate dosage which should enable intubation to be performed under light anaesthesia (i.e. full paralysing dose); the time taken following injection for that degree of relaxation to develop; the duration of action of the drug concerned; and finally certain characteristic properties of each drug.

d-tubo-curarine (Curare).—Ampoules for intravenous injection. Colourless fluid, non-miscible with barbiturates, 15 mg in 1·5 ml
Dosage—0·4 mg/kg body weight
Achievement of adequate relaxation—3 minutes
Duration of action—45 minutes
Side effects—Moderate fall in blood pressure, particularly when associated with halothane. Occasionally produces histamine-release, therefore not ideal in the presence of asthma and other allergies. Action potentiated by ether, halothane and diazepam.

Gallamine (Flaxedil).—Dosage—2 mg/kg body weight
Achievement of adequate relaxation—2 minutes
Duration of action—30 minutes
Side effects—Produces tachycardia, which may be accompanied by increased
bleeding. Does not cause hypotension or histamine-release.

Pancuronium (Pavulon).—Dosage—0·08 mg/kg body weight
Achievement of adequate relaxation—1·5 minutes
Duration of action—60 minutes
Side effects—Transient hypertension but no tachycardia or histamine-release.
Occasional difficulty in reversal.

Alcuronium Chloride (Alloferin).—Dosage—0·2 mg/kg body weight
Achievement of adequate relaxation—2 minutes
Duration of action—20 minutes

Reversal of Non-Depolarizing Relaxants

The action of all the non-depolarizing relaxants can be reversed by neostigmine—
a drug with powerful anticholinesterase activity. The basis of this action is as follows.
Normal voluntary muscular contraction is initiated by the nicotine-like action of
acetyl choline which is released at the motor end-plate (neuromuscular junction)
during motor nerve stimulation. Curare acts by blocking this nicotine-like action.
Such a block can be reversed by allowing an excess of acetyl choline to build up at
the neuromuscular junction, and replace curare quantitatively from its common
receptor substance. Since the accumulation of excess acetyl choline is normally
prevented by its immediate destruction by the enzyme cholinesterase, administration
of an anticholinesterase such as neostigmine allows sufficient build-up of acetyl
choline for displacement of curare to occur. The administration of neostigmine will
allow an increase of acetyl choline concentration at sites other than neuromuscular
junctions, and therefore it is necessary to block its unwanted muscarine-like actions
(e.g. bradycardia, salivation, intestinal colic) at these sites by the prior administration
of atropine. The standard reversal of curarization is therefore accomplished by the
administration intravenously of atropine 1·2 mg followed by 1–2·5 mg of neostigmine.

The second group of drugs which is used to produce voluntary muscle paralysis
acts by causing a spread and prolongation of depolarization at the neuromuscular
junction. This prevents contraction of the muscle under all normal circumstances.
The onset of depolarization is marked by a varying degree of muscular fasciculation,
which has been claimed to be directly related to the incidence and severity of postoperative muscle pain (Scoline after-pains). The two members of this group in
common use are suxamethonium chloride and decamethonium iodide.

Suxamethonium Chloride (Scoline).—Dosage—1 mg/kg body weight—intravenous
2 mg/kg body weight—intramuscular
This dosage produces complete paralysis of all voluntary muscles including laryngeal and respiratory.
Onset of paralysis—About 30 seconds—intravenous
                    2 minutes—intramuscular
Duration of paralysis—About 1–3 minutes—intravenous
                    7–10 minutes—intramuscular
N.B.—The duration of action with any given dose may be increased by prior administration of (a) Epontol, (b) 'The Pill', (c) Tacrine.
Side effects—Muscle fasciculation and salivation frequently follow immediately after injection. Pronounced bradycardia may occur, particularly after second and subsequent injections. Histamine-release and the very rare and usually fatal 'malignant hyperpyrexia' may be associated with the use of Scoline. By far the most important side effects are Scoline after-pains and Scoline apnoea.

Scoline After-Pains

Occurrence—24–48 hours postoperatively
Duration—6 hours to 3 days
Distribution—Chest, abdomen, shoulders, neck and pharyngeal muscles
Incidence—Men: 20%–30%
             Women: 30%–40%
             Children: Very rare
Treatment—Rest, aspirin, local heat
Prevention—Avoidance of Scoline. It is also claimed that a small dose of a non-depolarizing relaxant administered prior to the Scoline will reduce the incidence and severity of this symptom. We have been unable to substantiate the claim that the administration of Vitamin C in large doses reduces the incidence of these pains.

Scoline Apnoea

This is the term applied to the occasional prolonged action of the drug which results in a period of apnoea lasting for hours rather than the customary 2 minutes. It is due to a shortage of pseudocholinesterase in the patient's blood, this enzyme being normally responsible for the rapid breakdown of suxamethonium in the body. This disability is usually familial but may be a consequence of liver damage resulting from disease or chemical poison. The only essential treatment is the performance of adequate artificial ventilation, until such time as satisfactory spontaneous breathing is resumed. This usually occurs naturally, but it is possible to assist matters by the transfusion of fresh blood (assumed to contain normal pseudocholinesterase content), or the administration of the relevant extract 'cholase', if available.

Scoline and Hyperkalaemia

Scoline should only be given with caution to patients suffering from any condition associated with hyperkalaemia (high blood potassium level), in view of the recorded association between this condition and cardiac arrest. The most common of these conditions are severe burns, advanced renal disease and, occasionally, paraplegia.

Decamethonium.—Dosage—2·5–5 mg
Onset of paralysis—1–2 minutes
Duration of paralysis—15–20 minutes
Side effects—Mild fasciculation, salivation, occasional prolonged action, muscular
         after-pains—usually mild.

Decamethonium After-Pains.—Not as severe as those following suxamethonium. Pains are usually confined to calf and jaw muscles.

Decamethonium Apnoea.—Prolonged action may be reversed by the administration of pentamethonium which, however, has such serious hypotensive side effects that its use is not considered justified.

CHOICE OF ANAESTHETIC METHOD FOR INTUBATION

There are a number of ways of achieving conditions suitable for endotracheal intubation, and we will now describe five methods in common use.

1. **Blind Nasal Intubation** (See page 370)

This is the only method of intubation which does not require profound relaxation of jaw and laryngeal musculature, since the tube is introduced *via* the nose 'blindly' into the trachea without the use of a laryngoscope. The method is of particular value for patients in whom jaw opening is limited, and therefore laryngoscopy difficult or impossible to perform. Also the avoidance of laryngoscopy in patients with delicate upper incisor crowns can be valuable. For ordinary routine use, the method carries the disadvantage that any foreign material picked up by the tip of the tube in its passage through the nose will be carried, unbeknown to the anaesthetist, into the trachea. In addition, even in highly skilled hands, the failure rate is higher than that encountered in the direct-vision methods. There are several ways of performing blind intubation, but the following has proved the most successful in our hands. Induction of anaesthesia designed to give minimal respiratory depression is continued with nitrous oxide, oxygen, 1% halothane and 7–10% carbon dioxide until marked hyperventilation occurs. In response to this respiratory stimulus, the glottis opens widely during inspiration and the tube can be passed readily through the abducted vocal cords into the trachea. Success depends largely upon the achievement of the correct position of the patient's head in relationship to the curvature of the tube selected (Fig. 120). Mastery of this technique can only be obtained by constant practical experience. Once intubation has been achieved, the carbon dioxide is discontinued and anaesthesia deepened by increasing the halothane concentration in order to facilitate pharyngeal packing. Subsequently, anaesthesia is at a light level, but deep enough to avoid coughing on the tube; this level can usually be achieved with nitrous oxide, oxygen and 0·5–1 % halothane.

2. Light Anaesthesia and Scoline

The onset of anaesthesia is immediately followed by administration of a paralysing dose of suxamethonium (usually 50–100 mg). As soon as muscle fasciculation commences, an oropharyngeal airway is inserted, and the patient's lungs are inflated with oxygen five or six times. Any resistance to such inflation indicates either an upper respiratory obstruction which must be corrected, or more rarely, bronchospasm (page 148). The pharyngeal airway is now removed and the endotracheal tube passed through the nose until the tip lies in the pharynx, from whence, under direct vision laryngoscopy and sometimes with the aid of Magill's Introducing Forceps, it is manipulated through the paralysed vocal cords into the trachea. The lungs are inflated with nitrous oxide, oxygen and 2% halothane until spontaneous respiration returns, so long as this period does not exceed 3 minutes, after which time the halothane concentration should be reduced to not more than 0·5%. Anaesthesia can subsequently be maintained in the manner described previously. The use of Scoline carries the advantage that with the minimum delay, the anaesthetist is presented with ideal conditions (complete muscular paralysis) under which to perform laryngoscopy and intubation; thus the method is of particular value whenever any technical intubation difficulty is anticipated. It does, however, carry the disadvantages associated with the use of depolarizing muscle relaxants, namely the commonly occurring Scoline after-pains, and the much less common Scoline apnoea.

3. Light Anaesthesia and Non-Depolarizing Relaxant

With this technique, the use of suxamethonium is avoided by the administration of a paralysing dose of a non-depolarizing muscle relaxant. Good, but not always perfect, intubating conditions will be achieved within 1·5–4 minutes, the exact time depending upon the relaxant chosen. Since this technique will achieve paralysis, or gross impairment, of the respiratory musculature for a considerable period of time, adequate manual or mechanical ventilation of the lungs throughout the operative procedure is mandatory. In the average subject, maintenance can be achieved at a light level of anaesthesia with nitrous oxide and oxygen only, but the addition of 0·5% halothane may be necessary in resistant cases. Postoperative reversal of the relaxant by neostigmine is essential after using the full paralysing dose, and occasionally, when the operation is completed within 15–20 minutes, full reversal may prove difficult to achieve.

4. Deep Anaesthesia with Halothane

It is possible to produce sufficient muscular relaxation for laryngoscopy and intubation with nitrous oxide, oxygen and halothane. To achieve the necessary depth of anaesthesia will frequently take 5–7 minutes using 4% halothane. The great advantage of this technique is that it avoids the use of both types of muscle relaxant. Thus, on the one hand the patient is spared the discomfort of Scoline after-pains, and on the other, the anaesthetist is spared the problems sometimes associated with the reversal of non-depolarizing relaxants.

Maintenance is achieved with nitrous oxide and halothane, the latter being reduced to 0·5%.

The method is particularly suitable for children, in whom a 3–4 minute induction period usually suffices.

5. Halothane and Non-Depolarizing Relaxant

It is possible to shorten the induction period described in the preceding technique, by administering a non-depolarizing muscle relaxant in about one half its full paralysing dose, followed by a rapid increase in halothane concentration using assisted respiration. An oropharyngeal airway is inserted as soon as jaw relaxation will permit, and the patient's lungs are inflated with nitrous oxide, oxygen and up to 4% halothane *via* a facemask; conditions suitable for laryngoscopy and intubation are obtained within a total induction time of two to four minutes. Successful inflation of the lungs—without the production of gastric distension—can be achieved with a face mask provided such inflation is only attempted in the presence of a completely unobstructed airway, and when a considerable degree of muscular relaxation has been achieved. Following even small doses of non-depolarizing relaxant, the patient will require artificial ventilation after intubation, until such time as full spontaneous respiration is resumed. Anaesthesia is maintained with nitrous oxide, oxygen, and 0·5% halothane. Provided the operation takes 20 minutes or longer, we have found that a dose of 5–7 mg Alloferin does not usually require reversal, full spontaneous respiration being resumed on the cessation of manual or mechanical ventilation. Spraying the vocal cords with 4% lignocaine may facilitate intubation, but the consequent impairment of the laryngeal protective reflexes for about 30 minutes must be taken into consideration.

SUMMARY OF METHODS

The choice of method of intubation and maintenance must be the anaesthetist's individual decision, depending upon his experience and the type of conditions he requires. We favour either the combination of Alloferin and halothane or the deep halothane method for minor oral surgery of short duration in the uncomplicated adult out-patient, as these techniques avoid the use of suxamethonium, and do not require the administration of neostigmine; for the inexperienced anaesthetist and the technically difficult intubation, the use of suxamethonium may be justified in spite of the incidence of after-pains.

The technique which entails the use of a full paralysing dose of a non-depolarizing relaxant carries the advantages of avoidance of halothane, extubation which is usually unaccompanied by signs of laryngeal irritation, and rapid symptom-free recovery; the disadvantages are those inherent in the routine use of neostigmine in the out-patient, occasional difficulties in achieving full reversal, and any purely technical problems which may be associated with the use of controlled ventilation. In short procedures (less than 30 minutes) on children, hand-ventilation with unsupplemented nitrous oxide and oxygen using a Jackson-Rees circuit and intermittent Scoline has been used successfully (see page 272).

Nasotracheal intubation is usually used in dentistry for obvious reasons, but either nasal or oral methods can be employed with the techniques outlined, except for the 'blind' method which is confined to the nasal route.

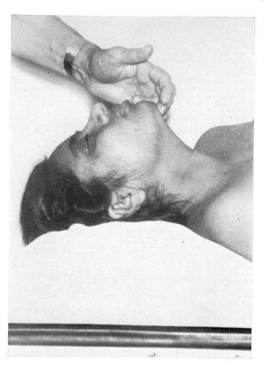

FIG. 120—Position of head in 'sniffing air' position with shoulders and head supported by pillow

Technique of Laryngoscopy and Intubation

Laryngoscopy can only be satisfactorily learned by practical instruction and experience, and therefore in the succeeding paragraphs we will attempt only to draw attention to certain aspects of technique which we feel are occasionally neglected.

1. Before preparing the patient for laryngoscopy, it is essential to ensure that the laryngoscope is working properly and that the under surface of its blade is lubricated; that a pair of Magill forceps, the necessary equipment for inflating the lungs, and suction apparatus are all immediately to hand.

2. Correct positioning of the patient's head in the 'sniffing air' position (Fig. 120) should be ensured.

3. Before attempting laryngoscopy, it is essential that good jaw relaxation is obtained.

4. When performing laryngoscopy, it is important to take the following precautions:

(a) The lips and tongue must be protected from trauma sustained by catching them between the teeth and the blade of the laryngoscope,

(b) The upper incisor teeth must be protected from damage by pressure from the laryngoscope blade, for the tooth enamel can easily be chipped or expensive crowns broken, unless some form of protection is used (Fig. 121).

5. When lifting the tongue and associated structures to visualize the glottis, care must be exercised not to overstretch the pillars of the fauces on the right side and thus damage the overlying mucous membrane; this is particularly likely to occur when using a Macintosh laryngoscope.

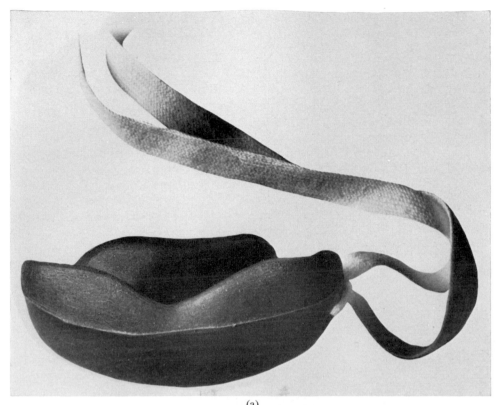

(a)

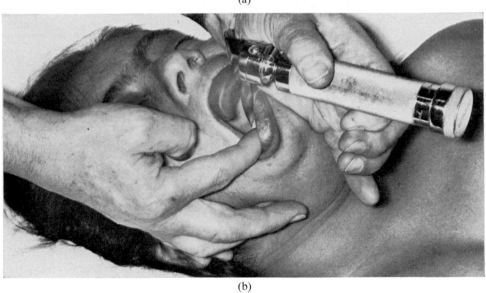

(b)

FIG. 121—A O'Leary dentgard   B Laryngoscopy

NOTE—1. Upper teeth protected by dentgard.   2. Lower lip has been prevented from being caught
between teeth and laryngoscope blade by right index finger

265

6. Care must be taken to select the correct size of tube for the patient. In nasal intubation, the largest tube which will pass freely through one or other nostril should be used. In adults, this size will readily pass the normal glottis, but very occasionally in children, the glottis may be smaller than the nasal passage. The passage of a tube through the nose may be facilitated by lubrication of the tube and by prior spraying of the nasal mucosa with 10% cocaine—or other vasoconstrictor. The length of the tube should be predetermined by measuring it against the side of the neck from nares to 2·5 cm beyond the lower border of cricoid cartilage. In oral intubation, the largest tube which will, without the use of any force, readily pass the glottis, should be used.

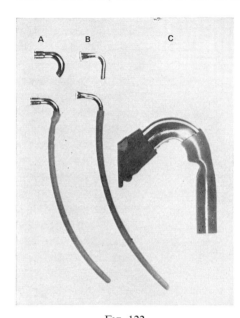

FIG. 122

A   Magill nasal connection
B   Doughty nasal connection
Potential point of kinking with highly
curved Magill connection

Its length is predetermined by measuring it against the distance from mouth to 2·5 cm beyond the lower border of cricoid cartilage.

7. Having intubated the trachea, it is essential to make sure that the tube remains *in situ* and cannot be advanced further into the right main bronchus. This can be confirmed, after fixing the tube in its final position, by inflating the lungs, and checking that both sides of the chest move equally; if in doubt, good air entry into both lungs should be confirmed with a stethoscope.

8. Finally, having fixed the tube and packed the pharynx, it is important to be satisfied that there is no kinking or obstruction in the tube to restrict the passage of gas through it. Whilst kinking of a soft nasal tube may occur anywhere in its course, special attention should be paid to the vulnerable site of junction of tube and connection (see Fig. 122). In particular, fixation at the nostril should ensure no drag or distortion. Kinking may also occur when the oral route is selected, for which many anaesthetists routinely employ some type of reinforced tube.

Attention will now be drawn to two difficulties which may be encountered.

(a) In spite of normal positioning of the head for nasal intubation, the tube will sometimes approach the glottis from the nasopharynx in such a way that the tip of the tube impacts at the anterior commissure of the cords. In the adult, this can usually be rectified by removal of the laryngoscope, and flexion of the head and neck whilst exerting gentle pressure on the tube. Occasionally, however, and particularly in the child, it may be necessary to manipulate the tube through the glottis with the aid of Magill's forceps.

(b) In certain subjects, in spite of perfect relaxation and positioning, it is extremely difficult or even impossible to visualize the larynx. This situation may be encountered in patients with one or more of the following features: small receding chin, prominent upper teeth, poor mouth opening, fixed or short neck, rigid epiglottis. In these patients, it is usually possible to see the arytenoid cartilages directly, and the view of the glottis may be improved if an assistant applies gentle external pressure to the thyroid cartilage. It is nearly always possible to manipulate a nasal tube into the glottic opening with the assistance of Magill's forceps, but when anatomical difficulty is extreme, the introduction of an oral tube may require the aid of a lubricated malleable copper or lead introducer, which should, therefore, always be readily

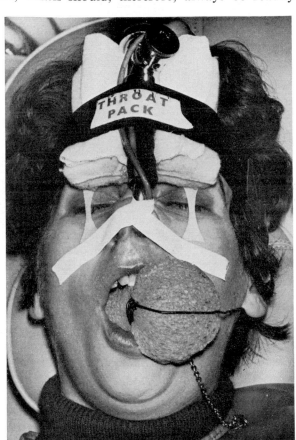

FIG. 123.—Method of fixing nasotracheal tube

It is possible to dispense with the strapping fixing the tube provided that the head-towels are correctly secured, and there is no 'drag' on the tube from the unsupported weight of the expiratory valve mount

NOTE.—Use of cuffed tube to allow artificial ventilation
Throat pack label
Protection of eyes by using butterfly sutures which do not stick to eye lashes
Use of flanged cellulose mouth pack to minimize soiling of pharyngeal pack and protect tongue from trauma

available. It should be remembered that the use of such an introducer will require that a suitable open ended connection (e.g. Nosworthy or Cobb) is employed from the outset.

Miscellaneous Technical Points

We recommend that the tube is fixed in the manner shown in Fig. 123, and that the eyes are protected by ensuring that the lids remain closed. It is beneficial to lubricate the lips with petroleum jelly.

Pharyngeal Packing (see page 345)

Although the presence of an endotracheal tube facilitates airway control, contamination of the lungs by foreign material from the operation site can only be prevented by the use of either a cuffed tube or pharyngeal pack. We consider it advisable to introduce the pack under direct vision laryngoscopy with the use of Magill's forceps, rather than blindly with the finger, since this latter method is clearly less controlled. It cannot be stressed too strongly that the delicate pharyngeal mucosa should always be treated with the utmost care if severe sore throat and other more serious types of trauma are to be avoided. Gauze soaked in a water soluble grease such as polyethylene glycol, and wrung out until damp, may be used. It is neither necessary nor advisable to pack the pharynx tightly. The minimum possible material should be used to 'surround' the endotracheal tube, in conjunction with a mouth pack as described on page 123, the pharyngeal pack thus acting as a last line of defence. If a cuffed tube (Fig. 123) and mouth packing are used, it may be possible to dispense with the pharyngeal pack altogether. Not only should gentleness be shown in placing the pack in the pharynx, but also in removing it at the conclusion of the operation, and this we prefer to do under direct vision laryngoscopy. There is a real danger that the pack may be forgotten and the tube removed with the pack *in situ*. This oversight may lead to a potentially fatal obstruction, as the jaws may be very difficult to open in light anaesthesia. The routine performance of pre-extubation laryngoscopy will not only ensure that this catastrophe never occurs, but will enable the anaesthetist to suck out the pharynx efficiently with a rigid pharyngeal sucker (Fig. 26). Other recommended safeguards against leaving a pack in the pharynx are that the end of the pack should be left protruding from the mouth throughout the operation, and that a suitable label be affixed to the face (Fig. 123). **Extubation and Recovery.**—Extubation should be performed following removal of the pharyngeal pack and gentle suction. Insertion of an oropharyngeal airway may prove necessary. It is most important to apply haemostatic packs over the operation sites in order to prevent any trickle of blood reaching the pharynx after removal of the pharyngeal pack and tube. These haemostatic packs should always be secured outside the mouth.

Extubation can be a worrying phase owing to the risk of it provoking laryngeal spasm. This risk is said to be minimized if withdrawal of the tube coincides exactly with either an inspiration or an expiration, but we consider the depth of anaesthesia to be a more important factor. Anaesthesia should be either sufficiently deep to avoid hyperactivity of the larynx, or sufficiently light for an active swallowing reflex to be present. If the former level of anaesthesia is employed, extubation should be carried out with the patient lying on his side, and it is under these conditions that an oropharyngeal airway will be tolerated. With the latter method, the patient will not need or tolerate an artificial airway, but should be placed on his side at the earliest possible opportunity. If extubation provokes spasm or breath-holding, oxygen should be administered *via* a face mask.

The patient should recover lying down undisturbed. By adopting this procedure, the incidence of nausea and vomiting is reduced. Since all anti-emetic drugs are to some extent sedative and thus delay recovery, it is wiser to reserve their use for the out-patient with a history of severe post-anaesthetic nausea, rather than give them routinely. When used, the dose should be small, e.g. perphenazine 1mg intravenously. After at least half an hour's recumbency, the patient may be allowed to sit up, receive all postoperative instructions, and finally to leave as soon as he is judged fit to travel home. The total time required until discharge varies widely, but most patients are ready to leave for home within an hour of the operation being completed.

Final Instructions

Before final discharge, it is necessary to make certain that the patient knows exactly what to do should any complication arise. He should be told that postoperative pain can be treated with simple analgesics; Scoline after-pains with analgesics and rest; sore throat with soluble aspirin gargle; and haemorrhage with local pressure. In addition, the patient should be warned that he may suffer some non-specific malaise during the ensuing 48 hours or so, and should be prepared to miss work or school for 2 or 3 days if this proves necessary; also, a period of postoperative bed rest may be advisable. Under no circumstances should the whole surgical and anaesthetic procedure be 'underplayed', for if it is, any postoperative sequelae will come as a shock and a disappointment to the patient who will then assume that something has gone wrong. Out-patient treatment of the minor oral surgical case, particularly that requiring intubation, is a most valuable facility to be able to offer, but such treatment should never be undertaken lightly or approached casually, for if it is, the method will surely fall rapidly into disrepute. In particular, the occasional sequelae of intubation such as pharyngitis, laryngitis, tracheitis, bronchitis or traumatic damage to teeth, lips or respiratory mucosa dictate that the method should only be used when it is considered unavoidable.

MANAGEMENT OF ANAESTHESIA IN THE IN-PATIENT

It is proposed now to consider the routine management of the normal patient admitted to hospital for minor oral surgery. The special management of patients admitted for medical reasons will be described separately.

The Healthy Patient

Admission

It is customary and often convenient to admit the patient on the afternoon or evening prior to operation, so that a medical examination, including necessary investigations may be carried out. However, should circumstances dictate, there is no objection to admission on the day of the operation, provided sufficient time is allowed for the normal routine preparation.

Routine Assessment

The routine medical assessment of these patients will not necessarily differ from that described for the out-patient (page 257). A detailed medical history must always be taken, and since physical examination is both expected by the patient, and easily carried out, we suggest that it should be routinely performed.

Night Sedation

Most patients, in the unfamiliar surroundings of hospital welcome a mild night sedative such as nitrazepam (Mogadon) or one of the suitable barbiturates. Very nervous patients will benefit from a course of tranquillizers (e.g. diazepam 5 mg t.d.s.) commencing several days prior to admission.

Premedication

Admission to hospital does not render premedication mandatory, and each case demands individual assessment. It should be borne in mind that the major disadvantage, namely that of delayed recovery is not so potent a consideration in the in-patient as in the out-patient, and therefore powerful premedicant drugs may be used with greater freedom. The range of drugs available for use is very wide (see Chapter 2), and below are given but a few examples of commonly used methods together with suitable dosage for the healthy adult.

1. *Papaveretum (Omnopon) and hyoscine (Scopolamine).*—This time honoured mixture is still widely used for the nervous patient. Given as a single intramuscular injection, (Omnopon 20 mg, Scopolamine 0·4 mg), within 20 minutes it will produce a pleasant sense of relaxation, drowsiness, euphoria, and amnesia. Postoperatively, the analgesic effects of Omnopon will often be an advantage. On the other hand, the incidence of post-anaesthetic nausea and vomiting is undoubtedly increased by the use of Omnopon, which should either be avoided or accompanied by a powerful anti-emetic in patients with a tendency towards nausea. Scopolamine is itself a mild anti-emetic, and as such is a valuable constituent of the mixture, but its powerful drying effect doubtless contributes to both the incidence and severity of post-operative sore throat. Omnopon is, of course, a powerful respiratory depressant, but in normal dosage, this is seldom a significant disadvantage, and the depressant effect on glottic reflex activity usually assists in smooth intubation and subsequent toleration of the tube. This depressant effect may interfere slightly with the efficacy of the 'protective' reflexes in the immediate postoperative period—hence the necessity for strict adherence to the post-extubation procedure described on page 268. This combination of drugs is poorly tolerated by the elderly, debilitated and shocked patient, and if used, the dose must be reduced accordingly.

2. *Pethidine and Promethazine (Phenergan).*—This combination given intramuscularly (Pethidine 50 mg, Phenergan 25 mg) can be conveniently prescribed as Pamergan P 100, 1 ml, and is particularly useful for bronchitic patients. Phenergan is not only a bronchodilator, but also a powerful anti-emetic. If analgesia is not required, Phenergan may be used by itself in dosage up to 50 mg.

3. *Oral Premedication.*—For the less nervous patient, or the patient who wishes to avoid an injection, any sedative or tranquillizer can be given orally with a sip of water one hour preoperatively. The combination of butobarbitone (Soneryl) and promethazine (Phenergan) can be conveniently prescribed as Sonergan, each tablet of which contains Soneryl 75 mg, Phenergan 15 mg. Two such tablets comprise a satisfactory premedicant dose. Diazepam 10 mg is a suitable mild tranquillizer which does not appear significantly to delay recovery, but some claim that it should be avoided if the use of a non-depolarizing relaxant is contemplated. It will be noted that atropine has not been recommended in any of these premedications. We hold the view that this drug should be given intravenously immediately prior to induction when it is used, as unpleasant subjective symptoms result from its intramuscular administration.

Induction, Maintenance and Recovery

Management does not differ materially from that described for the out-patient. Thiopentone may be freely used for induction, since rapid recovery to ambulation is not of paramount importance. Likewise, both analgesics and anti-emetics can be used if indicated, with less regard to their prolonged sedative properties.

It has been suggested that if suxamethonium has been used to accomplish intubation, the patient should remain in bed postoperatively for 48 hours, in order to minimize the incidence and severity of after-pains. We believe that this is an unjustifiable restriction, since in the majority of patients suxamethonium can be avoided by using one of the other methods of induction described earlier in this chapter.

TABLE XXIII.—*A Guide to Endotracheal Tube Size in Children*

Age Years	Weight kg	lbs	Magill No.	B.S. Diameter Internal
1	10	21	1	4·5
2	13	28	2	5·0
3	15	33	2	5·0
5	18	40	3	5·5
7	23	50	4	6·0
8	26	53	5	6·5
10	30	66	6	7·0
11	36	80	7	—
12	40	88	7·5	—
14	45	100	8	8·0
16	54	120	8 or 9	9·0

The Magill No. can be based on formula $\frac{Age}{2} + 1$

The B.S. internal diameter size can be based on the formula $\frac{Age}{4} + 4.5$

These figures are for non-cuffed plain tubes.

Discharge from Hospital

When circumstances permit, it is advisable to give the patient one clear day in hospital between operation and discharge, but ultimately, the length of stay will be a matter for individual assessment.

Special Considerations in Child Intubation

Children tolerate out-patient intubation very well, provided adequate recovery facilities are available.

The dentition should be carefully checked for the presence of any loose teeth.

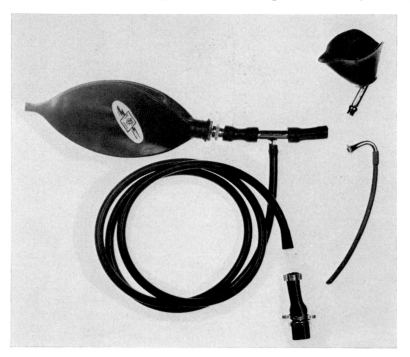

FIG. 124.—Mapleson (E) Circuit. (Jackson Rees)

It is sometimes taught that nasal intubation should be avoided in children owing to the risk of provoking haemorrhage from adenoidal tissue. We have not ourselves found this to be a particular problem, but we recommend that blind intubation should be avoided owing to the risk of a foreign body (e.g. button) being carried by the tip of the tube from the nose into the trachea. It is important that the correct size of tube should be selected, since in children a tube small enough to enter the nares may be too large to pass through the glottis. Table XXIII will act as a rough guide to the size suitable for the child's age. It cannot be emphasized too strongly that great care must be taken to fasten the nasal tube in such a way that kinking does not occur

TABLE XXIV

	Age Years	Weight kg	Weight lbs	Tidal v. ml	Resp. rate Resp/min	Min. vol. 1/min	Recommended minimal flow-rate 1/min
	1	10	21	78	45	3·5	7·0
A	2	13	28	136	30	4·0	8·0
	5	18	40	215	28	5·0	10·0
	7	23	50	300	22	6·5	6·0
B	10	30	66	400	18	7·0	6·5
	14	45	100	450	16	7·2	6·5
	16	54	120	500	15	7·5	7·0

This table gives a guide to the minimal gas flow-rates which should be employed at various ages. *Note.* Age 1–5, a T-piece circuit, such as the Jackson Rees (Fig. 124) should be used and the flow-rate should be twice minute volume (A).

Age 5–adult, a Magill circuit may be used and the flow-rate can be just below the minute volume (B).

within the nares at the point of junction of the connection and tube. We favour the use of a long Doughty oral connection firmly secured in such a way that the weight of the expiratory mount does not drag on the tube.

Owing to the relatively anterior position of the larynx in children, the nasal tube usually has to be lifted forward with Magill forceps into the glottis. This manipulation may be facilitated by the use of Scoline which very rarely gives rise to after-pains in children.

For maintenance, children may be allowed to breathe spontaneously using nitrous oxide, oxygen and halothane. Alternatively, they may be paralysed using curare for long (over 40 minutes) cases, or intermittent suxamethonium for shorter cases; when relaxants are used, anaesthesia is maintained by artificial ventilation with nitrous oxide and oxygen using a high flow-rate, hyperventilation and a suitable non-rebreathing circuit. Whichever technique is selected, it is essential in the under 4-year old to use a special paediatric circuit (Fig. 124) if anaesthesia is to be prolonged, and this will demand the use of gas flow-rates approximately twice the expected minute volume (see Table XXIV).

Intubation in the child on an out-patient basis has sometimes been held to be unjustifiable on the grounds that post-extubation laryngeal oedema could develop after discharge home. If the child is supervised until he is able to speak and swallow normally, we believe that this risk does not exist.

RECOMMENDED READING

BROWNE, D. (1969) A Guide to Tracheal Tubes. *Anaesthesia*, **24**, 620.
ELLIS, F. R. (1973) Malignant Hyperpyrexia. *Anaesthesia*, **28**, 245.

CHAPTER FOURTEEN

GENERAL ANAESTHESIA FOR THE MEDICALLY UNFIT

It is proposed in this chapter to discuss certain medical conditions which influence the nature of anaesthetic care in dentistry.

A. CARDIOVASCULAR DISEASE

Patients suffering from cardiovascular disease may be divided into two categories; those with healed cardiac lesions and normal cardiovascular function; and those with cardiovascular disease resulting in the signs and symptoms accompanying circulatory insufficiency.

1. Disease with Normal Function

Healed valvular and congenital cardiac disease renders the patient a potential victim of subacute bacterial endocarditis following exposure to bacteraemia. The scarred valve and congenitally abnormal heart are particularly susceptible to infection with *Streptococcus viridans*, which may be released into the blood-stream following extraction and scaling of teeth, or root canal therapy. Whilst not requiring any special consideration in anaesthetic management these patients require full antibiotic cover during the period of dental treatment, in addition to special care in extraction technique.

The antibiotic cover must be bactericidal rather than bacteriostatic, and whilst penicillin is the drug of choice, there are certain circumstances in which other agents must be used.

We suggest the use of one of the following regimen.

(i) **When penicillin is not contraindicated.**—Benzylpenicillin 600 mg (1 mega unit) given by intramuscular injection half an hour preoperatively, and followed by the oral administration of phenoxymethyl penicillin (Penicillin V), 250 mg six-hourly for 3 days.

(ii) **When penicillin is contraindicated, other than because of hypersensitivity.**—Cephaloridine, 500 mg given by intramuscular injection half an hour preoperatively, and followed by the oral administration of erythromycin estolate, 250 mg six-hourly for 3 days. This regime is most commonly indicated when the patient has received penicillin therapy within the previous 8 weeks; or when he has been treated with small doses of penicillin as an intended prophylaxis against the recurrence of rheumatic fever.

(iii) **When the patient is hypersensitive to penicillin.**—Erythromycin estolate, 500 mg by mouth two hours preoperatively, followed by 250 mg six-hourly for 3 days. In these cases, cephaloridine is avoided since there is some degree of cross allergenicity between penicillin and the cephalosporins.

It should be noted, that in no circumstances is the administration of antibiotics on the day prior to operation recommended, since sensitive strains of *Streptococcus viridans* may be rapidly replaced by resistant ones.

If dentistry is multiquadrant, the use of general anaesthesia, by enabling it to be completed under one antibiotic course, may be considered especially indicated.

2. Disease with Circulatory Impairment

Many important factors relevant to initial assessment of the cardiac case have already been discussed on page 2. The conclusion reached was that cardiac disease *per se* does not usually constitute a contraindication to general anaesthesia, provided that the anaesthetic is administered by an experienced physician. The first duty of the anaesthetist is to assess whether the cardiac state of the patient can be improved by treatment, for if it can, the dental procedure should be delayed until optimum medical conditions have been achieved. Both the treatment required, and the assessment of its maximum efficacy should be matters for full consultation with the patient's general physicians or cardiologist.

Preparatory treatment may often involve admission of the patient to hospital for a short period of observation, bed-rest, and any other therapy indicated. But admission to hospital for purely medical reasons must never be allowed to dictate the anaesthetic technique, which should always be the simplest possible to achieve safely the requisite surgical conditions. Moreover, it is sometimes said that a cardiac patient should be admitted to hospital in order to have a 'proper anaesthetic'—i.e. one in which the airway is protected by endotracheal intubation. We disagree with this approach, for it ignores the many practical hazards which may arise unexpectedly during the intubation and extubation procedures. Thus, any case, in which intubation is not justified on surgical grounds (see page 253), should certainly not be subjected to these hazards on the grounds of cardiac disease.

There are many reasons for undertaking general anaesthesia on the cardiac case in the hospital environment, and often as an in-patient. These reasons include the ready availability of full resuscitation and nursing facilities, and the frequent necessity for preoperative medical care, as described. The hospital which undertakes treatment of these cases should provide facilities for every type of dental anaesthetic, including the simple unintubated variety so often most satisfactorily undertaken in a conventional dental chair, in which the full posture range can be readily achieved.

The following account draws attention to the points in anaesthetic management which we consider to be of particular importance in these patients, assuming that the necessary treatment to achieve maximum improvement in the circulatory state has already been undertaken.

Premedication

If there is no contraindication to treatment as an out-patient, the close personal contact which exists under these circumstances between patient and anaesthetist will generally render premedication unnecessary. Likewise, the in-patient who can be treated in the dental chair with a simple anaesthetic, rarely requires premedication, but occasionally a simple sedative may be of value.

The in-patient who has to be taken on a trolley to the operating theatre and who will subsequently require endotracheal anaesthesia, is easier to manage following premedication with papaveretum 20 mg and hyoscine 0·4 mg, although this dose may have to be reduced (page 270). The anxiolytic effect of this combination is of particular importance in the cardiac case, and outweighs the disadvantages associated with the slight resultant respiratory depression. Drugs known to be powerful circulatory depressants (e.g. the phenothiazines) are best avoided, but diazepam given intravenously by the anaesthetist immediately before the journey from ward to theatre may prove a useful alternative to papaveretum and hyoscine, provided the risk of postural hypotension and the profound effect of a small dose on the elderly is borne in mind.

Pre-oxygenation

Inhalation of 100% oxygen for at least 2 minutes prior to the induction of anaesthesia is always advisable provided that the patient does not find this distressing.

Induction of Anaesthesia

General Principles

Since the induction of anaesthesia should not be unduly prolonged or accompanied by any excitement, an intravenous method is preferable. However, most intravenous anaesthetic agents may cause both a fall in peripheral resistance and a decrease in cardiac output. Thus it is most important that these drugs should always be administered slowly and cautiously to the cardiac case, particularly if limited output is a feature of the disease (e.g. severe mitral stenosis). The same precaution applies when the diastolic blood pressure is abnormally low (i.e. aortic regurgitation), for any further fall may seriously imperil the coronary circulation. These principles do not infer that anaesthesia should be kept at a lighter level than is customary. Indeed, it is particularly important that cardiac patients should not be subjected to surgical stimulation at an inadequate level of anaesthesia; nor does slow injection imply a tedious induction, but simply that none of the quick methods of induction (e.g. 'surge' technique, page 210) with a predetermined weight based dosage should ever be used. The intravenous drug should be titrated against effect, the pulse being continuously monitored or palpated, and injection should cease as soon as the desired level of anaesthesia is adjudged to have been reached.

The posture of the cardiac patient during induction is of particular importance. The factors influencing choice of posture have been fully discussed in Chapter 8. Here, it must be stressed that pulmonary congestion of cardiac origin usually gives rise to breathlessness when lying flat (orthopnoea), and in these cases such a posture is contraindicated. The majority of cardiac cases are best anaesthetized in the posture in which they themselves are most comfortable. Any alteration in posture required by the surgeon following induction, must be achieved gradually and only after due consideration of its possible effects on the circulatory state.

Induction for the Intubated Case

The foregoing principles apply in equal force irrespective of whether or not intubation is to be performed. The method of induction for intubation will, in part, depend upon the intended method of maintenance. If a technique which permits spontaneous respiration is to be used, intubation is best accomplished with the aid of suxamethonium. We justify the use of this drug in cardiac cases on the following grounds:

  (i) Optimal conditions for intubation are produced, thus reducing the risk of encountering technical difficulty likely to result in a hypoxic episode.

 (ii) The 'blind' method is unsuitable because there is a risk of provoking cardiac dysrhythmia during or immediately following intubation under light anaesthesia.

(iii) Deep halothane is undesirable on account of its cardiotoxic properties.

The dose of suxamethonium should secure paralysis of sufficient duration to enable surgical anaesthesia to be achieved prior to the return of spontaneous respiration, thus preventing the breath-holding and straining which may result from the presence of a tube in the trachea of an inadequately anaesthetized patient.

If the method of maintenance incorporates controlled respiration, intubation may be achieved with the aid of a full paralysing dose of a non-depolarizing muscle relaxant. Pancuronium or Curare for the long case, Alloferin for the shorter case, will provide good intubating conditions with minimum circulatory disturbance. It is important to allow sufficient time to elapse to achieve these conditions (2 to 3 minutes), during which respiration is manually assisted and anaesthesia maintained with nitrous oxide, at least 30% oxygen and 1% halothane.

Induction for the Unintubated Case

The induction in these cases should follow the general principles laid down earlier, using an intravenous agent followed by nitrous oxide, at least 30% oxygen, and halothane.

Maintenance

General Principles

Since cardiac arrest is more likely to result from minor anaesthetic imperfections in the cardiac than in the normal patient, the anaesthetist is well advised to monitor the heart or pulse continuously irrespective of the anaesthetic technique used. In addition, a high oxygen content in the inspired mixture (30%–50%) should be a feature of any chosen technique.

The Intubated Case

The anaesthetist has a choice between two main methods of maintenance.

 (i) **Spontaneous Respiration.**—Provided that there is no central or peripheral depression of respiratory activity, spontaneous respiration may be permitted following intubation.

Anaesthesia should be maintained at a light level, but sufficiently deep to prevent reaction to both surgical stimulation and the presence of tube in trachea. Halothane is the agent most commonly used, but it must be remembered that when administered in the presence of a raised pCO_2, cardiac dysrhythmias are likely to result. Thus, if spontaneous respiration is allowed, special care must be taken to avoid undue respiratory resistance which might result from the use of a nasal tube of restricted calibre or an ill-designed connection. Moreover, if the slight respiratory depression which can result from heavy premedication persists in spite of surgical stimulation, it is wiser to paralyse the patient and proceed with controlled ventilation.

This technique is chiefly of value in the short (20 minutes) case.

(ii) **Controlled Respiration.**—It is possible to avoid the use of halothane altogether, or at least restrict the quantity used to 0·5 %, by employing an anaesthetic technique in which peripheral respiratory paralysis is achieved with the assistance of a long-acting muscle relaxant, and respiration is controlled throughout. Such a technique will achieve optimal pulmonary ventilation, and in so doing will ensure both a high pO_2 and low pCO_2-conditions highly desirable for the cardiac case, particularly in the presence of a dysrhythmogenic drug such as halothane. It is necessary to use a cuffed endotracheal tube in order to carry out efficient mechanical ventilation of the lungs, and this may rarely necessitate oral intubation which carries the disadvantage that the tube so placed often encroaches upon the operating field. It should be remembered that controlled intermittent positive pressure ventilation (I.P.P.V.), halothane and curarization are all factors which tend to lower the blood pressure.

Achievement of controlled respiration by the use of a non-depolarizing relaxant, will usually require reversal of the relaxant with neostigmine (see page 259) in order to establish adequate spontaneous respiration at the conclusion of the operation.

The Unintubated Case

Maintenance should follow the general principles laid down earlier, perfect airway control being essential at all times. Liberal oxygenation and a stable level of anaesthesia with halothane should enable smooth, incident-free operating conditions to be achieved in the vast majority of straightforward short extraction cases.

Recovery

All cases should receive oxygen supplementation during the recovery period.

Extubation

The principles enumerated on page 268 should be strictly adhered to, and since the cardiac case will normally be undertaken as an in-patient, we recommend that extubation should be performed at a level of anaesthesia in which the laryngeal reflexes are still depressed. 0·5% halothane in oxygen may be administered for a minute or so prior to extubation, which should be performed with the patient in the lateral position. Extubation is immediately followed by the administration of 100% oxygen *via* a face mask, and as soon as the anaesthetist is satisfied that adequate spontaneous respiration has been firmly established, this oxygen therapy may be continued with an air-oxygen mixture delivered from a standard venturi mask. As soon as the patient is fully conscious, he should be allowed to resume the posture of maximum comfort, and oxygen therapy may be discontinued unless the patient's condition demands more prolonged administration.

The foregoing account summarizes the general principles governing the management of all cardiac cases. The following specific conditions warrant special mention:

Coronary Insufficiency

A clear history of coronary infarction within the past 6 months is normally taken to indicate that general anaesthesia should be avoided whenever possible.

The presence of anginal pain on effort indicates a severe degree of coronary insufficiency, which may constitute a special anaesthetic hazard. All anaesthetic techniques tend to produce vasodilatation and if the coronary arteries are prevented by disease from participating in this dilatation, uncompensated hypotension will inevitably lead to coronary insufficiency. It is therefore those patients whose anginal pain is not normally adequately relieved by vasodilator drugs such as glyceryl trinitrate, who are at special risk, and for whom it is important to avoid general anaesthesia whenever possible. The patient who obtains ready relief from anginal pain, can be expected to tolerate carefully administered general anaesthesia, for his coronary arteries are likely to participate in the overall vasodilatation produced by the anaesthetic, cardiac perfusion thus being maintained. Premedication may, with benefit, include the patient's usual coronary dilator drug.

It should be further noted that aortic valvular disease which frequently results in constriction of the orifices of the coronary arteries, may be associated with occult coronary insufficiency.

Fixed Cardiac Output Disease

A number of cardiac diseases, such as severe valvular disease, constrictive pericarditis and certain cardiomyopathies, prevent the heart from increasing its stroke volume in response to changes in circulatory dynamics, particularly sudden vasodilatation.

Special caution has to be exercised with these patients during the intravenous induction of anaesthesia, as the resultant sudden vasodilatation may cause circulatory failure and death. General anaesthesia is best avoided.

Heart Block

Heart block may be congenital or ischaemic in origin, and is due to varying degrees of atrioventricular dissociation. Complete dissociation may produce a heart rate as low as 35/min, and is often characterized by bouts of sudden loss of consciousness due to gross reduction in cardiac output leading to cerebral ischaemia (Stokes-Adams Attack). Severe degrees always constitute a serious anaesthetic hazard, and merit full consultation with a cardiologist regarding the advisability of pre-anaesthetic treatment with drugs such as ephedrine. These cases should be anaesthetized in hospital with a full cardiac team and equipment (e.g. pacemaker) readily available.

So far as anaesthetic management is concerned, the general principles already outlined must be meticulously observed. In addition, inhalation agents such as cyclopropane, halothane and trichlorethylene should only be used in minimal dosage and with extreme caution; ether is the only inhalational supplement devoid of special risk. In consequence, full muscular paralysis with controlled respiration is the anaesthetic method of choice.

Hypovolaemic Shock

This condition is rarely associated with dental surgery, but may result from severe postoperative haemorrhage which requires general anaesthesia to establish control of the bleeding.

We do not consider that a detailed account of this complex subject is within the scope of this book, but the following points must be borne in mind:

1. Whenever possible the blood volume should be corrected by transfusion before anaesthesia is induced. Whole blood (warmed to body temperature by a suitable blood warmer) is ideal, but plasma or Macrodex 70 may be used in an emergency.
2. It must be remembered that whatever method is employed to induce anaesthesia, the patient will be extremely sensitive to the drug used, and will thus require a greatly reduced dose. This sensitivity will apply particularly to the intravenous hypnotic drugs, and is due to the intense peripheral vasoconstriction which accompanies hypovolaemia, thus increasing the relative proportion of the cardiac output (and hence the injected drug) which initially goes to the brain as compared with the rest of the body (see page 183). Liberal oxygenation is essential.
3. Ideally the external environmental temperature should be maintained at 33°C.
4. Careful use of the alpha adrenergic blocking agents may be justified in severe hypovolaemic shock, provided adequate fluid replacement is immediately available and its administration controlled by central venous pressure monitoring.
5. Very rarely, Isoprenalin 1 mg/100 ml at 8–10 drops/min may be indicated as a cardiac stimulant, but must only be administered under E.C.G. control, after correction of the hypovolaemic state. The same principles apply to the newer inotropic agents Glucagon and Dopamine.
6. Massive steroid therapy has been recommended.

B. RESPIRATORY DISEASE

The overall significance of respiratory disease, and the desirability of avoiding general anaesthesia have been briefly discussed on page 4. The following conditions merit further comments.

1. Upper Respiratory Infection

Whenever possible patients suffering from acute upper respiratory infection, such as the common cold or sinusitis, should wait for the infection to subside before a general anaesthetic is given, particularly if intubation is contemplated. We nevertheless consider that the common cold is not a contraindication to general anaesthesia in an emergency. Chronic sinusitis or catarrh often results in a continuous post-nasal mucus drip, which may result in laryngeal irritation. If general anaesthesia cannot be avoided, it is best carried out with the patient supine so that mucus tends to remain in the upper pharynx.

2. Lower Respiratory Infection

(a) **Acute Bronchitis and Pneumonia.**—These conditions constitute an absolute contra-indication to general anaesthesia for dental purposes.

(b) **Chronic Bronchitis and Emphysema.**—Chronic bronchitis is characterized by excessive secretions which may produce bouts of coughing, and a tendency towards the development of bronchospasm. General anaesthesia is thus difficult, and should be avoided whenever possible.

If intubation is not considered necessary, anaesthesia may be induced by the intravenous route, but must be maintained at a stable level of adequate depth with halothane and liberal oxygenation.

If intubation is necessary, the patient should be admitted to hospital. Premedication with promethazine will serve both to reduce respiratory secretions and to minimize the likelihood of bronchospasm. The excessive drying effect of atropine may result in the production of highly viscous secretions which are difficult to eliminate. Intubation under light anaesthesia may be followed by bouts of coughing and bronchospasm, and we therefore recommend the establishment of an adequate depth of anaesthesia before intubation, and its subsequent maintenance throughout the operation. Emphysema is frequently associated with chronic bronchitis and is characterized by structural lung damage which may result in severe limitation of respiratory function. If general anaesthesia cannot be avoided, respiration may have to be assisted or controlled. The chief problem lies in the recovery phase, when it may be necessary to continue artificial ventilation owing to the difficulty frequently encountered in the re-establishment of adequate spontaneous breathing.

In both these conditions, whenever possible, anaesthesia should be postponed until maximum benefit has been obtained by preoperative therapy. This may include physiotherapy, antibiotics and bronchodilators. Ideally, choice of antibiotic should depend upon sensitivity tests, but both ampicillin and tetracycline are widely used. Heavy smokers frequently suffer from chronic bronchitis, but even if not classified as bronchitics, they usually present the same anaesthetic problems.

(c) **Bronchiectasis.**—It is particularly desirable to avoid the use of general anaesthesia in this condition, since it may encourage the spread of purulent sputum into unaffected segments of lung.

(d) **Tuberculosis.**—Healed pulmonary tuberculosis with negative sputum requires no special management. The presence of positive sputum carries the risk of spread of disease, which can be lessened by the use of appropriate chemotherapy cover.

A.A.D.—10

Contamination of anaesthetic apparatus may lead to cross-infection, and must be rigorously avoided. General anaesthesia for dental purposes is thus usually contra-indicated.

(e) **Pneumothorax and Lung Cysts.**—A history of spontaneous pneumothorax or lung cysts constitutes a relative contraindication to general anaesthesia. Should this, however, prove essential, positive pressure ventilation, coughing, and straining should be avoided.

3. Asthma (see page 148)

Asthmatics usually tolerate general anaesthesia well, and contrary to past teaching, the intravenous barbiturates are not contraindicated. Halothane, accompanied by liberal oxygenation is suitable for maintenance. It is most important to avoid all forms of stimulation under light anaesthesia. If the patient is under treatment with bronchodilator drugs, this treatment should not be interrupted. If bronchospasm should be present immediately prior to the proposed anaesthetic, the patient may, with benefit, be allowed to use his usual inhaler.

Established bronchospasm may be relieved by one of the following drugs.

  (i) Ephedrine 15–20 mg intravenously
 (ii) Aminophylline 250 mg (in 10 ml) intravenously
(iii) Promethazine 25 mg intravenously
(iv) Hydrocortisone 100 mg intravenously
 (v) Adrenaline 1 : 1000, 0·2–0·5 ml subcutaneously
(vi) Isoprenaline Spray B.P.C. 1%.

4. Ludwig's Angina

The dangers associated with this condition have already been stressed (see pages 4 and 143). If general anaesthesia is unavoidable, induction should be inhalational, a mixture of oxygen (30%), helium and either cyclopropane or halothane being used. This induction should proceed with great care to a depth which will enable intubation under direct vision to be attempted. Should this prove impossible, it may be necessary to perform emergency tracheostomy.

If preoperative respiratory distress is severe, general anaesthesia must not be undertaken unless it is preceded by endotracheal intubation or tracheostomy in the conscious state.

C. BLOOD DYSCRASIAS

1. Anaemia

(a) **Hypochromic Anaemia.**—Whenever possible, patients suffering from severe hypochromic anaemia should be treated in an attempt to raise the haemoglobin level to at least 70% (11 g%) before operation is considered. Iron therapy usually suffices, but if blood transfusion is indicated, packed cells should be used, and the transfusion given at least 48 hours prior to surgery. One pint (568 ml) of packed cells or two pints of whole blood may be expected to raise the haemoglobin level by 15%. Should it be necessary to administer anaesthesia in the presence of severe anaemia, the following points must be stressed:

(i) Adequate oxygen must be ensured at all times, and it should be remembered that cyanosis will not develop as a warning sign of hypoxaemia as readily as when the haemoglobin level is normal (see page 132).

(ii) The myocardium may be weakened by anaemia, and the heart thus unable to compensate for circulatory changes initiated by the anaesthetic. The patients should therefore be treated with the same caution as those suffering from fixed cardiac output disease (see page 279).

(b) **Hyperchromic Anaemia.**—The most commonly encountered hyperchromic anaemia is pernicious anaemia, which will always be under specific treatment when encountered in the dental environment. Any operative treatment should be delayed until medical control is optimal, and the anaesthetic management follows the general principles described under Hypochromic Anaemia.

(c) **Thalassaemia** (see page 6).—The management of anaesthesia in patients suffering from this rare type of anaemia is similar to that described under Hypochromic Anaemia, but there are two additional problems. Firstly, the anaemia may prove difficult to treat, since it does not respond readily to iron therapy. Secondly, these patients develop an abnormal hypertrophy of the bone marrow, which leads to a characteristic overgrowth of the maxilla, making intubation very difficult and sometimes impossible.

(d) **Sickle Cell Anaemia** (see page 6).—Patients suffering from homozygous (SS) sickle cell anaemia should not be given a general anaesthetic, unless this is unavoidable, since the risk of producing haemolysis or multiple infarction is considerable, following exposure to minor degrees of central or peripheral hypoxaemia or hypercarbia.

Patients with heterozygous (AS) disease (sickle cell trait), are at less risk and general anaesthesia, in the presence of a good indication, is not contraindicated provided hypoxic episodes are meticulously avoided. These patients have less than 50% abnormal haemoglobin S in their blood, and a fairly severe degree of deoxygenation is required to produce sickling. Their admission to hospital for general anaesthesia is not considered obligatory. If, however, sickle cell trait is accompanied by thalassaemia, the risks are comparable to those associated with homozygous disease. Also, the rare SC heterozygous disease is associated with an increased sickling risk.

Should a general anaesthetic prove unavoidable in the case of homozygous sickle cell anaemia, the following precautions must be taken:

(i) The patient must be admitted to hospital
(ii) A period of pre-oxygenation before induction of anaesthesia is advisable

(iii) Pre-anaesthetic administration of sodium bicarbonate to establish a base excess may be considered necessary. This may be given by intravenous infusion of 50–100 ml of 8·4% solution.

(iv) Hypoxia, acidosis or hypotension during anaesthesia must be scrupulously avoided.

(v) Oxygen therapy should be continued postoperatively until recovery is complete.

Treatment of Sickling Crisis

(i) Continue oxygen therapy and the administration of bicarbonate to maintain a slight base excess.

(ii) Haemolysis may lead to severe anaemia which should be treated with transfusion of packed cells if haemoglobin level falls below 50%.

(iii) Infarction will be heralded by pain in the limbs, chest or abdomen. This should be treated with analgesics and the intravenous infusion of dextrose or Macrodex 40 to reduce blood viscosity. It has also been suggested that magnesium sulphate 2 ml of 50% solution should be administered intravenously every 4 hours.

One of the common causes of death in these patients is pulmonary embolism, and it is therefore suggested that all patients who complain of limb or abdominal pain should be immediately heparinized. An initial dose of 12,000 units should be given intravenously, followed by 10,000 units at 4 to 6-hourly intervals to keep the clotting time at about three times the preoperative level.

Routine Screening of African and West Indian Patients

There is no general agreement on the correct procedure. Ideally, all patients at risk should have a sickle cell test, haemoglobin estimation and blood film, before commencing dental treatment. Should the Sickledex test prove positive and the haemoglobin be below 11 g%, on no account should a general anaesthetic be administered until electrophoresis has eliminated the possibility of both SS (homozygous) or SC disease being present. If the Sickledex is positive, but the haemoglobin near normal, provided examination of a blood film fails to disclose the presence of Target Cells, it can be assumed that the disease is heterozygous of the AS as opposed to the SC variety, and a careful anaesthetic may be administered without further examination. In practice, this routine is seldom carried out, and the anaesthetist is usually faced with a patient to anaesthetize who may be at risk. Dental treatment may be urgent, and although the Sickledex test may be performed at the chairside, it is often undesirable to subject a nervous child to this ordeal immediately prior to an anaesthetic. Provided neither the child's history, nor that of his family, suggests the presence of this disease, it is common practice to administer a *careful* anaesthetic with liberal oxygenation, and whilst such a course of action is not totally devoid of risk, we cannot condemn it under the inescapable conditions of everyday practice. However, we consider that every attempt should be made to postpone the anaesthetic until full screening has been carried out.

2. Bleeding Diatheses

A history of abnormal bleeding in the dental patient must always be treated seriously, and a correct diagnosis made before any treatment is undertaken. Frequently, a carefully taken history will reveal that the reported excessive bleeding is not associated with disease, only having occurred on an isolated occasion in association with an abnormal degree of trauma. However, if doubt exists, the cause of the bleeding must be established. Two major groups of disease may be recognized clinic-ally—namely those due to capillary defects or platelet disorders, and those due to defective clotting. The former require meticulous haemostasis, not normally accom-panied by specific pre-anaesthetic management; the latter, specific preparation and the special operative and anaesthetic technique described below. Although the ulti-mate diagnosis depends upon laboratory investigations, a clinical diagnosis can usually be made from the history (see Table XXV).

The following laboratory tests should be carried out.

Full blood count, including platelets.
Bleeding time.
Clotting time.
Prothrombin time.

Should a clotting deficiency be revealed, special tests will be carried out by the haema-tologist to identify the precise nature of the factor defect.

The following are the bleeding diatheses likely to be encountered.

TABLE XXV.—*Differential Bleeding*

(Anscombe, *Annals of Surgery*, July 1970)

Signs and symptoms	Capillary and Platelet defects (e.g. Purpura)	Clotting abnormalities (e.g. Haemophilia)
Petechiae	Common	Rare
Bruising	Spontaneous	Minor Trauma
Bleeding from Mucus Membranes	Common	Rare
Deep Tissue Haemorrhage	Rare	Very Common
Joint Haemorrhage	Very rare	Very common
Pin prick	Bleeding $++$	Bleeding normal

Disorders of Clotting

(a) **Haemophilia.**—Haemophilia is an inherited sex linked disease manifest only in the male and due to the absence or deficiency of antihaemolytic globulin (A.H.G.—Factor VIII) in the plasma. Clinically the patients may be separated into three groups according to the A.H.G. blood levels.

(i) A.H.G. plasma level over 25%
   These patients can lead normal lives and only suffer excessive bleeding following major trauma. They seldom present problems to either surgeon or anaesthetist following dental extractions.
(ii) A.H.G. plasma level 5%–25%
   These patients are subject to excessive bleeding following minor trauma, so that dental treatment must always be preceded by transfusion with fresh frozen plasma. One litre

of plasma will raise the A.H.G. level by 10%–15%, and clearly treatment should be aimed at the achievement of an A.H.G. plasma level of at least 25%.

(iii) A.H.G. plasma level less than 5%

These patients are classified as severe haemophiliacs and are usually grossly handicapped. Even minimal trauma may carry grave consequences. The A.H.G. plasma level must be raised to at least 25% by the use of freshly thawed cryoglobulin which is normally only obtainable from special haemophiliac centres. The value of antiplasmins such as aminocaproic acid (EACA, Epsikapron) is not universally accepted.

Having described the detailed specific preparation, it is necessary now to stress the broad principles of management which should be observed in all haemophiliacs.

Choice of Anaesthetic.—The use of local infiltration and nerve block is strictly contra-indicated and thus general anaesthesia should always be preferred.

Preoperative Preparation and Premedication.—An intravenous infusion should always be commenced prior to the induction of anaesthesia. This may be used for the administration of A.H.G. and for premedication. No intramuscular injections should be given. The use of aspirin—with its tendency to provoke gastric haemorrhage—should be avoided.

Management of Anaesthesia.—Drugs may be administered intravenously *via* the drip. All patients should be intubated unless the interference associated with intubation is adjudged to exceed that inherent in the surgical procedure. Optimal intubating conditions must be achieved, usually necessitating the use of suxamethonium. Nasal intubation, with its attendant risk of haemorrhage, must be avoided, and the use of a cuffed armoured latex oral tube is recommended. The position of such an armoured tube can be readily altered, without the risk of kinking, thus allowing the surgeon access to all areas of the mouth and enabling him to apply haemostatic splints, should these prove necessary. A pharyngeal pack is essential, but must not be applied too tightly. Extubation should be delayed until satisfactory haemostasis has been established, and careful observation in the postoperative period is essential.

(b) **Von Willebrand's Disease.**—This disease affects both sexes, and although the bleeding diathesis is associated with the presence of large, tortuous, fragile capillaries, patients frequently also have a low plasma A.H.G., and therefore exhibit many of the characteristics of haemophilia.

(c) **Christmas Disease.**—This disease is characterized by a deficiency in Factor IX (Christmas Factor or Plasma Thromboplastin Component), so that although the disease clinically resembles haemophilia, its correction requires the administration of Factor IX rather than A.H.G. (Factor VIII). Unlike haemophilia, the female carrier has a tendency to bleed.

Capillary and Platelet Disorders

This group of diseases includes hereditary haemorrhagic telangiectasia and the thrombocytopenic purpuras. The problems which confront the anaesthetist are those associated with the very low haemoglobin and platelet content of the blood so often present in these patients. Provided any gross abnormality is corrected (e.g. by fresh blood transfusion), no special anaesthetic management is required. The anaesthetist must, however, bear in mind that preservation of the patient's veins for a possible emergency transfusion is vital.

3. Polycythaemia (see page 92)

The raised haemoglobin sometimes allows the patient to exhibit cyanosis in the absence of hypoxaemia; in addition, cyanosis due to peripheral stasis is often present, owing to the increased blood viscosity. These factors mean that special care must be taken, especially with the use of drugs liable to cause a reduction in cardiac output, or hypotension.

D. METABOLIC DISORDERS

1. Porphyria

A full description of this disease will be found on page 26.

Except for the avoidance of barbiturates preoperatively or during the anaesthetic, a standard anaesthetic technique may be used. As a precaution, general anaesthesia should always be administered in hospital where full resuscitation equipment is available.

2. Diabetes (see page 4)

(a) **In Minor Oral Surgery of Short Duration.**—General anaesthesia for minor oral surgery in the controlled diabetic presents few problems and does not require hospitalization or alteration of diabetic regime, provided the following precautions are taken:

 (i) Anaesthesia is administered 4 hours after the last meal, which should preferably be a light breakfast of normal calorie content.
 (ii) Premedication, other than atropine if required, is omitted
(iii) Anaesthesia is maintained at a light level, preferably avoiding the use of agents such as cyclopropane and ether which tend to cause nausea and vomiting postoperatively.
(iv) To assure that severe dental infection has not upset the diabetic balance.

Occasionally, the performance of minor oral surgery of short duration will prove necessary on a diabetic out of control. Usually, the acute inflammatory process in the mouth, together with restricted food intake, will have rendered the previously controlled patient unstable. Sometimes, however, the presence of diabetes will have been revealed *de novo* by routine urine-testing in a patient presenting with a dental abscess. In any event the uncontrolled diabetic patient should always be admitted to hospital, and if operative interference is a matter of urgency, 50 g of dextrose accompanied by 24 units of soluble insulin may be given intravenously preoperatively, and further treatment controlled by urine and blood sugar estimations. In the presence of ketosis, the initial quantity of insulin may have to be increased.

(b) **In Major Oral Surgery.**—Hospitalization is essential under these conditions, since alteration in feeding may be necessary and postoperative blood sugar estimation may be required.

As in the out-patient, anaesthesia should be kept light, and a technique using a minimum of anaesthetic with a relaxant and controlled respiration is recommended.

Alteration in the preoperative diet and insulin is often unnecessary but some physicians prefer to reduce both calorie intake and insulin by about one third. If prolonged feeding difficulties after the operation are anticipated, as with the treatment of jaw fractures, an intravenous drip of 5% dextrose is essential in the postoperative period.

The following intravenous routine is recommended. One litre of 5% dextrose followed by 500 ml 0·9% saline every 12 hours. This should be accompanied by 4-hourly urine tests and the administration of insulin as follows:

If urine is blue or green in Benedicts test — no insulin
    ,,   ,, ,, yellow   ,,   ,,   ,, — 10 units of soluble insulin
    ,,   ,, ,, orange   ,,   ,,   ,, — 15 units of soluble insulin
    ,,   ,, ,, red   ,,   ,,   ,, — 20 units of soluble insulin

Blood sugar estimations should be carried out at regular intervals as a check.

E. RENAL DISEASE

Patients with severe renal disease on chronic dialysis may occasionally present for general anaesthesia associated with dental treatment. Anaesthesia presents surprisingly few problems in these patients provided the following precautions are taken:

1. The operation should be performed within 24 hours of the last dialysis.
2. Premedication, if necessary, should not consist of drugs which depend primarily on renal excretion for elimination. Pethidine or pentobarbitone with hyoscine or atropine have proved satisfactory.
3. Anaesthesia with methohexitone or thiopentone, followed by nitrous oxide and halothane is recommended. If a muscle relaxant is required, suxamethonium is the drug of choice, unless the serum potassium is raised, when it may be preferable to use a non-depolarizing agent, such as pancuronium.
4. Care should be taken with patients on peritoneal dialysis, since accumulation of fluid in the stomach may occur, with the accompanying risk of regurgitation.

F. HEPATIC DISEASE

It is unlikely that patients with severe liver disease will present for major oral surgery, but they may require general anaesthesia for the extraction of septic teeth when local anaesthesia is impracticable.

The following precautions should be taken:

1. Analgesics should be used with caution, particularly the opiates, to which there may be extreme sensitivity. Aspirin and panadol are safe in reduced dosage. Pethidine and phenoperidine appear to be tolerated adequately.

2. The barbiturates are not strictly contraindicated, but may have to be used in reduced dosage. Methohexitone and thiopentone may be used for the induction of anaesthesia, but repeated doses should be avoided. Propanidid is considered unsuitable in severe cases.

3. Nitrous oxide and halothane may be used with safety, provided that liberal oxygenation is ensured and hypotension avoided. There is no evidence that halothane or its breakdown products are hepatotoxic.

4. Absorption of Vitamin K may be impaired, thus necessitating its administration by injection prior to surgery.

5. These patients may be very sensitive to suxamethonium which is therefore best avoided.

6. The toxicity of local anaesthetics is considerably increased in severe liver disease.

7. Severe cases may suffer from hypoproteinaemia which may be responsible for an increased sensitivity to certain drugs.

G. DISEASES OF THE NERVOUS SYSTEM

There are a number of neurological disorders, which although rare, may present problems in the management of dental anaesthesia, either because of sensitivity to anaesthetic drugs or a general difficulty in management. Many of these disorders occur predominantly in children, and have been discussed on page 233. Here, will be described briefly the management of those conditions seen mostly in adult life.

1. Senility

The very elderly or those who are prematurely old due to cerebral arterio-sclerosis, need special care under general anaesthesia. The briefest period of hypoxaemia may just 'tip the balance' and considerably shorten their useful life. It is worth noting that these patients are sometimes unexpectedly resistant to the intravenous hypnotic drugs (page 183), owing to a reduction in cerebral circulation.

2. Porphyria

A full discussion of this disease will be found on page 26. Induction of anaesthesia with propanidid or Althesin followed by nitrous oxide, oxygen and halothane is safe. Facilities for prolonged artificial ventilation should, however, always be available making hospitalization, but not necessarily in-patient treatment, essential.

3. Myasthenia Gravis

In this disease all muscle relaxants must be avoided. If muscle relaxation is required for intubation this is easily achieved with halothane. Diazepam is probably best avoided.

A.A.D.—10*

4. Dystrophia Myotonica

These patients have a very limited respiratory reserve, and any central depressant drugs may render respiration inadequate; thus general anaesthesia should be avoided whenever possible, and it must be remembered that such patients are often extremely sensitive to the barbiturates, and depolarizing muscle relaxants are said to be contra-indicated.

5. Epilepsy

The management of the average epileptic patient is described on page 219. The severe epileptic may rarely develop convulsions during induction of, or recovery from, anaesthesia. Treatment consists in the maintenance of a clear airway, protection of the patient from trauma, liberal oxygenation and artificial respiration if necessary, and the intravenous administration of sufficient diazepam or thiopentone to control the convulsions.

H. PATIENTS ON SPECIFIC DRUGS

1. Corticosteroids (see page 9)

Before discussing the management of patients on steroid therapy, it is necessary to summarize the actions of this complex group of drugs.

In general, the adrenal corticosteroids, of which hydrocortisone will be taken as an example, act as catalysts to various physiological processes. The effects of chief relevance are as follows:

(a) Improvement of Circulatory Efficiency

(i) There is an inotropic effect on the heart (increased strength of contraction) which leads to an improvement in stroke volume.

(ii) Peripheral resistance in the microcirculation is reduced, thus improving tissue perfusion. The exact mechanism of this response is obscure, but it is thought to be other than by adrenergic blockade.

(iii) By restricting the renal excretion of sodium ions, restoration of blood volume is facilitated.

(b) **Anti-Inflammatory.**—Cortisone inhibits hypersensitivity responses to antigen-antibody reactions. By this mechanism, anaphylactic shock in guinea-pigs may be prevented. In man, the chief sphere of usefulness of this property lies in the treatment of bronchial asthma. The benefit produced is probably due to a reduction in the oedema of the bronchial mucosa, rather than bronchial muscular relaxation.

Where the deleterious effects of an inflammatory response outweigh the usefulness of that response, hydrocortisone will be of value, *e.g.* angioneurotic oedema. However, when that response is an essential component of the defence mechanism against a harmful process, *e.g.* infection, the administration of hydrocortisone may be dangerous.

(c) **Metabolic Changes.**—The metabolic effects of the steroids are widespread, and vary with the actual preparation used. The effect which leads to sodium retention and potassium excretion is the most important.

In addition to its use in the various medical conditions listed on page 9, cortisone is used intravenously by the anaesthetist in certain emergency situations, e.g. anaphylaxis (see page 26). Care should be taken that the drug, when administered by the intravenous route in an emergency, is the correct preparation for this purpose, i.e.

Hydrocortisone Sodium Phosphate

> Trade name—Efcortesol
> Ampoules—1 ml contains equivalent of 100 mg hydrocortisone

Hydrocortisone Sodium Succinate B.P.

> Trade name—Efcortelan
> Vial—Powder containing the equivalent of 100 mg hydrocortisone to be dissolved in water immediately before use.
> It is advisable to avoid these drugs in the first trimester of pregnancy.

Management of Patients on Steroid Therapy

The necessity to increase or re-establish steroid therapy in patients about to undergo anaesthesia or surgery, who have been, or are on steroid therapy, is still a matter of controversy; however, some suggestions may be helpful.

The following patients should receive hormone therapy preoperatively and during operation:

(i) Patients with Addison's Disease
(ii) Those patients currently on steroid therapy
(iii) Patients who have had continuous therapy for more than one month in the 6 months prior to operation, and who have had a total dose of more than 1·0 g of cortisol or its equivalent.

The regime shown in Table XXVI is suitable when major oral surgery is being performed on patients in the above categories.

TABLE XXVI.—*Method of Preparation for Elective Cases*

Time	Cortisone dose	Route
Day before operation	100 mg night and morning	Intramuscular
With premedication	100 mg	Intramuscular
During operation	100–200 mg	Intravenous in 500 ml dextrose
Immediately post operation	100 mg	Intramuscular

During the postoperative period, the daily dose should be gradually reduced until the normal maintenance dose has been reached.

Table XXVII shows a suggested scheme.

TABLE XXVII.—*Postoperative Administration of Steroid for Patients Previously on Steroid Therapy*

Date	Total dose	Intramuscular Injection (mg) 8 a.m.	3 p.m.	8 p.m.
1st Day	200	100	50	50
2nd Day	150	75	50	25
3rd Day	100	50	25	25
4th Day	50	25	25	0
5th Day	25	25	0	0
6th Day	25	25	0	0
7th Day	0	0	0	0

No patients other than those in one of the above categories require active steroid therapy, but hydrocortisone should be at hand should a collapse suggestive of hydrocortisone insufficiency occur. Indeed it is doubtful whether patients in category (iii) require coverage, particularly when the operative procedure is of a minor nature; suprarenal response tests have indicated that depression of suprarenal function is, in fact, rare in these patients.

2. Hypotensive Agents

Patients with high blood pressure may be under treatment with a number of hypotensive agents (page 11, Table III), and the drugs which are in current use may be divided into three groups. Firstly, central sedatives (e.g. phenobarbitone), which are used only in mild hypertension and present no special anaesthetic problems; they will not be further discussed. Secondly, those drugs which act on the autonomic nervous system and are the most likely to influence the course of anaesthesia. Thirdly, those which act on the peripheral blood vessels, directly relaxing arteriolar tone.

(a) Drugs acting on the Autonomic Nervous System

(i) **The 'Anti-Adrenergic' Drugs.**—Guanethidine and bethanidine are the two drugs in common use, guanethidine being the longer acting. Both drugs cause depletion of noradrenaline at post-ganglionic sympathetic nerve-ending, and give rise to side-effects associated with the inevitable instability of blood pressure which results from their use. These take the form of severe postural and exertional hypotension usually manifested as faintness or dizziness on standing, or following strenuous exercise. It is therefore vital that such patients should not be subjected to any similar influence during the course of an anaesthetic. The posture selected should normally be supine, but if a particular patient's blood-pressure is controlled to such a limited degree that he experiences *hyper*tensive symptoms when lying flat, then it is sensible to adopt a comfortable reclining posture for anaesthesia, but on no account should the legs be dependant. All anaesthetic drugs with hypotensive properties (e.g. halothane, barbiturates) must, of course, be administered with the greatest possible care, accompanied by frequent monitoring of the blood pressure.

(ii) **Methyldopa** (Aldomet).—Methyldopa has both a central and peripheral autonomic effect. Although the peripheral action is similar to that of guanethidine, postural changes have less effect on the patient's blood pressure, and it should therefore never prove necessary to anaesthetize these patients in any but the fully supine posture. The effects of the drug are slow in onset, and may persist for several days after it has been discontinued.

(iii) **Reserpine** (Serpasil).—Reserpine has both a central sedative and mild peripheral hypotensive action, the latter being due to depletion of noradrenaline.

(iv) **Ganglion-Blocking Drugs.**—These drugs are now seldom used in the routine control of hypertension, but are of value in anaesthesia to produce controlled hypotension for surgical purposes. The same precautions as described in association with guanethidine, apply to patients under treatment with ganglion blocking agents.

(v) **The Adrenergic Blocking Drugs**

Alpha Blocking Agents.—These drugs, of which phenoxybenzamine is the most commonly used, act by blocking alpha (vasoconstrictor) receptors. Chiefly of value in the control of hypertension associated with phaeochromocytoma, they have more recently been used to augment the effect of guanethidine (Ismelin) in resistant cases of hypertension.

Beta Blocking Agents.—The beta blocking agents (e.g. propranolol and practolol) are capable of lowering the blood pressure, but since their mode of action depends chiefly upon a reduction in cardiac output, their place in the treatment of hypertension is, at present, controversial.

(b) **Drugs acting directly on the Peripheral Blood Vessels**

(i) **Thiazides and Chlorthalidone.**—Whilst the thiazides and chlorthalidone are used primarily as diuretic agents, they also exert a mild hypotensive effect. The site of their action is thought to be directly on the peripheral blood vessels. The principal side effect of these drugs is potassium depletion, which may lead to muscular weakness.

(ii) **Hydrallazine.**—Hydrallazine is sometimes used orally in combination with the thiazides in the control of mild hypertension. Its site and mode of action are not known for certain, but postural hypotension is a possible consequence of its use. The drug has been used parenterally to achieve 'controlled' hypotension.

All these drugs complicate anaesthesia in that they tend to potentiate the circulatory effects of many anaesthetic agents, thus giving an unstable blood pressure. This instability of blood pressure has led many anaesthetists to insist that specific hypotensive therapy is discontinued well in advance of the administration of an anaesthetic. With this view we disagree. If the symptoms and risks associated with the illness are sufficient to warrant active blood pressure reduction by drugs, then it would appear to us unwise to expose the patient to these risks prior to the stress of an operative procedure and general anaesthetic. Indeed, such preparation, to be effective, may necessitate withdrawal of the controlling drugs a week or more before the intended surgery. Successful hypotensive therapy is often extremely difficult to establish in terms of dose adjustment, and to interrupt a satisfactory maintenance regime for any reason requires most careful consideration, in view of the hazards to which the patient may be subjected by drug withdrawal, and the difficulties it may present to the physician in terms of subsequent re-establishment of adequate control. This is not to suggest that the administration of an anaesthetic to a patient receiving hypotensive therapy is devoid of special risk; but we believe that this risk is less than that of discontinuing the treatment, provided that the choice of drugs, technique and posture is carefully controlled by an experienced anaesthetist. If, in spite of these considerations, the anaesthetist feels that treatment should be discontinued, this decision should not be finalized until he has discussed the specific problems involved with the physician in charge of the case.

Anaesthesia should, whenever possible, be induced with the patient in that posture in which he normally sleeps most comfortably. All drugs which are known to affect the blood pressure (e.g. methohexitone, halothane) should be administered slowly and carefully. Some method of monitoring the cardiovascular state is obligatory, and all 'episodes' likely to produce sudden alteration in circulatory dynamics in general, and blood pressure in particular, must be avoided.

3. Anti-Depressant Drugs

The clinical significance of these drugs in relation to anaesthesia is fully discussed on page 7.

The treatment of adverse interactions between the anti-depressants and other drugs will depend upon whether the dominant circulatory change is hypertensive or hypotensive in nature. If the former, the cautious intravenous administration of chlorpromazine or an alpha blocking agent such as phentolamine may prove necessary. If the latter, hydrocortisone rather than a vasopressor amine, should be used in conjunction with other supportative measures.

RECOMMENDED READING

Prophylactic Chemotherapy in the Heart Case
WALTON, J. G. & THOMPSON, J. W. (1970), Chemotherapeutic Agents; including their Prophylactic Use. In *Pharmacology for the Dental Practioner.* London: British Dental Association. p. 88.

CHAPTER FIFTEEN

LOCAL ANAESTHESIA IN DENTAL SURGERY

BY

KENNETH RAY

The control of pain during routine dental treatment is readily achieved for the majority of patients by the use of local anaesthesia.

Modern local anaesthetic drugs are very efficient and rarely cause systemic complications. Local side effects due to injection of the drugs into the tissues are uncommon and when they do occur are rarely serious.

INDICATIONS FOR USE OF LOCAL ANAESTHESIA IN DENTAL SURGERY

The main indication for use is the prevention or relief of pain.

Most patients will accept periods of an hour or more of conservative dental treatment under local anaesthesia. For more traumatic oral surgical procedures, it is wise to limit treatment to that which can confidently be performed within 30 minutes, without distress to the patient.

Local anaesthesia is also of value in the diagnosis of facial pain. Patients and their dental surgeons often have difficulty in locating the cause of facial pain which, although originating from a single tooth, may be widely distributed over the upper and lower jaws. Diagnostic injections which selectively anaesthetize parts of the jaws may enable the tooth involved to be determined.

CONTRAINDICATIONS TO THE USE OF LOCAL ANAESTHESIA

Absolute contraindications to the use of local anaesthesia are few, but there are several limiting factors.

1. General limitations

The dental surgeon depends upon the patient's co-operation when giving local anaesthetic injections. Therefore it is unwise to attempt the use of local anaesthesia alone for control of pain in mentally confused, hysterical, or very apprehensive patients. The sudden uncontrolled athetoid movements of severe spastics make safe injection difficult. The coarse regular tremor of the lower jaw seen in Parkinsonism may also present a problem. However, the above general limitations can often be overcome by premedication with drugs having tranquillizing and muscle relaxing properties (page 36). It is difficult to reason with the suspicious very young child particularly if the first experience of dental treatment is for the relief of severe pain. General anaesthesia should be used for such a patient.

Cardiovascular Diseases.—In the six months after an episode of myocardial infarction dental treatment should be limited to that necessary for the relief of pain and resolution of acute infection. Patients with such a history, and those with symptoms of myocardial ischaemia revealed by attacks of angina pectoris, may be at risk from local anaesthetic injections containing adrenaline or other sympathomimetic vasoconstrictors. Fortunately, felypressin is now available as an effective alternative vasoconstrictor which is devoid of cardiac irritant properties.

Minor dental treatment of short duration for patients with cardiovascular disease is best undertaken with local anaesthesia. However, any form of stress brought about by pain, or even fear of pain and dental treatment, is harmful for these patients. Premedication with sedatives or tranquillizers prior to giving the local anaesthetic is advisable, and treatment should be carried out as expeditiously as possible. If extensive dental treatment is necessary, such as multiple extractions, the patient should be admitted to hospital to permit all the extractions to be carried out at one time under endotracheal anaesthesia. This causes less stress than a series of visits for one or two extractions at a time under local anaesthesia.

Hypertension.—Patients suffering from hypertension may usually be safely given local anaesthetics. A solution containing felypressin rather than adrenaline or noradrenaline as vasoconstrictor is recommended. Many hypertensive patients take hypotensive drugs such as methyldopa (Aldomet), guanethidine sulphate (Ismelin), or bethanidine sulphate (Esbatal). These drugs can cause postural hypotension. To avoid cerebral ischaemia and fainting, the patient should be placed lying down before being given the local anaesthetic injection. On completion of treatment the patient should rise slowly and a watch be kept for fainting caused by the fall in blood-pressure on standing up.

Hyperthyroidism.—Uncorrected overactivity of the thyroid gland produces a nervous irritable patient subject to tachycardia and arrhythmias. Sedatives should be prescribed prior to dental treatment. A characteristic of this disease is the patient's marked sensitivity to catecholamine drugs such as adrenaline and noradrenaline. Local anaesthetic solutions containing these vasoconstrictors are therefore contraindicated. A solution containing felypressin as vasoconstrictor is safe, since this drug is not a catecholamine.

Major Haemorrhagic Disorders.—Haemophilia and Christmas disease are disorders of blood coagulation. Local anaesthetic injections should be avoided, particularly deep block injections which may cause haemorrhage and extensive haematoma formation. Extractions in these patients are usually carried out under general anaesthesia in hospital after replacement of the missing coagulation factor. For conservative dental treatment, local anaesthetics should only be injected superficially at sites where the soft tissues are firmly attached to the underlying bone, e.g. at the interdental papilla.

Similar precautions should be taken in patients suffering from the vascular disorder, Von Willebrand's disease, and platelet disorders, the thrombocytopenic purpuras. The danger of a haemorrhagic state in patients taking anticoagulants must also be remembered. Warfarin sodium (Marevan) and phenindione (Dindevan) are the commonest anticoagulants in use at present. Fortunately neither haematoma formation after local anaesthetic injections, nor postextraction haemorrhage, commonly occur in patients whose anticoagulant dosage has been carefully controlled by regular prothrombin time estimations.

Antidepressant Drugs.—The tricyclic antidepressants are a group of drugs used in the treatment of endogenous depression. Those in common use are amitriptyline (Tryptizol), imipramine (Tofranil), and protriptyline (Concordin). These drugs potentiate the effect of adrenaline and noradrenaline. Although only very small quantities of these vasoconstrictors are used in local anaesthesia for dental surgery it would seem wise to avoid their use. A solution containing felypressin (Octapressin) is a safe alternative.

2. Local limitations to the use of Local Anaesthesia

Local anaesthetics must not be injected into acutely infected tissues for this may lead to spread of the infection to produce a cellulitis of the soft tissues or osteomyelitis of the mandible. Abscessed teeth may be extracted where a nerve block injection can be given well clear of the infected area. Otherwise general anaesthesia is used or surgical treatment under local anaesthesia delayed until resolution of the acute infection is obtained by drainage of pus and use of antibiotics. Infected teeth with apical periodontal infection, as demonstrated by tenderness on percussion, may prove difficult to anaesthetize to a sufficient degree to permit extraction.

The incidence of delayed healing of extraction sockets due to 'dry socket', i.e. localized osteitis of the socket walls with breakdown of the bloodclot, is greater with local anaesthesia than general anaesthesia. The reason for this is probably the effect of the vasoconstrictor in the local anaesthetic. Therefore, solutions containing vasoconstrictors are best avoided in patients giving a history of 'dry socket', and also in all patients whose jawbones may have a reduced blood supply or be densely sclerosed. These latter conditions occur in Paget's disease, osteopetrosis, and occasionally following irradiation of the jaws or adjacent structures in the treatment of malignant disease. Fortunately, efficient local anaesthetic solutions such as prilocaine (Citanest) without added vasoconstrictor are now available.

THE PHARMACOLOGY OF LOCAL ANAESTHETICS

Mode of action in producing local anaesthesia

Local anaesthetics act by causing a temporary reversible block of conduction in nerve endings and axons. Stimulation of pain-receptor nerve endings leads to the passage of an impulse along the nerve axon to the central cell body. The conduction of this electrical impulse along the axon of the nerve fibre depends on the movement of ions across the nerve cell membrane which surrounds the axon. A local anaesthetic blocks conduction of the impulse by interfering with the movement of sodium ions across this membrane.

The size of a nerve fibre is a factor in the speed of onset of blocking of conduction by local anaesthetics. The speed appears to be inversely proportional to the fibre diameter. This is of functional significance, since the smaller sensory fibres are more rapidly affected than the larger motor fibres. Many pain fibres are very narrow and non-myelinated, and are thus very susceptible to local anaesthetics. Larger myelinated sensory fibres are less susceptible, for the local anaesthetic only acts readily at the nodes of Ranvier where the layer of myelin separating the nerve axon from its sheathing neurilemma is absent.

Pain is commonly the first modality of sensation to be blocked by a local anaesthetic, followed by temperature, light touch, and pressure. However, in a peripheral nerve trunk consisting of fibres of mixed diameter, the smaller fibres are often situated centrally and will, therefore, be reached by the anaesthetic agent later than the larger fibres at the periphery of the trunk. This may be of clinical significance in explaining why after dental nerve block, the more peripherally situated soft tissues such as the lower lip become anaesthetized before the pulp of a lower molar.

Local anaesthetics only act as such when applied directly to peripheral nerves. Systemically their pharmacological effect is different. The plasma levels of the local anaesthetic agents reached when used in dental surgery in the recommended dose, are very low. Systemic effects only occur when inadvertent vascular uptake of a significant quantity has taken place.

Other effects of Local Anaesthetics

(a) **The central nervous system.**—Rapid achievement of high blood levels of local anaesthetic may result in stimulation causing restlessness, muscle twitching, and finally convulsions. This state of excitation may be followed by depression, particularly of the respiratory and cardiovascular centres. However, with some agents, e.g. lignocaine, the initial excitatory phase does not occur. Very rarely a normal dose may provoke these reactions, when an idiosyncrasy to the drug exists.

(b) **Cardiovascular system.**—With sufficiently large doses, myocardial excitability is lessened, the refractory period lengthened, and impulse conduction through the cardiac muscle slowed. These properties are utilized by physicians, who use intravenous lignocaine to correct some cardiac arrhythmias.

The effects in (a) and (b) above are unlikely to occur with the doses used in dental surgery, even allowing for the mishap of intravascular injection.

(c) **Muscle.**—Smooth muscle is relaxed, which accounts for the vasodilating properties of most local anaesthetics. Depression of neuromuscular conduction in skeletal muscle also occurs but is rarely of clinical significance in dental surgery.

THE CHEMISTRY OF LOCAL ANAESTHETIC DRUGS

There are many compounds of diverse chemical structure capable of producing local anaesthesia. However, there are but a few of these that possess the properties to make them effective and safe enough for clinical use.

Ideally, the compound should be capable of producing a reversible state of local anaesthesia without damaging the tissues, or causing systemic toxic effects. It should produce anaesthesia of rapid onset and consistent duration, and be available in a stable, sterilizable aquaeous solution for injection, and also in a form that will readily penetrate mucosal surfaces for topical anaesthesia.

Most local anaesthetics used for injection are hydrochloride salts of organic bases. In this form a stable aquaeous solution can be prepared, whereas the base itself is almost insoluble in water. The bases have a common pattern, with molecules composed of three parts. At one end of the molecule is the aromatic hydrocarbon residue, radical 1, which is connected by an intermediate chain, radical 2, to a substituted amino group at the other end, radicals 3 and 4. The intermediate aliphatic chain, R2, is joined to the aromatic hydrocarbon group, R1, by either an ester or amide link in the majority of local anaesthetics currently used. Thus the two main types of local anaesthetics used in dental surgery can be represented by the diagrammatic formulae:

(a) Ester type   R1—COO—R2 (with R3 and R4 branching)

(b) Anilide type   R1—NHCO—R2 (with R3 and R4 branching)

The degree of local anaesthetic activity of a particular drug depends on a complex series of factors and is conditioned by its chemical structure and physical properties. All local anaesthetics possess varying degrees of lipid and water solubility. The aromatic hydrocarbon, R1, part of the molecule is lipophilic, whereas the amino-

group N (with R3 and R4 branching) is hydrophilic. This combination of properties influences the diffusibility of the anaesthetic agent through tissue fluids and lymph, and its ability to penetrate the highly lipid nerve membranes, thus enabling it to reach, and act at, the receptor site on or within the individual nerve fibre.

In aquaeous solution, local anaesthetics, which are weak bases, occur in two forms—uncharged free base, and the cationic form. In the latter, the base molecule has a positively charged hydrogen ion. The degree of ionization will depend upon the inherent dissociation constant for the agent in question, and the pH of the fluid medium. This pH will be that of the prepared solution, modified by the buffering effect of the alkaline tissue fluids. An increase in pH increases the proportion of the uncharged free base molecules of the local anaesthetic. It was formerly thought that local anaesthetic activity depended solely upon this uncharged form of the free base molecule, but more recent research has tended to indicate that it is the water soluble, ionized, charged form of the molecule that has the main activity on or within the single nerve fibre, to produce the agent receptor bond. However, in addition to activity at the receptor site, the factor of penetration of the anaesthetic from the point of injection to the receptor site must be considered. In this context, there is little doubt that it is the uncharged form of free base that readily penetrates the lipid barriers of the whole nerve sheath, since only this form of the molecule is lipid soluble.

It is of interest to note that benzocaine has no terminal hydrophilic amino-group, (Table XXVIII) and being insoluble in water does not exist in the charged ionized molecule form. However, it is a potent local anaesthetic agent but can, of course, only be used topically and not for injection, as the foregoing theoretical concept would lead one to expect. On the other hand, injections of local anaesthetic solutions into acutely inflamed tissues, which have a relatively low pH, are often not fully effective in controlling pain. The decrease in the proportion of uncharged free base available in such an acid environment may be an explanation of this undoubted clinical fact.

Absorption, Distribution and Metabolism

In clinical practice local anaesthetics are either used topically on mucous membranes, or injected. Absorption through intact skin does not occur. The rate of absorption is dependant on the chemical structure of the drug, the concentration in which it is used, and the vascularity of the tissues. A comparison of the topical anaesthetic activity of two para-aminobenzoic acid esters, procaine and amethocaine illustrates the relevance of the first factor. Procaine has a low lipid solubility, and is so poorly absorbed from mucous membranes as to be useless for topical anaesthesia. Amethocaine, however, has a high lipid solubility and is so rapidly absorbed from vascular mucous membranes that a plasma level may be reached approaching that caused by an intravenous injection of an equivalent dose.

The more vascular the site of injection the more rapid is the absorption of the anaesthetic into the plasma. As in clinical practice the object is to keep as much of the anaesthetic drug as possible in the vicinity of the peripheral nerve branches, vasoconstrictor drugs are often added to reduce the vascularity at the injection site.

Ultimately, all the local anaesthetic is absorbed into the blood plasma and the plasma level will be related to the rate of absorption and the total dose absorbed rather than merely the concentration of the injected solution. From the plasma it is distributed to tissues and organs throughout the body.

The major site of metabolism is the liver, where biotransformation to inactive breakdown products by enzymes takes place.

Those local anaesthetics with an ester linkage in the molecule (Table XXVIII) are also broken down by the plasma enzyme pseudocholinesterase which, although produced in the liver, is also active in the blood stream and tissues. Once again, the chemical structure of the particular 'ester type' drug is important. Procaine, for example, is rapidly broken down whereas amethocaine takes four or five times as long.

The anaesthetically inactive metabolites of local anaesthetics are excreted by the kidney.

TABLE **XXVIII.**—*Illustrates how the Structure of Some Common Local Anaesthetics fit into these general formulae*

Name	Aromatic hydrocarbon residue R1	Intermediate chain R2	Amino group R3 + R4	Type
procaine (Novocaine)	NH_2—⬡—	—C—O—CH_2—CH_2—N— (C=O)	C_2H_5 / C_2H_5	para-aminobenzoic acid ester
amethocaine (tetracaine (U.S.P.)	H—N / C_4H_9 ⬡—	—C—O—CH_2—CH_2—N— (C=O)	CH_3 / CH_3	para-aminobenzoic acid ester
propoxycaine (Ravocaine)	OC_3H_7 / NH_2—⬡—	—C—O—CH_2—CH_2—N— (C=O)	C_2H_5 / C_2H_5	para-aminobenzoic acid ester
benzocaine	NH_2—⬡—	—C—O—CH_2—CH_3 (C=O)		para-aminobenzoic acid ester
metabutethamine (Unacaine)	NH_2 / ⬡—	—C—O—CH_2—CH_2—N— (C=O)	H / C_4H_9	meta-aminobenzoic acid ester
lignocaine (Xylocaine, Xylotox)	CH_3 / ⬡ \ CH_3	—NH—C—CH_2——N— (C=O)	C_2H_5 / C_2H_5	anilide
prilocaine (Citanest)	CH_3 / ⬡	—NH—C—CH—— N— (C=O) (CH₃)	H / C_3H_7	anilide

The Properties of Specific Local Anaesthetic Drugs

Cocaine

Methyl benzoylecgonine is an ester of benzoic acid. This drug is mentioned first for historical reasons. It is obtained naturally from the leaves of the tree, Erythroxylum coca, which grows in South America. Cocaine was the first drug used as a local anaesthetic and was introduced in 1884. However, it was found to be extremely toxic, so that early research concentrated on the synthesis of less toxic related compounds by altering the cocaine molecule. Cocaine has a marked vasoconstrictor effect on small vessels, a property not found in any of the local anaesthetic drugs subsequently synthesized, most of which are active vasodilators. Due to the systemic toxicity of cocaine it is now only used for surface anaesthesia. The vasoconstrictor effect is of particular value on the highly vascular mucous membranes of the nose. Application of a 5–10% solution of the hydrochloride salt or a 20% paste produces good local anaesthesia and marked shrinkage of the mucous membranes prior to nasal surgery. These preparations have been used by dental surgeons to provide anaesthesia of the floor of the nose during removal of cysts, and for apicectomy operations on upper incisors when dental infiltration and block injections have failed to control pain.

Idiosyncrasy to the drug has been reported, rapid onset of toxic symptoms having occurred with small topical doses. Since there are now safer alternative topical anaesthetics, there is no longer any indication for the use of cocaine in dental surgery.

Lignocaine—Lidocaine (U.S.P.)—(Trade names—Xylocaine, Xylotox, Lignostab)

This was the first successful local anaesthetic of the anilide group (Table XXVIII) to be synthesized. It was introduced for clinical use in 1948 and soon became the most widely used local anaesthetic, taking over the role of procaine as the standard against which all new drugs are compared. The base is almost insoluble in water and a solution is prepared from the hydrochloride salt, the concentration used for dental surgery being 2%. This solution is extremely stable and may be autoclaved. It has a shelf life of at least $2\frac{1}{2}$ years. A plain 2% solution is not very efficient and to ensure that the frequency of successful injection approaches 100%, as is expected of modern local anaesthetics, a vasoconstrictor must be added. Commercial preparations in this country contain either adrenaline or noradrenaline 1:80,000. The 2% lignocaine with adrenaline 1:80,000 solution is the standard solution for most dental surgeons in the U.K. at the present time.

This solution gives a rapid onset of anaesthesia with good spread from the site of injection, and a duration of pulp anaesthesia varying from 30 minutes to over 2 hours, depending on the type of injection and the dose given. Systemic toxicity and allergic reactions to lignocaine are rare, particularly in the field of dental surgery. Once absorbed into the blood plasma, lignocaine is rapidly distributed to tissues. Biotransformation takes place mainly in the liver.

For an adult, the recommended maximum dose of the 2% solution with a vaso-constrictor is 25 ml, which contains 500 mg of the hydrochloride salt. With the 2% plain solution without vasoconstrictor this should be reduced to 10 ml, owing to the more rapid absorption, and thus greater possibility of systemic effect of this solution. Lignocaine is also a potent topical anaesthetic, producing surface anaesthesia within 2 minutes and lasting up to 20 minutes (see Topical Anaesthetics, p. 313).

Prilocaine—(Trade name—Citanest)

This drug, which was introduced in 1960, is closely related chemically to ligno-caine, and shares its effectiveness as a local anaesthetic, but has some definite advantages. It has a slight but significant vasoconstrictor action which aids in local-ization at the injection site, thus delaying absorption. Once absorbed, however, it leaves the circulation and is redistributed to the tissues more rapidly than lignocaine, and is also metabolized at a greater rate. From animal experiments the toxicity of prilocaine is estimated to be 60% that of lignocaine. The low toxicity and the vaso-constrictor property of prilocaine permit the use of more concentrated solutions than of lignocaine, with a reduction in the amount of added vasoconstrictor. Whilst the resultant anaesthesia is of the same rapid onset, spread, and profound degree, the duration time with infiltration injections is shorter.

The standard commercial preparation for dental surgery, when adrenaline is used as the vasoconstrictor, is 3% prilocaine with 1:300,000 adrenaline. A plain 4% solution is also very effective with an onset time of half to 1 minute. As would be expected with no vasoconstrictor, the duration time of pulp anaesthesia following infiltration is limited to 15 minutes, but with block injections is up to 90 minutes. This solution may advantageously be used for patients for whom vasoconstrictors may be contraindicated (see Vasoconstrictors, page 305). The third commercial preparation of prilocaine for use in dental surgery is a 3% solution containing, as vasoconstrictor, felypressin which is free of some of the potentially harmful side effects of the catechol amine vasoconstrictors, adrenaline and noradrenaline (see Vasoconstrictors, page 305). This solution is as efficient as 2% lignocaine with 1:80,000 adrenaline, or 3% prilocaine with 1:300,000 adrenaline but gives a duration time of pulp anaesthesia roughly between the two.

The maximum recommended doses of prilocaine hydrochloride are 400 mg when used in plain solution, and 600 mg with a vasoconstrictor present. Plasma levels produced by dosages much above those recommended can give rise to cyanosis caused by methaemoglobinaemia.

Mepivacaine—(Trade name—Carbocaine)

This drug is another of the anilide group and has properties very similar to lignocaine. In the U.K. the very stable hydrochloride salt is used in a 3% solution without a vasoconstrictor. In North America 2% solutions with either adrenaline 1:80,000 or levonordefrin 1:20,000 are also available. Mepivacaine shares with prilocaine a slight vasoconstrictor effect which allows it to be used without adding a vasoconstrictor drug. On injection it is readily absorbed, redistributed to the tissues, and metabolized. Anaesthesia is therefore rapidly produced, and is similar in degree to that associated with 2% lignocaine with 1:80,000 adrenaline but, with infiltration, is of shorter duration, giving pulp anaesthesia of 15 minutes. Toxicity is similar to lignocaine. The recommended maximum dose for injections in the jaws is 400 mg.

Butanilicaine—(Trade name—Hostacain)

The commercial preparation Hostacain uses a 2% solution of the phosphate salt of this anilide type local anaesthetic in a mixture with a 1% solution of procaine phosphate. Hostacain Sp. has adrenaline 1:50,000 as a vasoconstrictor and Hostacain Nor has noradrenaline 1:25,000. Butanilicaine has the same degree of anaesthetic activity as the other members of the anilide group mentioned previously. It is, however, metabolized far more rapidly than lignocaine which accounts for the high maximum dose of 1g which is permissible. This is equivalent to 50 ml of the 2% solution, a quantity never required in dental surgery, nor indeed recommendable with such high concentrations of vasoconstrictor as these commercial solutions contain.

Procaine—Procaine hydrochloride (B.P. and U.S.P.)—(Trade names—Novocain, Novutox)

From 1905, when this ester of para-aminobenzoic acid was synthesized, until the introduction of the more effective lignocaine in 1948, it was by far the most extensively used local anaesthetic.

Procaine replaced cocaine for injection anaesthesia because, although less potent, it was much less toxic. However, it did not replace cocaine as a surface anaesthetic, since its poor absorption through mucous membranes made it useless for this purpose. Procaine is an active vasodilator, and is rapidly absorbed into the blood stream on injection. The low toxicity is explained by the equally rapid metabolism of this drug, which occurs mainly in the plasma by pseudocholinesterase as soon as it is absorbed, and also by esterases in the liver. To be effective in the vascular situation of the jaws, the addition of a vasoconstrictor is essential, and adrenaline 1:50,000 is used in most commercial preparations.

The maximum dose of this preparation should be 400 mg, i.e. 20 ml.

Although no longer used as a sole agent in local anaesthetic solutions for dental surgery, it is still a popular agent for surgical situations where a large quantity of local anaesthetic needs to be injected for, with its very low toxicity, up to 1 g may be used in dilute solutions of 0·5%.

A disadvantage is that patients and dental surgeons may become hypersensitive to procaine and other drugs of the ester type (Table XXVIII).

Propoxycaine—(Trade name—Ravocaine)

This drug is another para-aminobenzoic acid ester, much more potent than procaine, but in equal dose more toxic. However, it is potent at a concentration of 0·4%

and at this strength its toxicity is not much greater than procaine. Commercial preparations used for dental surgery in North America are a mixture of the hydrochloride salts of propoxycaine 0·4% and procaine 2%. The vasoconstrictors used are levonordefrin (Neo-Cobefrin)1 : 20,000 or noradrenaline 1:30,000. The dose should be kept below 10 ml.

Metabutethamine—(Trade name—Unacaine)
2-isobutylaminoethyl meta-aminobenzoate.

An ester of meta-aminobenzoic acid, this is a potent local anaesthetic with rapid onset time but short duration, since it has a slight vasodilator action. The North American commercial preparation is a 3·8% solution with adrenaline 1:60,000.

Metabutethamine has a very low toxicity, being less than procaine. The dosage of the commercial solution is limited by the adrenaline content rather than the amount of metabutethamine and should not exceed 12 ml.

Amethocaine (B.P.)—Tetracain (U.S.P.)—(Trade names—Anethaine, Pontocaine)

This is a very potent drug of the ester type which is very toxic when compared with procaine in equal dosage. However, the extreme potency allows it to be used at a dilution of 0·15% of the hydrochloride salt, which is safe in the quantity required for dental surgery. It has a slow onset time on injection, but long duration when used with added vasoconstrictor. To overcome the slow onset time, commercial solutions in North America where, unlike the U.K., amethocaine is used for injection purposes, contain a mixture of amethocaine 0·15% and procaine 2%. Noradrenaline 1:30,000 or levonordefrin (Neo-Cobefrin) 1:20,000 are used as vasoconstrictors.

In the U.K. the use of amethocaine in dental surgery is mainly as a topical anaesthetic in concentrations of 0·5–2%. It readily penetrates the oral mucous membrane to produce effective surface anaesthesia very rapidly.

VASOCONSTRICTORS

Vasoconstrictors are added to local anaesthetic solutions to retard the absorption of the anaesthetic into the blood plasma. Since an effective quantity of local anaesthetic will in consequence stay longer at the site of injection, the duration of anaesthesia will increase. This effect is more marked on giving infiltration injections than with nerve block injections. Local spread of the anaesthetic drug from the injection site by diffusion through the tissues is not markedly affected. The total dose of anaesthetic drug required to produce effective anaesthesia for a given period of time will be reduced on adding a vasoconstrictor. The possible occurrence of systemic toxic effects of the local anaesthetic is, therefore, reduced by decreasing both the total dose and the rate at which it enters the circulation. The dangers of systemic absorption have, however, been exaggerated in the past, for even with accidental intravascular injection of the doses of local anaesthetics used in dental surgery toxic effects are unlikely to occur. However, in the event of an intravascular injection the added vasoconstrictor may well produce a systemic effect, particularly if the injection has been given rapidly. With many commercial local anaesthetic solutions it is the vasoconstrictor content which limits the total volume that may safely be injected.

To a varying degree vasoconstrictors are also useful in restricting haemorrhage during oral surgical procedures, thus providing a relatively blood-free field for the operation and avoiding unnecessary blood loss.

Adrenaline (B.P.) —Epinephrine (U.S.P.)

Adrenaline is the most common vasoconstrictor in use with local anaesthetics. This catechol amine is one of the hormones of the adrenal medulla, but can be synthesized. Its pharmacological action is generally sympathomimetic showing both α and β adrenergic actions. The concentrations present in local anaesthetic solutions for use in dental surgery are from 1:300,000 to 1:50,000. In the doses used the effect should be purely the local one of vasoconstriction. However, cardio-vascular disturbances, presumably resulting from systemic absorption, have been recorded.

The action of adrenaline on the cardiovascular system is complex, but the small amount likely to be absorbed in dentistry may cause a rise in systolic pressure following increased cardiac output which results from an increase of rate and force of beat. Larger amounts may cause cardiac arrhythmias leading to ventricular fibrillation. These complications can also occur with quite small doses, such as might be used in dental surgery, if the heart is unduly sensitive to catechol amines as a result of the concurrent action of other drugs such as the general anaesthetic agent halothane.

It is obviously wise to mitigate the effect of systemic absorption of adrenaline by reducing the concentrations in local anaesthetics to a minimum. It has been suggested that the concentration of 1:80,000, that is currently used in the U.K. with the most popular local anaesthetic, lignocaine, is too great. However, published evidence is conflicting, Gangerosa and Halik (1967) could find no clinical advantage of 2% lignocaine with 1:100,000 adrenaline compared with 2% lignocaine with 1:300,000 adrenaline. Cardwell and Cawson (1969), however, in a double blind trial of 2% lignocaine 1:80,000 adrenaline against 2% ligocaine 1:250,000 adrenaline found a significant increase in the number of failed injections with the lower adrenaline concentration.

Noradrenaline (B.P.) —Levarterenol (U.S.P.)

Noradrenaline is also a naturally occurring hormone of the adrenal medulla, but can be synthesized. This catechol amine, unlike adrenaline, has a pharmacological action limited almost entirely to α receptor effects. It is the chemical transmitter released by postganglionic sympathetic fibres and controls normal vasomotor tone.

As a vasoconstrictor it is less effective than adrenaline and is often used in concentrations as high as 1:30,000, although in the U.K. the commercially available 2% lignocaine solutions usually contain 1:80,000. At this concentration local vasoconstriction should occur without systemic side-effects. However, as with adrenaline, the mishap of intravascular injection could possibly cause cardiovascular disturbance. Systemically noradrenaline causes constriction of all peripheral vessels, with marked increase in the overall peripheral resistance and a consequent rise in systolic and diastolic pressures. Heart rate slows secondarily to the rise in blood-pressure but there is little effect on cardiac output.

Noradrenaline is less likely to cause disturbance of cardiac rhythm than adrenaline, but it is not absolutely safe to use as a vasoconstrictor in dental surgery whilst patients are under general anaesthesia with agents such as halothane. It must also be used with caution in hypertensive patients.

Intravascular injection of noradrenaline in patients taking tricyclic antidepressant drugs, e.g. imipramine (Tofranil) can lead to a marked rise in blood-pressure. This group of drugs also potentiates the effect of adrenaline, but to a lesser degree.

Adrenaline and noradrenaline are only stable in acid solution, and the pH of the local anaesthetic must therefore be reduced from that of the alkaline plain solution. This may lead to a minor increase in irritation on injection into the alkaline environment of the tissue fluids.

Both these vasoconstrictors are readily oxidized and therefore sodium metabisulphite is added to the solutions as a preservative anti-oxidant.

Other Vasoconstrictors

In addition to adrenaline and noradrenaline, which are the commonly used vasoconstrictors in the U.K. and Europe, other sympathomimetic amines are used in North America. They appear to have no major advantages over adrenaline, and precautions in use are similar.

Nordefrin—(Trade name—Cobefrin)

This drug is chemically similar to adrenaline but has less marked vasoconstrictor activity and to be effective must be used at a concentration of 1:10,000. Its systemic toxicity on intravascular injection is lower than adrenaline.

Levonordefrin—(Trade name—Neo-Cobefrin)

A development from nordefrin this drug is the levo isomer which has most of the vasoconstrictor activity of the nordefrin molecule. It is used in a concentration of 1:20,000 with propoxycaine and tetracaine.

Phenylephrine—(Trade names—Neosynephrine, Neophryn)

This drug is also structurally similar to adrenaline but has less action on the heart, and is unlikely to produce arrhythmias on accidental intravascular injection. Its vasoconstrictor activity is comparatively weak and it must be used at the higher concentration of 1:2500. However, it is more stable than adrenaline and, being metabolized more slowly, has a longer vasoconstrictor effect in equivalent dosage.

Felypressin—(Trade name—Octapressin)

Following the extraction of the hormone vasopressin, which was found to have antidiuretic and vasoconstrictor properties, from the posterior lobe of the pituitary gland, synthesis of various analogues of this polypeptide was carried out to produce a hormone having vasoconstrictor action without the other effect.

Felypressin (2-phenylalanine-8-lysin vasopressin) was found to have a marked constrictor effect on small vessels and was therefore investigated as a vasoconstrictor. Berling (1966) reported on his investigations of the use of felypressin as a vasoconstrictor for dental local anaesthesia, and subsequently a solution of 3% prilocaine with felypressin in a concentration of 0·03 International Units per ml (1 iu = 0·18 mg) was introduced.

This combination was found to be more effective than lignocaine with felypressin.

Felypressin has a very low systemic toxicity and in the concentration used does not affect the coronary circulation or cause myocardial irritability when used together with general anaesthetics. In contrast to adrenaline therefore, there is no risk of ventricular fibrillation. Felypressin can also be used safely in patients taking anti-depressant drugs.

The 3% prilocaine with felypressin solution does, therefore, seem to be a safe alternative for those patients who may be at risk from systemic effects of even small doses of catechol amine vasoconstrictors. The weaker vasoconstrictor activity of felypressin when compared with adrenaline makes the only available 3% prilocaine felypressin solution less effective in providing a blood free field for oral surgical procedures than 3% prilocaine with 1:300,000 adrenaline.

The maximum vasoconstrictor effect is reached some 10–15 minutes after infiltration, whereas the solution with adrenaline takes only 3–5 minutes.

CHOICE OF LOCAL ANAESTHETIC SOLUTION

An ideal solution for use in dental surgery would produce complete anaesthesia of rapid onset, which should last for a predictable time period. Wide variation in duration of the painful stage of operative procedures will necessitate a range of such solutions with varying lengths of action. They should be without toxic or other side-effects in the doses required for any operation, and therefore be usable for all patients without restriction by age or state of general health. A close examination of the modern local anaesthetic solutions commonly available, will show that a sensible choice can be made which will fulfil most of the theoretically ideal criteria.

Clinical testing of local anaesthetic solutions in dental surgery is complicated by the many variable factors that must be taken into account. There is variation in response between individuals, and even variation in response by the same individual on different occasions. Some teeth are more difficult to anaesthetize than others. The type of injection is important, for infiltration and block injections are not comparable and must be assessed separately. With apprehensive patients, a considerable factor, difficult to express scientifically, is the dental surgeon's ability to gain their confidence, and thereby the ability of the anaesthetic solution to prevent pain.

Björn (1947) and Cowan (1964) describe in detail methods of determining the comparative clinical efficiency of local anaesthetics for dental surgery.

The main parameters for assessment are frequency of success; onset time; extent of anaesthesia; duration; toxic and side effects. These parameters will be considered with particular relation to the following list of currently available proprietary solutions:

2% lignocaine—adrenaline 1:80,000
2% lignocaine—noradrenaline 1:80,000
3% prilocaine—adrenaline 1:300,000
3% prilocaine—felypressin 0·03 iu/ml
4% prilocaine plain
3% mepivacaine plain
2% butanilicaine + 1% procaine—adrenaline 1:50,000 (Hostacain Sp.)

(a) Frequency of success

Unless a solution gives successful results of well over 90% it is not worth considering for standard use. Published reports suggest that Hostacain Sp. and 3% mepivacaine do not reach this requirement. However, a 2% mepivacaine solution with added vasoconstrictor does so, but the preparation is not freely available in the U.K. and would, in any case, be unlikely to challenge the more efficient 2% lignocaine-adrenaline solution.

(b) Onset time

The time taken from start of injection until pulp anaesthesia is obtained should be as short as possible, but an arbitrary maximum period of 5 minutes would be reasonable. All the solutions listed produce anaesthesia within this period.

(c) Extent of anaesthesia

The property of local spread of anaesthesia from the site of injection to adjacent teeth, bone, and soft tissues is valuable. In surgical operations this permits the painless reflection of broad based mucoperiosteal flaps without the necessity for multiple infiltration injections. If, on completing a cavity preparation in one tooth, interstitial caries is discovered in the adjacent tooth, it is useful to be able to treat this without a further injection. With block injections, particularly for the inferior dental nerve, because there is anatomical variation of both injection landmarks and the path of the nerve to the mandibular foramen, there may be lack of certainty in placing the solution correctly; the excellent spreading power of modern local anaesthetics compensates for this. The degree of spread may be assessed clinically by testing for anaesthesia of adjacent teeth pulps and soft tissues, after an infiltration injection over one tooth.

Of the solutions listed 2% lignocaine-adrenaline 1:80,000 gives the greatest spread on infiltration and this is one factor that has established it as the most popular solution for oral surgery.

(d) Duration of anaesthesia

The painful stage of operative procedures on the teeth and jaws varies from less than 1 minute for a simple extraction to up to 60 minutes for complicated restorations and surgical operations. However, the vast majority of painful procedures are completed within 25 minutes. Ideally, anaesthesia should last as long as the painful part of the operation. A disadvantage of all the current local anaesthetic solutions is the persistence of soft tissue anaesthesia for far longer than tooth anaesthesia, particularly with solutions containing the highest vasoconstrictor concentration. With block injections, 2% lignocaine-adrenaline 1:80,000 may give soft tissue anaesthesia for over 3 hours. The most valuable information given by clinical tests is the minimum duration figure that can confidently be expected for pulp anaesthesia, on injection of a standard dose of the chosen solution at each particular site.

In practice, using the commercial preparations readily available, it is possible to vary the duration of anaesthesia in four ways.

1. Choice of anaesthetic drug
2. Variation of concentration of the drug in the solution
3. Variation of the vasoconstrictor content
4. Variation in the dose given

Lignocaine is only effective for dental anaesthesia with added vasoconstrictor. The duration figures for the two available solutions, i.e. 2% lignocaine with either adrenaline or noradrenaline 1:80,000, are very similar. Although adrenaline is the more powerful vasoconstrictor, there is only a marginal increase in duration time of pulp anaesthesia compared with that for the noradrenaline solution, but the difference is rather more marked for duration of soft tissue anaesthesia. With infiltration injections, a minimum pulp anaesthesia duration of 30 minutes can confidently be expected, with a mean figure of 47 minutes. The minimum duration of soft tissue anaesthesia is 2 hours, and mean duration 3 hours.

Infiltrations of 3% prilocaine-adrenaline 1:300,000 give a mean duration figure of 22 minutes, but a minimum nearer to 10 minutes. The duration of soft tissue anaesthesia is markedly reduced, for whereas 100% of cases infiltrated with 2% lignocaine-adrenaline 1:80,000 had soft tissue anaesthesia after 2 hours, with 3% prilocaine-adrenaline 1:300,000 the figure falls to only 45%.

When 3% prilocaine is used with felypressin 0·03 iu/ml, duration times for infiltration injections are a minimum of 15 minutes, with a mean of 40 minutes. Soft tissue anaesthesia is prolonged up to 4 hours. Infiltrations of a 4% prilocaine solution without vasoconstrictor produce anaesthesia of rapid onset but short duration. The minimum period for which pulp anaesthesia can confidently be expected is 5 minutes, with a mean figure of 13 minutes. A 3% mepivacaine solution gives very similar figures.

TABLE XXIX.—*Duration of Anaesthesia—Infiltration Injections (in mins.)*

	Pulp anaesthesia Minimum	Mean	Soft tissue anaesthesia Mean
2% lignocaine-adrenaline 1:80,000	30	47	190
3% prilocaine-adrenaline 1:300,000	10	22	90
3% prilocaine-felypressin 0·03 iu/ml	15	40	240
4% prilocaine	5	13	85
3% mepivacaine	5	17	80

Cowan (1964, 1965), in using his minimal dosage technique for the clinical comparison of local anaesthetic agents, has shown that duration time after infiltration injections may be reduced by giving smaller doses. Between 0·25 ml and 1 ml are recommended depending on the duration required and whether the tooth is easy to anaesthetize such as an upper premolar, or more difficult as with an upper central incisor or first molar.

There is much less variation in the duration time of anaesthesia when inferior dental block injections with the various solutions are compared. They will all give pulp anaesthesia for a minimum duration of 30 minutes, with the mean duration close to one hour. The duration of soft tissue anaesthesia is in the same time range of 100 minutes to 270 minutes for all the solutions. There will be a greater percentage of injections giving duration figures in the upper part of the range when 2% lignocaine-adrenaline 1:80,000 and 3% prilocaine-felypressin 0·03 iu/ml are used.

(e) Toxicity and side-effects

Most of the 'reactions' that occur in dental local anaesthesia are due to the patient's apprehension. They are, therefore, more a reflection of the operator's failure to cope with the patient's stress, than of the effects of the anaesthetic solution. Toxic reactions to the local anaesthetic base in any of the modern solutions in the quantities used, are so unlikely to occur that this is not a factor to consider when making a choice of solution. However, reactions to the vasoconstrictor content must be considered. Although adrenaline or noradrenaline in the concentrations used are unlikely, with slow absorption, to cause systemic effects, inadvertent intravascular injection may cause them to do so. Therefore, since equally effective alternative solutions are available, those containing these catecholamines should not be used on patients who may be at risk if systemic absorption occurs (page 296).

It has been observed that the immediate pain on injection is significantly greater for some patients when solutions containing adrenaline 1:80,000 are used. This may be explained by the ischaemia produced by the adrenaline, or possibly by the irritant effect of the low pH of the solution which is necessary when adrenaline is present. The sensation of pain as the anaesthetic and vasoconstrictor effect diminishes, may be due to the reactive hyperaemia that is reported following vasoconstriction with adrenaline. Both adrenaline and noradrenaline are reported to produce cyanosis with tissue hypoxia on infiltration into skin, but it is doubtful whether this effect is ever produced by submucous injection in the mouth.

Indications and contraindications for use of specific solutions

The 2% lignocaine-adrenaline 1:80,000 solution is very efficient. It is the solution of choice for long operative procedures, and those such as removal of impacted teeth and gingivectomy, where vasoconstriction is desirable to provide a bloodless field. Its main disadvantage for routine use as a sole anaesthetic, is the long duration of anaesthesia, which is too long for most restorative procedures although use of a minimal dose technique reduces the excess period (*vide supra*). The lengthy soft tissue anaesthesia is unpleasant, and in children may lead to self inflicted trauma to the cheeks and lips. The shorter duration with infiltrations of 3% prilocaine-adrenaline 1:300,000 makes it a useful alternative for shorter procedures where ischaemia of the soft tissues is not required for surgical reasons.

The 3% prilocaine-felypressin 0·03 iu/ml solution gives a duration of anaesthesia sufficient for most operations. The main advantage and indication for its use is in those patients for whom adrenaline may be hazardous, e.g. cardiovascular disease and hyperthyroidism. Felypressin is a safe and efficient alternative vasoconstrictor, provided profound haemostasis is not a prime requisite.

Formerly some dental surgeons used 2% lignocaine-noradrenaline 1:80,000 in patients for whom adrenaline was contraindicated, and many still use it as a standard solution for all patients. It is certainly an efficient preparation but noradrenaline is also not without hazard as a vasoconstrictor (page 307), particularly for patients on tricyclic anti-depressants.

For short infiltration, where a mean duration of 13 minutes is acceptable, 4% prilocaine solution gives an excellent degree of anaesthesia with rapid onset. In block injections it can be used as a general purpose solution for restorative procedures (Brown and Livingstone Ward, 1969). It is safe for use on 'cardiac patients'. However, the short minimum duration of 5 minutes on infiltration should be remembered, and if there is any doubt that the painful stage of the procedure would take longer, a wise choice would be the solution containing felypressin.

The plain solution of 3% mepivacaine offers no advantages over 4% prilocaine and may be marginally less efficient as judged by frequency of successful anaesthesia.

Allergy

All the solutions that have been considered are of the anilide type (with the exception of Hostacain which is a mixture of the anilide butanilicaine and the ester procaine). Allergy to drugs of this group is almost unknown, but if it occurs, one of the ester type could be used. However, their overall efficiency as local anaesthetics is not as good as the best of the anilide group. In the ester group, 0·4% propoxycaine—2% procaine mixture with levonordefrin as vasoconstrictor (Ravocaine) would be suitable for long procedures, and 3·8% metabutethamine-adrenaline 1:60,000 (Unacaine) for short cases.

A history of so-called 'allergy' is often given by a patient who has in fact had a vasovagal attack due to imperfect management on a previous occasion.

TOPICAL ANAESTHESIA

The application of local anaesthetic agents to the surface tissues of the mouth may be of value in the following circumstances: prior to injections, particularly in the palate; scaling and curettage of periodontal pockets; incision of a fluctuant abscess; removal of loose deciduous teeth and bone sequestra; symptomatic relief of oral ulceration; and suppression of retching whilst taking impressions.

The most effective and commonly used agents for oral topical anaesthesia are amethocaine, lignocaine, prilocaine and cocaine (page 302). Benzocaine although less effective is also used.

The drugs are prepared in various forms as solutions, water miscible pastes, aerosol sprays, viscous gels and lozenges.

Solutions of 4% lignocaine hydrochloride and 4% prilocaine hydrochloride may be applied by swabs or sprays up to a dose of 5 ml. Adrenaline is sometimes added to these topical solutions with the object of increasing the duration of anaesthesia.

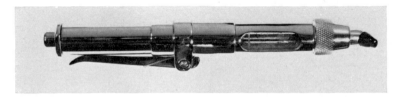

Fig. 125.—The 'Panjet' instrument (*Wright Dental Group*)

However, this vasoconstrictor does not have the same effect topically as when injected. The duration of anaesthesia is not prolonged, and disadvantageously the onset is delayed, for the addition of adrenaline hydrochloride increases the acidity of the preparation, which retards penetration of the mucous membrane. Prior to injections, a more useful preparation is a water miscible paste which can be applied to the small area of mucosa involved on a pledget of cotton gauze. These may contain a pleasant flavouring agent which makes them particularly acceptable to children.

Xylotox-Normal paste (Pharmaceutical Manufacturing Co.) contains 5% lignocaine, whereas Xylotox-Extra contains, in addition, the more potent 2% amethocaine. Xylodase (Astra) ointment contains 5% lignocaine plus hyaluronidase 0·015%. This enzyme is added in an attempt to facilitate the spread of the anaesthetic agent into the tissues. Hyaluronidase hydrolyses hyaluronic acid, a component of the ground substance of connective tissues, which limits the passage of fluids in the tissue spaces. However, Adriani *et al.* (1964) state that topical application of hyaluronidase is without significant effect. These pastes produce surface anaesthesia within 2 minutes and lasting for up to 20 minutes.

A useful method of obtaining surface anaesthesia of the periodontal tissues is with an aerosol spray giving a metered dose at each depression of the spray nozzle. Proprietary preparations are available with either lignocaine or amethocaine as the anaesthetic agent.

A.A.D.—11

Xylocaine (Astra) 10% spray gives a metered dose of 10 mg at each release of the valve. Twenty spray doses is the recommended maximum which gives a total dose of 200 mg. The contents of the aerosol are the lignocaine plus cetylpyridium chloride which is a bacteriostat, in a vehicle of a mixture of polyethylene glycol and ethanol. A pleasant flavour is added. The propellant gases are di- and tri-chlorfluormethanes.

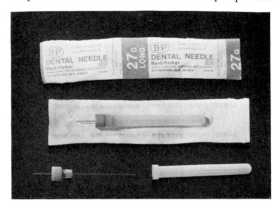

Fig. 126.—Pre-sterilized disposable cartridge syringe needle (*Bard-Parker*)

The similar Gingicain (Hoechst) aerosol contains amethocaine gentisate, chlorbutol, and benzalkonium chloride as bacteriostat. Each spray dose gives 0·8 mg of amethocaine gentisate. The maximum recommended 25 sprays is equivalent to 20 mg of the anaesthetic agent.

Another method of applying anaesthetic solutions for surface anaesthesia is with the Panjet (Fig. 125), a compressed air gun which produces a high velocity stream of droplets which penetrates into the submucosal tissues. A metered dose of 0·06 ml is given at each firing. It is especially useful on the palate and attached gingivae which, being well keratinized, are not so readily anaesthetized by simple surface application. The 'Panjet' may produce small mucosal tears on thin non-keratinized mucosa.

A very effective and convenient method of producing a circumscribed area of surface anaesthesia prior to injection, is by application of an Anaestho-Tab (Voco-Chemie of West Germany). This is a 5 mm diameter paper disc impregnated with amethocaine which adheres to the wet mucosa. It is dyed with methylene blue which transfers to the mucosa thus pinpointing the spot for injection. The methylene blue also has an antiseptic effect.

Benzocaine compound lozenges B.P.C. which

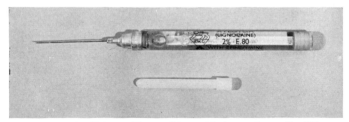

Fig. 127.—The 'Disposall' cartridge with integral needle (*Pharmaceutical Manufacturing Co.*)

contain benzocaine 100 mg, menthol 3 mg, and borax 50 mg have been used to prevent retching on taking impressions. However, benzocaine is not so effective as one of the aerosol sprays mentioned above. Another alternative used for the above purpose and also to give temporary symptomatic relief in oral ulceration is the proprietary product Xylocaine viscous (Astra). This contains 2% lignocaine hydrochloride with 2·5% carboxymethylcellulose in a flavoured viscous gel prepared for use in anaesthesia of the gastrointestinal tract. Its properties of high viscosity and low surface tension enable it to disperse over the mucous membrane to form an even film which adheres to the mucosa for long enough to produce surface anaesthesia. Five-15 ml held in the mouth for a few minutes gives anaesthesia of the mucosa lasting for 15 minutes. It is particularly useful for children with acute ulceration as the effect lasts long enough for a meal to be eaten without distress.

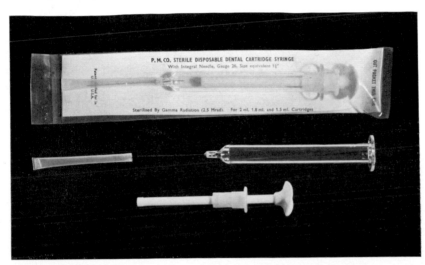

FIG. 128.—Disposable cartridge syringe and needle unit. Supplied in sealed plastic film pack sterilized by gamma radiation (*Pharmaceutical Manufacturing Co.*)

Probably the oldest method of producing anaesthesia of superficial tissues is by lowering the surface temperature. A rapidly evaporating fluid sprayed on to mucosa or skin soon leads to refrigeration. Ethyl chloride was commonly used prior to the incision of a fluctuant abscess, but the effect in the mouth is short lived and there is considerable discomfort as the tissues return to normal temperature. Topical anaesthetic aerosol sprays are probably more effective for intra-oral use, although ethyl chloride still has a place for use on skin surfaces where topical anaesthetic agents are ineffective.

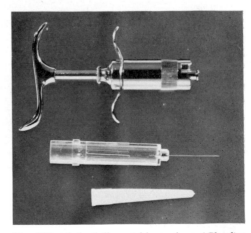

FIG. 129.—Ash sterile cartridge syringe. (*Claudius Ash, Sons & Co. Ltd.*) The disposable plastic barrel with bonded needle is supplied in a sterile pack.

EQUIPMENT FOR LOCAL ANAESTHESIA

The advantages of having a local anaesthetic solution stored sterile in a cartridge, in a suitable quantity and readily available for injection, led to the almost universal adoption of the cartridge syringe method of injection by dental surgeons. The more recent introduction of pre-sterilized cartridge syringe needles (Fig. 126) that are disposable after use on a single patient was another advantage, for this dispensed with the difficult task of sharpening and sterilizing needles, and reduced the chance of cross infection from one patient to another.

However, there are some disadvantages with the cartridge syringe system. Firstly, with most of the syringes in use, aspiration prior to, and during, injection of the solution is impossible. As most of the side effects of anaesthetic solutions, and many of the failures to produce anaesthesia are due to inadvertent intravascular injection,

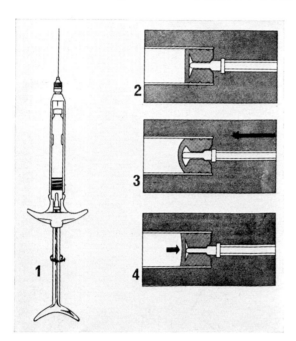

Fig. 130.—

1. The 'Astra' plastic disposable syringe with self-aspirating device.

2. The special cartridge has a modified rubber plunger with a recess into which the piston fits.

3. The thin rubber diaphragm stretches on applying injection pressure to the piston.

4. The plunger diaphragm recoils on release of pressure and so achieves aspiration.

(*Astra Chemicals Ltd.*)

the ability to aspirate blood, and thus detect if the needle is in a vessel, would be a valuable preventive measure. Secondly, the cartridge syringe must be sterilized between each patient even though disposable needles are used. A third factor is that the outside surface of the cartridge diaphragm or aluminium cap that is penetrated by the reverse point of the needle is a possible break in the chain of sterility.

These points could be overcome by reverting to the use of a Luer type syringe, as used for injections elsewhere on the body. The plastic disposable form of this syringe has the added advantage of being relatively cheap. However, this change would involve losing the advantages of the cartridge for the more tedious drawing up of solutions from ampoules or stock bottles, with the increased risk of contamination with the latter.

Accepting the entrenched position of the cartridge syringe in dental surgery, manufacturers have tried various ways of overcoming its disadvantages.

The Disposall Cartridge System (Graham Chemical Co., New York and Pharmaceutical Manufacturing Co.—Great Britain).

Each cartridge is supplied with the needle as an integral part (Fig. 127). The cartridge, with needle still protected by its plastic sheath, is dropped into the syringe barrel with no risk of contamination. A valve within the cartridge will only release the solution into the needle when the syringe piston exerts pressure on the plunger bung.

This system does not solve the problem of aspiration. It is relatively expensive, for if more than one cartridge is needed for one patient a new needle is used with each cartridge. It requires a simple modification to the end of existing syringe barrels. Only the type of solution supplied by the manufacturer can be used.

Sterile disposable cartridge syringes

The syringe illustrated in Fig. 128 does not permit aspiration and is rather expensive for routine use. The system in Fig. 129 has a disposable barrel plus needle supplied in a pre-sterilized plastic pack, and a non-disposable metal handle and piston rod

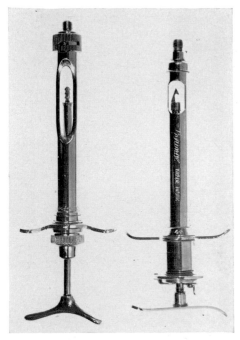

FIG. 131.—Aspirating syringes with pistons designed to engage the rubber plunger of standard cartridges

assembly. It does not provide for aspiration and the metal handle part requires sterilization between patients. The Astra (Sweden) model illustrated in Fig. 130

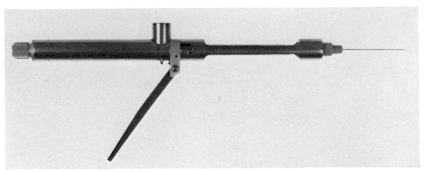

FIG. 132.—The 'Densco' gas actuated syringe (*Getz Dental Products, U.S.A.*)

is supplied sterile in a plastic pack. The great advantage is that it is an aspirating syringe to which any type of disposable needle can be fitted. Repeated aspiration can be achieved without changing the grip on the syringe and thus moving the needle point. Its main disadvantage is that only cartridges with the modified plunger bung supplied by the one manufacturer can be used. However, this is lessened by the range of solutions available, i.e. 2% lignocaine-adrenaline 1:80,000, 3% prilocaine-adrenaline 1:300,000, and 3% prilocaine-felypressin 0·03 iu/ml. This syringe system is likely to be expensive. (The cost is unknown for it is not yet marketed in the U.K.)

Other aspirating syringes

Many attempts have been made to provide for aspiration without modification of the plunger bung of the cartridge. Various designs of hooks (Fig. 131) have been added to the syringe piston rod. Many are not constantly effective.

The Densco automatic aspirating syringe (William Getz Dental Products, U.S.A.) illustrated in Fig. 132 is a very sophisticated and expensive apparatus. The syringe is actuated by a small 'gas' cylinder and injects very smoothly. Aspiration prior to injection can be achieved but there is no real advantage over simpler and far less expensive instruments. A simple hooked piston type of syringe that works well with most cartridges is produced by the Graham Chemical Co. of New York. It may readily be modified to accept the Disposall type cartridge with attached needle developed by the same manufacturer.

Needles

Cartridge syringe needles are usually supplied in two lengths—1 in. (25 mm) and 1⅝ in. (42 mm), and in gauges varying from 23 to 30.

Conventionally the short needles are used for infiltration and the long for nerve block injections. However, if it is accepted that needles should be used once only, and thereby the risk of breakage that follows repeated use is eliminated, all the commonly given intra-oral injections can be performed with a 1⅝ in. needle.

Since the introduction of pre-sterilized (by gamma radiation or ethylene oxide gas) disposable needles, the range of gauges readily available has become limited.

Dentists favour the finer needles, 27 and 30 gauge being the most popular, assuming that these cause less pain on penetrating the tissues. This is not necessarily so and, as the heavier 25 gauge needle has some important advantages, it is recommended for use in adults. The greater rigidity is a help in giving inferior dental nerve block injections, as the needle can be more positively directed to the deep site of injection. The needle can be used as a feeling probe, thus allowing any impedance to its insertion on encountering muscle or tendinous attachments to be readily perceived. This is not possible with narrower flexible needles. Aspiration is difficult to achieve through needles finer than 25 gauge, and there is little point in practising this technique if a high incidence of false negative aspirations is likely to occur as is so with finer needles. There is less likelihood of penetrating small vessels with the broader needle.

Cartridges

The volume of local anaesthetic solution in each cartridge may be 1·8 ml, 2 ml, or 2·2 ml. The contents of the cartridge are sterile, but the outside surface of the aluminium diaphragm penetrated by the cartridge syringe needle is not. Immersion of this end of the cartridge in a chemical antiseptic solution such as 1 % chlorhexidine (Hibitane I.C.I.) in 70% ethyl alcohol is an accepted method of dealing with common pathogenic organisms, although spore forms will resist this treatment.

In addition to the local anaesthetic agent and vasoconstrictor drug, the solution in the cartridge usually contains a bacteriostatic agent, e.g. methylhydroxybenzoate, a stabilizing antioxidant, e.g. sodium metabisulphite, and sodium chloride in pyrogen-free distilled water to make the solution isotonic with the tissue fluids.

Local anaesthetic cartridges should have a shelf life, without deterioration of the contents, of at least 2 years if kept cool and out of strong light.

INFILTRATION AND REGIONAL NERVE BLOCK ANAESTHESIA—INJECTION TECHNIQUES

There are two main methods of producing local anaesthesia by injection. In the first, usually termed 'infiltration anaesthesia', the solution affects only the nerve endings and terminal branches in the tissues at the site of injection. In the second method, usually termed 'nerve block anaesthesia' the solution is deposited around the trunk of a major nerve branch and, on diffusion into the trunk, blocks conduction from the regions it supplies peripheral to the site of injection. Both methods are used in local anaesthesia for dental surgery.

Dental surgeons require rather more extensive spread from infiltration injections to anaesthetize the teeth than is needed for purely soft tissue infiltration anaesthesia elsewhere in the body. To reach the fine nerves passing from the dental pulp through the apical foraminae of the teeth, the solution deposited in the soft tissues must diffuse through the periosteum, the cortical plate, and underlying spongy bone.

Infiltration injections can only be used to anaesthetize the teeth where over-lying bone is thin and porous enough to allow the anaesthetic solution to diffuse through the cortical plate. The outer cortical plate of the alveolus of the upper jaw is porous enough to permit successful infiltration anaesthesia of all the teeth. Occasional difficulty occurs due to the dense bone of the maxillary zygomatic process, which lies over the roots of the upper first molar (Fig. 134). However, by infiltrating a sufficient amount of solution just anterior and posterior to this buttress of bone, anaesthesia of the first molar may usually be obtained and only rarely is a nerve block injection necessary.

In the lower jaw, however, the thick, dense bone of the outer cortical plate over-lying the posterior teeth precludes the use of infiltration anaesthesia. Further anteriorly on the mandible, the bone of the outer cortical plate becomes thinner as the canine is reached and very porous in the incisive fossa, where on a dry specimen numerous foraminae may be seen overlying the roots of the lower incisors. Infiltration anaesthesia is therefore successful for the lower canine and incisors, whereas nerve block techniques are used for the lower molars and premolars.

In children, the outer cortical plate overlying the mandibular deciduous molars is porous, and thus infiltration injections are effective in the mandible, as in the maxilla.

The roots of deciduous teeth are shorter than permanent teeth and the depth of insertion of the needle will be less.

LOCAL ANAESTHESIA OF THE UPPER JAW AND TEETH

Anatomy.—The nerve supply to the maxilla is from the second division of the trigeminal nerve. The maxillary nerve leaves the base of the skull through the foramen rotundum to enter the pterygopalatine fossa where it divides. Soon after entering the fossa the sphenopalatine ganglion is suspended from the main trunk of the nerve by two or three roots. Sensory fibres of the maxillary nerve pass through the ganglion without synapsing, for the ganglion cells are purely parasympathetic. Leaving the ganglion these sensory fibres form several nerve branches, namely orbital, pharyngeal, short sphenopalatine to the nose, long sphenopalatine or nasopalatine, and the greater and lesser palatine branches. The nasopalatine nerve passes from the roof of the nasal cavity posteriorly to the floor anteriorly, running diagonally across the nasal septum which it supplies. The two nerves from the right and left sides then pass through the incisive canal and descend through to the oral cavity at the incisive foramen to supply the gingivae and mucoperiosteum of the anterior hard palate, roughly forward of a line joining the two upper canine teeth.

The greater and lesser palatine nerves descend in the pterygopalatine canal to reach the palate through the greater and lesser palatine foraminae. The greater palatine nerve (syn. anterior palatine nerve) leaves the greater palatine foramen (syn. anterior palatine foramen) which has a funnel shaped orifice situated medial to the upper third molar. It traverses forwards supplying the hard palate, mucoperiosteum, and gingivae, to anastomose in the canine region with terminal branches of the nasopalatine nerve thus forming with the latter the so called 'inner nerve network' of the maxilla.

The lesser palatine nerves (*syn.* middle and posterior palatine nerves) leave the lesser palatine foraminae which are situated immediately posterior to the greater palatine foramen (Fig. 135 (a)) to supply the soft palate and part of the tonsil.

Immediately after giving off the descending roots to the sphenopalatine ganglion the maxillary nerve provides first a zygomatic branch which, *via* the orbit, reaches the face to supply the skin of the temporal and zygomatic area, and then descending posterior superior dental branches, two or three in number, which traverse down the posterior wall of the maxilla. One small branch remains superficial and passes forward to supply the buccal mucosa and gingivae of the upper molars whilst the remainder pass through foraminae situated on the posterior wall of the maxilla about 1 cm above the alveolar margin of the third molar. From here they ramify through the bone to supply the upper molar teeth, excepting on some occasions the mesiobuccal root of the first molar. The maxillary nerve then passes forwards to enter the orbit through the inferior orbital fissure, where it is now called the infra-orbital nerve. It runs first in a groove and then a canal in the floor of the orbit to emerge on the face at the infra-orbital foramen, where it splits into terminal branches to supply the soft tissues of the lower eyelid, anterior face and side of nose, and the upper lip. Within the orbit it gives a middle superior dental branch which descends in the lateral wall of the antrum, which it also innervates, to supply the premolars and the mesiobuccal root of the first molar. Shortly before leaving the canal anteriorly a further branch, the anterior superior dental nerve, descends within bone to supply the canine, incisors, and overlying tissues on the labial aspect of the alveolus. Twigs from it also go to the lining of the antrum and the nasal vestibule.

The anatomical arrangement of this plexus of superior dental nerves, forming the so called 'outer nerve network' of the maxilla, is very variable and often the middle branch is absent, its function being shared by the other two branches.

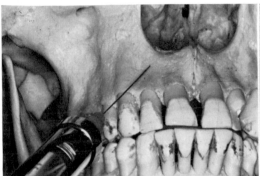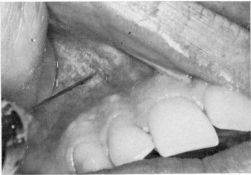

FIG. 133 (a and b).—*Infiltration injection*. The lip is firmly retracted. The needle is inserted through the taut mucosa. It enters at the reflection of the sulcus and is passed to lie supraperiosteally just below the level of the root apex.

Infiltration injection technique

From the above description of the nerve supply to the upper jaw it will be apparent that an infiltration of anaesthetic solution on the buccal aspect of the alveolus will anaesthetize the pulp of the tooth, and often adjacent teeth, plus the overlying bone and soft tissues on that side of the alveolus.

Thus treatment involving drilling of the teeth or even pulp removal would be painless. When extraction of the tooth is to be undertaken a separate injection on the palatal aspect would be necessary.

Although it is impossible to sterilize completely the oral mucosa prior to injection, the bacterial population at the injection site can be markedly reduced by first drying the mucosa with gauze and then applying an antiseptic such as 0·5% chlorhexidine (Hibitane, I.C.I.) in 70% ethyl alcohol, or povidone iodine solution (Betadine, Berk).

The upper lip and cheek is firmly retracted, which will make the surface mucous membrane taut so that the needle, with bevel facing towards the jaw, may pass through without causing pain (Fig. 133(a) and (b)). The prior application of a topical anaesthetic is rarely necessary for buccal infiltrations. The injections should be made well above the mucogingival junction towards the point of reflection of the sulcus. On penetrating the mucous membrane a few drops of solution should be deposited taking care to avoid ballooning the tissues. After pausing for a few seconds the needle is advanced to just below the estimated level of the apex of the tooth when, after aspirating to ensure the needle is not in a vessel, the requisite amount of solution is slowly injected. Pain is avoided by slow injection of the solution which should be at body temperature. The solution is deposited supraperiosteally and care should be taken to avoid stripping up the periosteum with the needle point, for this will cause pain at injection and also tenderness following the period of anaesthesia.

At the central incisor there is less lax soft tissue for the solution to pass into, and the fibro-muscular labial fraenum is firmly attached to the prominent nasal spine. It is difficult to give a pain-free injection here, and prior application of a topical anaesthetic is helpful. The injection should be just below the apex of this tooth, for the dense overhanging bone of the piriform rim and base of the nasal spine thicken the outer plate over the actual apex.

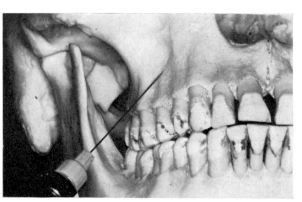

FIG. 134.—The buttress of bone formed by the zygomatic process of the maxilla may be up to 1 cm thick over the apices of the first molar. It is dense and few vascular foraminae are seen on its surface. Infiltration of solution anterior and posterior to this buttress, where the outer plate is thinner and more porous, may be necessary to anaesthetize the first molar

Similarly, the buccal apices of the upper first molar may be covered by dense bone of the zygomatic process of the maxilla to a depth of 1 cm, particularly in the child. The concavity of the surface produced by this buttress of bone means that the injection cannot be given at the level of the apices (Fig. 134), and if a lower injection fails to produce anaesthesia of sufficient degree, further solution should be deposited at the apical level just anterior and posterior to the zygomatic process.

The amount injected will depend on the type of solution and the duration of anaesthesia required, and will vary from 0·5 ml to 1·5 ml. In the central incisor and first molar regions, which are the most difficult to anaesthetize, a minimum quantity of 1 ml is necessary, whereas 0·5 ml will usually suffice for the easy areas such as the lateral incisor and premolar.

The spreading power of local anaesthetic solutions has been discussed earlier (page 309). It is often unnecessary to give more than one infiltration injection if adjacent teeth are being treated.

Palatal injection techniques

If anaesthesia of the palatal mucoperiosteum, alveolar bone and gingivae is required for the extraction of an upper tooth, a simple infiltration injection may be given at a point midway between the gingival margin and centre line of the palate. At this site, where the horizontal palatal bone joins the vertical alveolar process of the maxilla, the soft tissue is thickest and can more readily contain the injected solution than the thinner and firmly attached dense mucoperiosteum nearer to the gingival margin.

However, the greatest amount of loose areolar tissue is found just in front of the greater palatine foramen, adjacent to the second molar, and an injection made here (Fig. 135(b)) is more comfortable than further forward in the first molar and premolar areas. This injection will anaesthetize the tissues palatal to all three molars, the second premolar and usually the first premolar. The needle enters the mucoperiosteum at right angles to its surface and penetrates a few millimetres into the lax wedge of areolar tissue into which 0·25 ml of solution is very slowly injected. Since the solution is placed in front of the greater palatine foramen, it is unlikely to spread far enough posteriorly to anaesthetize the lesser palatine nerves which would produce loss of

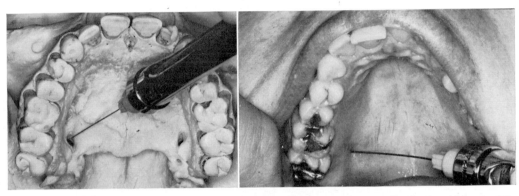

FIG. 135. (a).—*The greater palatine nerve injection* is given adjacent to the second molar just in front of the foramen and (b) midway between the gingival margin and centre line of the palate

sensation in the soft palate and fauces. This loss of sensation patients find unpleasant, and often follows attempts to block the greater palatine nerve by passing a needle into the foramen, when the lesser palatine nerves may also be anaesthetized.

In the canine region, where there is a cross innervation from the greater palatine and nasopalatine nerves, a local infiltration of solution is necessary unless both nerves are to be blocked for more extensive surgery.

The tissues palatal to the incisors can be anaesthetized by blocking the nasopalatine nerves as they leave the incisive foramen. The palatine papilla which overlies the incisive foramen is an extremely sensitive area. A topical anaesthetic is useful here, and the pain may be further reduced by injecting just lateral to the papilla (Fig. 136). With more extensive surgical procedures, such as removing buried maxillary canines or apical cysts on incisors, anaesthesia up to the level of the floor of the nose is often required. In these circumstances, following injection at the palatine papilla, the needle is passed 1 cm into the incisive canal, which runs parallel with the long axes of the central incisors. Whilst the needle is advanced, 0·5 ml of solution is slowly injected (Fig. 137(a) and (b)).

Nerve block injections for the upper jaw

There are two nerve block injections in common use in the upper jaw; the infra-orbital block injection, and the posterior superior dental block injection. The main trunk of the maxillary nerve can also be blocked in the pterygo-palatine fossa by either an intra-oral or extra-oral approach, but as these injections are not routinely used in dental practice they will not be described in detail.

(a) *Infra-orbital nerve block injection*

This injection is used when surgical procedures such as removal of cysts and apicectomies are to be carried out in the anterior maxilla, and when infiltration injections prove to be ineffective in the presence of periapical inflammation.

The position of the infra-orbital foramen may readily be determined. It lies directly below the pupil when the patient looks to the front, and 0·5 cm below the inferior rim of the orbit. The site of the zygomatico-maxillary suture on the rim can often be palpated as a notch and this lies immediately above the foramen. A perpendicular line dropped from the pupil of the eye passes through the infra-orbital foramen and coincides with the long axis of the second premolar (Fig. 138(a) and (b)). The index finger is placed over the foramen while the lip is retracted by the thumb. The entry point for the needle is just buccal to the reflection of the

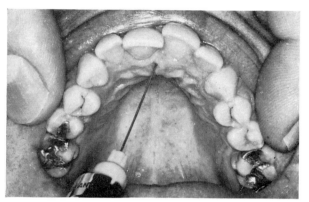

FIG. 136.—*Injection for the anterior part of the palate* given just lateral to the incisive papilla

sulcus, and further lateral than for infiltration injections. This point of entry allows the needle to pass up to the foramen in the loose areolar tissue lying between the levator anguli oris, which attaches below the foramen, and the levator labii superioris, which attaches above the foramen. If any impedance is felt to the passage of the needle, it is probably within the levator anguli oris fibres, and the solution will be deposited too low in the canine fossa. The needle is advanced slowly in the long axis of the second premolar, solution being injected at intervals until the point is just below the foramen, when the palpating finger will feel the solution being deposited. The needle point is advanced a further 0·5 cm to reach into the orifice of the foramen, where 1 ml of solution is injected very slowly whilst firm pressure is applied by the palpating index finger.

This injection will affect the anterior and, in most cases, the middle superior dental nerves, anaesthetizing the premolars, canine and incisors, the labial alveolus and soft tissues plus the skin of the lower eyelid, side of nose and upper lip. Occasionally, anaesthesia of the central incisor and tissues near the midline is incomplete. This may be due to some cross innervation from the other side. Infiltration of

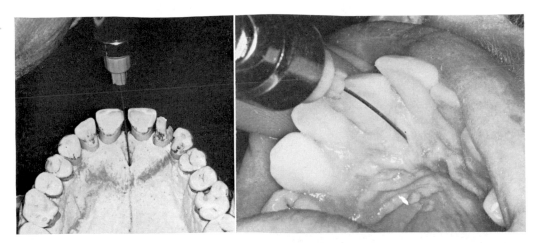

FIG. 137 (a and b).—*Nasopalatine or incisive nerve block injection* with the needle passed through the foramen into the canal

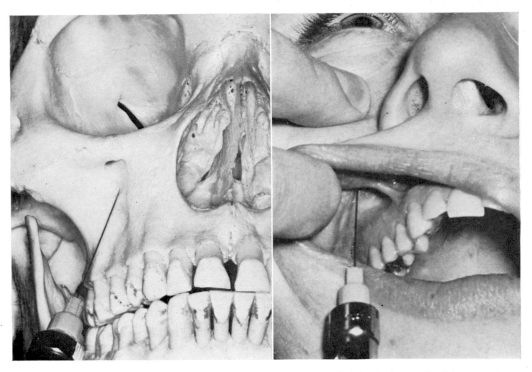

FIG. 138 (a and b).—*The infra-orbital nerve block injection.* The needle is in the long axis of the second premolar

0·25 ml of solution near the midline completes the anaesthesia. For surgical operations on the anterior maxilla, this injection is usually combined with the high nasopalatine block injection previously described.

(b) *The posterior superior dental nerve block*

With the excellent results achieved by infiltration injections using modern local
anaesthetic solutions, there is only rare need for this block injection. This is fortunate,
for it has the highest complication rate of all those commonly given in the jaws. Its
use should be restricted to cases where periodontal inflammation contraindicates an
infiltration injection, and on the few occasions when an infiltration will fail to produce
adequate anaesthesia.

For this injection, the patient's mouth should be half closed and the mandible
deviated to the same side to increase the space between the coronoid process and the

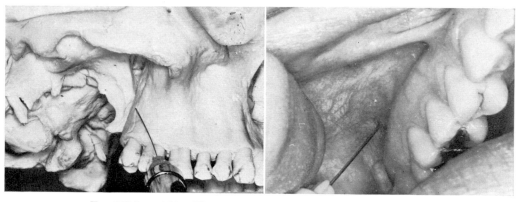

Fig. 139 (a and b).—*The posterior superior dental nerve block injection*

alveolus. The needle enters the reflection of the sulcus adjacent to the distal half of the
second molar at an angle of 45° to the alveolus laterally and 45° to the occlusal plane
(Fig. 139(a) and (b)). After infiltrating a few drops of solution and pausing for a few
seconds, the needle is advanced for 2 cm, keeping it close to the periosteum with the
syringe barrel kept as far laterally as the cheek and lips permit. This will ensure that
the needle point follows the curve of the posterolateral wall of the maxilla to the
point where the posterior superior dental nerves enter bone, and will avoid the
likelihood of damage to the pterygoid venous plexus or lateral pterygoid muscle.
Aspiration should be practised prior to injecting 1 to 1·5 ml of solution.

In patients below 15 years of age, the point of entry of the needle should be just
behind the zygomatic process of the maxilla, and in young children the angle from
the occlusal plane reduced to 30°.

This injection will give anaesthesia of the three upper molars, excepting sometimes the mesiobuccal root of the first molar, plus the alveolus and overlying soft
tissues on the buccal aspect.

LOCAL ANAESTHESIA OF THE LOWER JAW AND TEETH

Anatomy.—*The nerve supply* to the lower jaw is from the third or mandibular division of the trigeminal nerve, which leaves the base of the skull through the foramen ovale, at which point the sensory root is joined by the motor root fibres which supply the muscles of mastication. Immediately on entering the infra-temporal fossa a small motor branch is given to the medial pterygoid muscle after which the trunk divides into a predominantly motor anterior division and a predominantly sensory posterior division. The only sensory branch of the anterior division is the long buccal nerve which passes forwards and downwards from the infra-temporal fossa, running laterally to emerge from between the two heads of the lateral pterygoid muscle. Lower down it is in close relation to the temporalis muscle, and obliquely crosses first its deep tendinous attachment to the internal oblique ridge and then the superficial tendinous attachment to the external oblique ridge just below the occlusal level of the upper molars, where it is readily accessible for a nerve block injection. It then lies on the outer surface of the buccinator where it divides, sending some branches through this muscle to supply most of the mucous membrane of the cheek and buccal sulcus plus a variable area of the buccal gingivae from the second premolar distally. Other branches pass forwards and superficially to contribute to the sensory supply of the skin of the cheek.

The posterior division of the mandibular nerve first gives off two small roots which pass one each side of the middle meningeal artery, and unite posterior to it to form the auriculo-temporal nerve. This passes deep, then posterior, to the condyle of the mandible, supplying the temporo-mandibular joint, before becoming superficial and giving parasympathetic secretomotor fibres to the parotid gland and a sensory supply to part of the ear and scalp. The posterior division trunk then splits to form the lingual and inferior dental nerves, which leave the infra-temporal fossa, descending deep to the lateral pterygoid muscle into the pterygomandibular space. This is an inverted triangular shaped space with the roof formed by the lateral pterygoid and bounded laterally by the ramus of the mandible and medially by the medial pterygoid muscle. Posteriorly is the parotid gland. Anteriorly the entrance to this space is restricted laterally by the deep tendon of temporalis attached to the internal oblique line, and medially by the anterior border of medial pterygoid. This entrance is covered by the thin buccinator muscle and mucous membrane. The inferior dental nerve obliquely crosses the pterygo-mandibular space downwards and laterally to the mandibular foramen. Just before entering the foramen, the mylohyoid branch arises and perforates the spheno-mandibular ligament, and then descends in the mylohyoid groove to supply motor fibres to the mylohyoid muscle and anterior belly of digastric. The inferior dental nerve traverses the mandibular canal, supplying the molars and second premolar, and then divides at the mental foramen, a greater branch, the mental nerve, passing through the foramen, whilst the lesser branch, the incisive nerve, continues within bone to supply the first premolar, canine and incisors. The mental nerve splits on leaving its foramen to send fibres to the gingivae from the

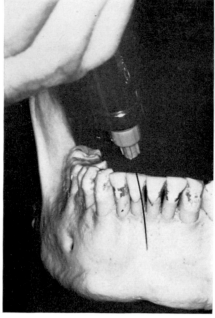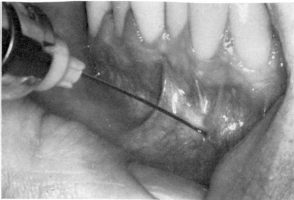

FIG. 140 (a and b).—Infiltration injection for the
mandibular incisors

first premolar to the midline, the mucosal and skin surfaces of the lower lip, and also
the chin.

As the lingual nerve descends into the pterygo-mandibular space between the
lateral and medial pterygoid muscles, it lies anterior and medial to the inferior dental
nerve. It runs downwards and forwards on the lateral surface of the medial pterygoid
muscle, turning sharply forwards into the floor of the mouth to lie on the mylohyoid
muscle, being at first just beneath the mucous membrane lingual to the third molar.
It supplies the gingivae on the lingual aspect of all the teeth, the mucous membrane
of the floor of the mouth, and the anterior two thirds of the tongue from which it
also conveys the taste fibres to the chorda tympani.

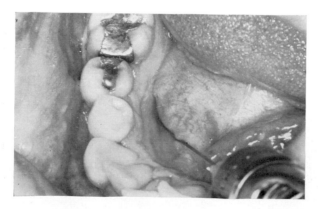

FIG. 141.—Infiltration injection to anaesthetize the lingual aspect of the mandibular
alveolus. The needle is kept close to the
surface of the mandible to avoid the sublingual gland and submandibular duct

Infiltration injection techniques

For reasons described above only the lower anterior teeth can be anaesthetized by this method. The injection technique is essentially the same as described for the upper teeth. The injection should be made just above the apices of the teeth to avoid, in so far as possible, injecting into the mentalis muscle (Fig. 140(a) and (b). The superficial fibres of the muscle are often penetrated, and to avoid pain the solution should be injected slowly and volume kept to the minimum necessary, i.e. 0·5 ml for lower incisors and 0·75 ml in the canine region where the bone is less porous. This injection will anaesthetize the tooth pulp plus bone and the soft tissues of the gingivae and sulcus on the labial aspect of the teeth. To anaesthetize the gingivae and mucoperiosteum on the lingual aspect of the teeth a separate infiltration injection is required. A volume of 0·25–0·5 ml should be deposited just below the muco-gingival junction keeping the needle close to the mandible to avoid injecting into the sublingual salivary gland or, near the midline, into the orifice of the submandibular duct (Fig. 141).

Nerve block injections for the lower jaw

There are two nerve block injections used for the lower jaw, the inferior dental nerve block and the mental and incisive nerve block. The main trunk of the mandibular nerve can be blocked *via* an extra-oral approach through the sigmoid notch, but as this injection is not in general use in dental practice it will not be described in detail.

(a) Inferior dental nerve block

As this is the only safe method of anaesthetizing the lower molars it is the most often used block injection in dental surgery. The aim of this injection is to deposit the anaesthetic solution around the trunk of the inferior dental nerve before it enters the mandibular foramen. The position of the foramen is variable and cannot be precisely determined in relation to bone and soft tissue landmarks. Fortunately the excellent spreading power of modern local anaesthetics compensates for this lack of precision and it is uncommon for even a beginner to fail to secure anaesthesia with this injection. Behind and above the mandibular foramen lies a depression in the medial surface of the ramus, the mandibular sulcus colli which funnels into the foramen (Fig. 142(a)). Anteromedially access to this sulcus from the opening to the pterygomandibular space is restricted by the lingula and the sphenomandibular ligament which, from its attachment to the lingula, passes upwards and medially. Provided the solution is deposited above the lingula and lateral to the sphenomandibular ligament it will flow upwards and backwards around the trunk of the inferior dental nerve. This spread has been demonstrated using injections of a radio-opaque fluid.

Many techniques have been described for this injection. The direct technique, which involves no change of direction of the needle once it is in the tissues, is advocated. A combination of soft tissue and bone landmarks is used, which allows for alteration in technique to accommodate known variations in position of the foramen with certain types of mandibular form. The beginner is advised to position the patient

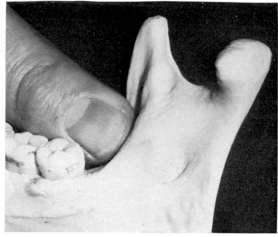

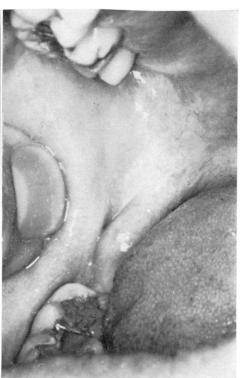

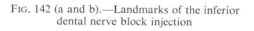

Fig. 142 (a and b).—Landmarks of the inferior
dental nerve block injection

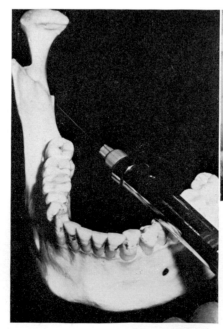

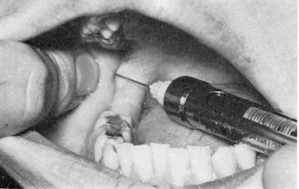

Fig. 143 (a and b).—*The inferior dental nerve block
injection.* The barrel of the syringe is kept over the
premolars on the opposite side. The needle is
inserted on a line bisecting the finger nail and at a
point lateral to the raised ridge of mucosa produced by the taut pterygo-mandibular raphe

so that, with the mouth wide open, the lower occlusal plane is horizontal. A 25 gauge long needle should be used (see Equipment, page 318). On opening the mouth widely the pterygo-mandibular raphe, a tendinous band extending from the medial wall of the mandible at the end of the mylohyoid line just behind and below the third molar up to the pterygoid hamulus, becomes taut to produce a prominent ridge in the overlying mucosa (Fig. 142(b)). To this raphe the buccinator muscle attaches anteriorly, and the superior constrictor of the pharynx posteriorly. For an injection on the right side the left index finger is passed along the buccal sulcus to palpate the external oblique ridge where the coronoid notch is found at the point of greatest concavity. For an injection on the left side, the left arm is passed behind the head of the patient, and the thumb used to retract the cheek and palpate the landmarks. The palpating digit is turned to point medially and the tip brought to lie in the retromolar fossa between the external and internal oblique ridges. A line, bisecting the finger nail and running parallel with the lower occlusal plane, will pass just above the lingula in the majority of patients (Fig. 142(a)). In the prognathic mandible, where the angle of the mandible is often obtuse, the lingula is usually above this line and therefore a higher injection should be given. In edentulous patients the line should be imagined parallel to the lower border.

The point of injection in the horizontal axis is determined (a) from palpation of the internal oblique ridge, for the needle must pass medial to the deep tendon of temporalis which is attached here, and (b) from the soft tissue landmark of the pterygomandibular raphe, for the needle must be inserted lateral to this to enter the pterygomandibular space avoiding the anterior border of medial pterygoid, which muscle forms the medial boundary of the opening to the space (Fig. 143(b)). The barrel of the syringe is placed over the premolars on the opposite side of the mandible, and is kept in this position throughout the injection (Fig. 143).

After penetrating the mucous membrane and the thin sheet of the buccinator muscle, a few drops of solution are injected and the needle slowly passed for a further 0·5 cm when it will lie medial to the lingual nerve which may readily be anaesthetized by injecting 0·25 ml here. One cm deeper the needle will lie over the lingula and even with slow injection the force of flow of 1 ml of the solution will carry it into the sulcus colli and around the nerve trunk.

To confirm the correct angulation of the needle, the beginner may pass the point deeper to make contact with the medial surface of the mandible distally in the sulcus, and then withdraw a few mm prior to injection. However, this step is not routinely necessary, and is a disadvantage, for the inferior dental vessels lie in the sulcus deeper and in closer relation to the bone surface than the nerve. Aspiration should be practised at both stages of the injection. Following introduction of the needle through the mucosa, if there is undue resistance to its further passage, it is likely to be too far laterally and impeded by the internal oblique ridge or the attached deep tendon of temporalis. This may be rectified by swinging the barrel of the syringe over the incisors to clear the needle from the obstruction, and then inserting it 0·5 cm to pass the muscle bundle, prior to returning the barrel to the original position over the premolars for the final part of the injection.

This nerve block injection will anaesthetize all the teeth to the midline, the body of the mandible, the lingual gingivae and soft tissues of the floor of the mouth and anterior two thirds of the tongue. On the buccal aspect, the soft tissues of the molar gingivae and buccal sulcus over the molars will not be fully anaesthetized as they are supplied by the long buccal nerve (*vide infra*).

Traditionally there has been a reluctance by dental surgeons to block the inferior dental and lingual nerves on both sides at one time. It appears to be widely believed that this procedure would lead to loss of control of the tongue. This is not so and most patients find little more discomfort from bilateral blocks than from a unilateral injection.

Bilateral inferior dental and lingual nerve blocks are particularly valuable in the following situations: (a) Fractures of the mandible, particularly anterior alveolar fractures, where infiltration injections into the traumatized soft tissues of the sulcus are often ineffective; (b) operations at the midline of the mandible, e.g. for removal of

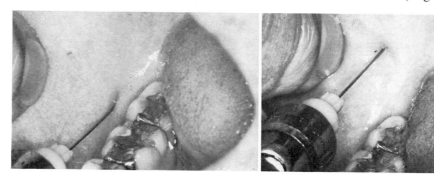

FIG. 144.—*Injections for the long buccal nerve.* (a) Infiltration in the sulcus adjacent to the molar to be extracted. (b) Block injection of the nerve as it passes from medial to lateral across the anterior border of the ascending ramus

a dental cyst and apicectomy, where infiltration and/or mental and incisive nerve block injections may not provide a satisfactory degree of anaesthesia.

Injections for the long buccal nerve are usually given by infiltration of the 0·25 to 0·5 ml of solution remaining in the cartridge after giving the inferior dental block injection, into the lax sulcus tissues adjacent to the molar which is to be extracted (Fig. 144(a)). However, if injection here is contraindicated by local infection, the nerve may be blocked as it crosses from medial to lateral across the anterior border of the ascending ramus just below the occlusal level of the upper molars (Fig. 144(b)).

(b) The mental and incisive nerve block

The mental foramen usually lies just below and between the apices of the two premolars. With firm pressure, the mental nerve can often be palpated as it curves out of the orifice to pass forwards over the rim of the foramen to supply the lip, sulcus and gingivae. In the edentulous patient, atrophy of the alveolus may bring the foramen to lie close to the crest of the alveolar ridge. The orifice of the foramen inclines posteriorly and therefore the injection should be given from behind the foramen with the needle inclined downwards and forwards (Fig. 145(a)). To facilitate this approach, the mouth should be half closed allowing greater retraction of the angle of the mouth (Fig. 145(b)). The needle penetrates the mucosa at the depth of the sulcus adjacent to the second premolar, and after infiltrating a few drops of solution, is passed forwards to enter the orifice of the foramen where 0·5–1·0 ml is slowly injected. This injection anaesthetizes the soft tissues supplied by the mental nerve, and the teeth supplied by the incisive nerve, i.e. the first premolar, canine and incisors. Often the second premolar and sometimes the first molar may be affected as the solution flows distally into the mandibular canal.

This injection will not anaesthetize the soft tissues on the lingual aspect and an infiltration lingually will be required if surgery involving these tissues is to be performed (Fig. 141).

It should be noted that there is a cross over of fibres at the midline extending to the opposite lower first incisor and overlying soft tissues. Therefore, to ensure freedom from pain when operating near to the midline, labial and lingual infiltrations may be necessary in addition to the mental nerve or inferior dental nerve blocks.

The following recommended choice of injection depends on the teeth to be treated and whether the treatment is restorative or surgical. (a) For lower incisors and/or canines—labial supraperiosteal infiltration for conservation, plus lingual infiltration for extractions; (b) for premolars alone or plus canine and incisors—mental and incisive block for conservation, as this will avoid unnecessary anaesthesia of the tongue, as would be produced by inferior dental nerve block. For extractions, the inferior dental nerve block is preferable, as one injection will include the lingual nerve territory whereas if a mental nerve block were to be given a separate lingual infiltration would be necessary; (c) when molars are involved in either conservative or surgical treatment, inferior dental nerve block supplemented by long buccal injection for extractions is indicated. For operations on the soft tissues of the floor of mouth and tongue, the lingual nerve may be blocked either as in the first part of the inferior dental nerve block injection, or at the site where it enters the floor of the mouth just medial to the lower third molar, where it lies superficially just below the mucosa. However, as local vasoconstriction is advantageous, infiltration injection at the operation site is commonly preferred to these block injections.

SPECIAL INFILTRATION TECHNIQUES FOR UPPER AND LOWER JAWS

(a) Papillary infiltration injections

These injections are commonly used to anaesthetize the gingivae for gingivectomy and gingivoplasty operations. By this method anaesthesia, plus excellent haemostasis of the vascular inflamed marginal gingivae, is achieved. However, the multiple injections into the rather dense tissue are painful. This may be helped by using topical anaesthetic aerosol sprays, or by infiltrating small amounts of solution into the laxer sulcus prior to the papillary injections. Only a few drops of solution are required in the base of each papilla which rapidly blanches (Fig. 146).

This technique is also of occasional use when supraperiosteal infiltrations or nerve block injections have failed to anaesthetize a tooth for extraction. Injection of the papillae anterior and posterior to the tooth, both buccally and lingually, with considerable pressure to force the solution into the periodontal membrane, often com-

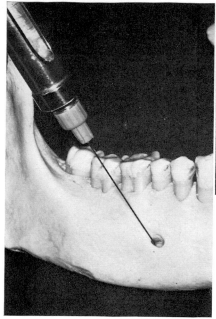

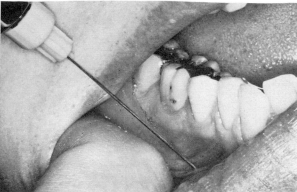

FIG. 145 (a and b).—*The mental and incisive nerve block*. The injection is given from behind the foramen with the needle inclined downwards and forwards.

pletes the anaesthesia. There is an increased risk of 'dry socket' following this procedure, and it is not recommended for routine use.

FIG. 146.—Papillary infiltration injection. A few drops of solution are injected slowly into the base of the interdental papilla which soon blanches

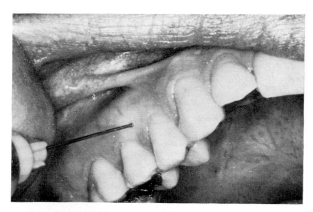

(b) Intra-osseous infiltration injections

Injection of local anaesthetic solution directly into spongy bone produces almost instantaneous anaesthesia of the adjacent teeth, as the solution rapidly diffuses around their roots. The duration of anaesthesia is relatively short, owing to rapid vascular absorption which may also lead to an increased incidence of side effects with adrenaline-containing solutions. A minority of dental surgeons use this technique routinely, for the incidence of failed injections is claimed to be lower than with infiltration and block injections, and prolonged soft tissue anaesthesia, which many patients dislike, is avoided.

The technique is particularly useful (a) where other injections have failed to anaesthetize the dental pulp adequately and (b) for the intra-septal alveolotomy technique of preparing the anterior alveolus for immediate replacement of upper teeth with a denture, where good anaesthesia and vasoconstriction is obtained without distortion of the soft tissues, which might interfere with placing the denture.

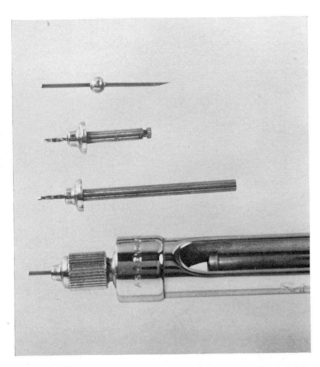

FIG. 147.—The Van Den Berg Intra-osseous Injection Kit which contains: Special cartridge syringe needle with one blunt end. Shoulder twist drills for contra-angle and straight dental hand-pieces; needle mounted in cartridge syringe with shouldered hub permitting penetration to depth of hole

The injections are often given at the interdental papilla to penetrate the interdental crest of bone. A disadvantage of this site is that the contents of infected periodontal pockets may spread deeply into the cancellous bone, and cases of osteomyelitis have been reported. Injections nearer to the apices give less chance of spreading infection, but increase the possibility of damage to the tooth roots if a drill hole is needed prior to the injection (*vide infra*). It is even possible to penetrate the outer cortex of the mandible in young children if a stout 25 gauge needle is used, and this may also suffice for the maxillary anterior teeth in adults. However, in the molar regions of adults a drill hole through the cortex must be made prior to the injection. This is best done with the special *Van Den Berg Intra-Osseous Kit* (Amalgamated Dental Co., London) illustrated in Fig. 147.

After infiltrating a few drops of solution at the mucogingival junction the twist drill is passed through the sterilized surface to tap through the cortical plate until the shoulder of the drill prevents further penetration. The special blunt ended cartridge syringe needle has the same diameter and length as the twist drill. On being placed firmly into the drill hole the shoulder of the needle hub must be pressed against the mucosa to prevent reflux of the solution. An injection of 0·5–1 ml is given slowly. The drill hole should be made on the attached gingival mucosa, for if placed on the sulcus side of the mucogingival junction the mucosa may move over the drill hole and make it difficult to locate with the needle (Fig. 148 (a and b)).

COMPLICATIONS OF LOCAL ANAESTHESIA IN DENTAL SURGERY

The incidence of serious complications of local anaesthesia in dental surgery is fortunately very low. Minor complications are of more frequent occurrence, but

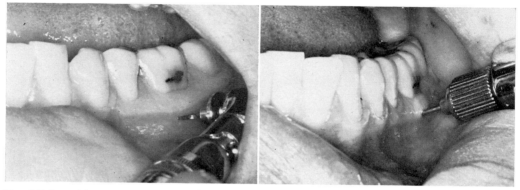

FIG. 148 (a and b).—Intra-ossous injection to obtain anaesthesia of the first mandibular molar prior to replacing a leaking buccal filling

often go unrecorded as the patient does not consider that the signs and symptoms warrant making a further visit to the dental surgeon. They are largely preventable by taking greater care with injection technique. Complications may conveniently be separated into those that are mainly systemic in effect, and those with signs and symptoms locally at the site of injection.

Systemic Complications

(a) **Fainting** (see page 167)

Fainting is the commonest complication and is due to the psychomotor effect of apprehension. Some patients have an irrational fear of injections and may even faint at the sight of the needle before the injection can be given. Many 'reactions' blamed on to the injected solution are in fact simple faints. An experienced operator will be able to recognize the apprehensive patient and prevent the faint by sympathetic management, avoiding display of instruments and unnecessary delay. A patient with a tendency to faint on being given injections will be helped by firm reassurance from a confident operator. He should be placed lying down in the dental chair with legs raised prior to the injection. A low blood sugar is not helpful in these circumstances, and the patient should therefore be advised to have a meal shortly before the appointment. In extreme cases of apprehension, premedication with a tranquillizer is useful.

The signs of an impending faint are pallor and sweating, and the skin feels cold and clammy. The patient may feel nauseated and eventually lose consciousness. If this is not noticed, and the patient is left sitting upright in the dental chair, the cerebral hypoxia consequent to the cerebral anaemia may cause jactitations. The pulse will be slow and may become weak. The treatment is to lie the patient down with legs raised, which should lead to rapid recovery of consciousness, but any dental operation should be delayed until the pulse is full and regular. Persistent bradycardia may require the administration of atropine. (See page 167).

(b) Toxic reactions (see page 311)

Toxic reactions to local anaesthetic solutions as used in dental surgery are extremely rare. To produce harmful central nervous system and cardiovascular effects, an overdose level must first be reached in the blood plasma. This can only occur with rapid intravascular injection of a large dose of local anaesthetic solution in normal patients. The very rapid absorption of potent surface anaesthetics, such as amethocaine and cocaine, from vascular mucous membranes, particularly when applied as a spray, should also not be forgotten.

Extremely rarely an individual may exhibit intolerance to a local anaesthetic drug, when toxic effects occur on injection of a standard amount of solution.

The sequence of toxic effects depends on the amount of the overdose and the type of anaesthetic solution. Cerebral stimulation manifested by excitement and confusion, with giddiness, nausea, headache and tinnitus, followed by muscle twitching and convulsions, may occur. With overdoses of anilide type drugs, e.g. lignocaine, this sequence may be missed and signs of the next stage, i.e. central depression, may occur immediately, with loss of consciousness, respiratory depression and circulatory failure. The immediate and most effective treatment of this crisis is to get the patient flat with legs raised, and give oxygen (page 290) .The convulsions were traditionally controlled by giving incremental intravenous doses of sod. thiopentone (Pentothal) in 2·5% solution, until they ceased. However, intravenous administration of diazepam is now considered the treatment of choice (page 36). If the blood pressure falls a vasopressor, e.g. metaraminol (Aramine) 1–5 mg should be given i.m. or i.v.

The vasoconstrictor content of the local anaesthetic solution, particularly adrenaline, can also cause systemic toxic effects on intravascular injection. The patient complains of palpitations due to the increased rate and force of the heart beat, a feeling of unease, and often headache due to the rise in blood-pressure. A fit patient will usually cope and recover in a few minutes but these effects could be dangerous if the patient had pre-existing cardiovascular disease.

The onset of these toxic effects could be prevented if intravascular injections were avoided by aspiration prior to injection. However, aspiration is frequently recommended but rarely practised by most dental surgeons. Not unreasonably these dental surgeons state that during many years in practice they have never witnessed a toxic reaction, and that the use of standard doses of solutions injected slowly is safe without aspiration. However, there are enough reports of untoward reactions, including several fatalities, to throw doubt on the wisdom of this attitude.

(c) Allergic reactions (see page 312)

Allergic or hypersensitivity reactions to injected local anaesthetic solutions are rare, now that the anilide type are in almost universal use. Procaine and other para-amino benzoic acid esters caused reactions more often.

The severe hypersensitivity reaction of anaphylactic shock is very rare, and in most cases of allergy due to local anaesthetics, milder immediate or delayed reactions, such as angioneurotic oedema of the lips, tongue or facies, urticarial skin rashes, or merely swelling and irritation at the site of injection, occur. The dental surgeon should be aware that repeated contact with 'ester type' topical anaesthetics, particularly those containing amethocaine, can produce an allergic contact dermatitis which may become very persistent and difficult to heal.

The treatment for acute serious reactions is intramuscular injection of 0·5–1 ml of a 1:1000 solution of adrenaline plus the administration of oxygen. An injection of hydrocortisone sodium succinate 100 mg intravenously may also be helpful. For treatment of milder angioneurotic oedema and urticarial rashes, antihistamines may be given, e.g. chlorpheniramine maleate (Piriton) 10–20 mg intramuscularly, or phenindamine tartrate (Thephorin) 25 mg t.d.s. orally.

(d) Interactions with other drugs

The only important reaction is that of the vasoconstrictor noradrenaline with tricyclic antidepressants, which may produce a significant rise in blood-pressure (page 307).

(e) Infection

Infection following local anaesthetic injections rarely causes marked systemic upset. An exception, however, may be the transmission of serum hepatitis from one patient to another by the use of contaminated needles or partly used local anaesthetic cartridges. This can obviously be avoided by using needles for one patient only and disposing of all partly used cartridges.

Local Complications

(a) Failure to obtain anaesthesia

Failure to obtain anaesthesia of teeth is an uncommon event. Periapical infection with consequent inflammation at the injection site is the most frequent reason for failure of infiltration injections (page 297). Failure with regional block injections may be due to incorrect placing of the injection, variation in the anatomy, or intravascular injection of the solution, and occurs most often with inferior dental nerve block injections. Using an aspirating technique, about 4% of all injections show evidence of intravascular injection but the figure rises to approximately 12% for inferior dental block injections alone. If most of the solution is injected into the vessel it is obvious that the nerve trunk will not be blocked.

(b) Pain

Pain at the time of injection is difficult to avoid completely. It can be minimized by using topical anaesthetics at particularly sensitive sites and by careful technique. All solutions should be warmed to body temperature. Injections should be given very slowly into dense tissues such as the palate. Injection into muscles and their tendons should be avoided. Entry into these structures can be felt, and thus injection into them prevented by using more rigid, 25 gauge, needles. The stripping of periosteum from bone by a needle point causes pain at the time of injection which often persists when the anaesthetic wears off.

Pain on injection may also be caused by irritation from the solution, usually due to contaminants. Prior to the introduction of presterilized disposable needles it was common practice to store cartridge syringes with attached needles in cold 'sterilizing' solutions. If this solution was not cleared from the lumen prior to injection, irritation of soft tissues, including nerve trunks, occurred. The incidence of after pain is greater when more concentrated, i.e. up to 1:50,000 adrenaline is used as a vasoconstrictor, and is probably due to the reactive hyperaemia that occurs after absorption of this drug. Low grade infection may be another cause of persistent discomfort at the injection site.

(c) Vascular complications

The formation of a haematoma at the site of injection occurs more often with nerve block than infiltration injections. The greatest incidence of this complication is with the posterior superior dental nerve block injection, owing to the close relation of the pterygoid plexus of veins and also the posterior superior dental artery to the site of injection (see page 326). Sometimes immediate swelling and sub-mucosal ecchymosis is obvious and further extravasation of blood should be prevented by applying firm pressure with a cotton wool roll in the sulcus. Haematoma formation is usually similarly obvious if it occurs after the mental and incisive nerve block and can be treated in the same manner. However, a haematoma following an inferior dental or infra-orbital nerve block injection is not so immediately apparent. Delayed discomfort and trismus (see section (e)) are symptomatic of inferior dental nerve block haematoma. Usually the haematoma is absorbed within a few days with no further complications but occasionally the extravasated blood becomes infected (see section (d)).

The possibility of reactionary haemorrhage into soft tissues, particularly following oral surgical procedures carried out under infiltration local anaesthesia with adrenaline containing solutions, should not be forgotten.

The systemic complications of intravascular injection and failure to obtain local anaesthesia have already been discussed. Rarely intra-arterial injection leads to other complications limited to the maxillo-facial region. Blanching of wide areas of mucosa or skin following inferior dental or posterior superior dental nerve block injections may be explained by vascular spasm caused by an intra-arterial injection of solution and vasoconstrictor, or by spasm induced by stimulation of sympathetic plexus fibres that travel with branches of the external carotid artery. Temporary disturbances of vision with blurring, double vision, or even blindness occur rarely and may be explained by intra-arterial injection (see section (i)).

(d) Infection

Infection at the site of injection is fortunately uncommon. It is unlikely that the local anaesthetic solution will be contaminated, but the practice of using a cartridge on more than one patient is to be deprecated. Infection, when it occurs, is most likely to originate from the needle, which may have been unsterile to start with, or have been contaminated by touching infected tooth surfaces or unprepared mucosa during injection. The mucosa should be dried and swabbed with an antiseptic prior to injection and care taken to avoid injections in close proximity to infected periodontal pockets or through other infected tissues. The formation of a 'needle track abscess' is rare and when it does occur is often secondary to haematoma formation. The injection involved is usually the posterior superior dental block. An abscess at this site is potentially dangerous owing to the paths of spread from the infratemporal fossa. Early drainage and antibiotic therapy is indicated.

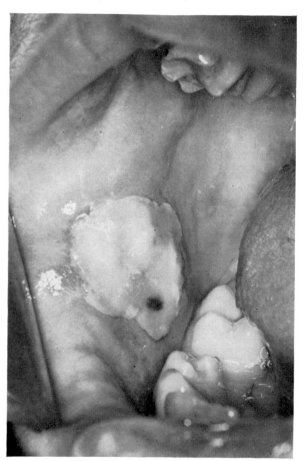

FIG. 149.—Ulceration of anaesthetized soft tissues in a child due to cheek and lip biting following inferior dental nerve block and long buccal nerve injections

(e) Trismus

Trismus is the commonest complication of inferior dental nerve block injections, and also occasionally occurs after posterior superior dental blocks. In the former, it is caused by spasm of the medial pterygoid or temporalis muscles following trauma by the needle, and in the latter, spasm of the lateral pterygoid muscle. Irritation by extravasated blood, or low grade infection may be a contributory factor. Usually the trismus is apparent soon after the anaesthetic effect wears off. Recovery to normal mouth-opening is within 5 or 6 days. However, another type of trismus less commonly occurs where the onset is gradual, over the 3 or 4 days after injection, progressing to almost complete closure which resists attempts to force the jaw open. This type may persist for several weeks until active treatment is sought. On giving the patient a general anaesthetic the trismus is not relieved, thus indicating mechanical obstruction to opening rather than simple spasm. On forcing the mouth open with gags a sudden marked snapping noise is heard, following which, manipulation of the mandible through a normal range of movement is possible. The explanation of this delayed type of trismus is probably that initial rupture of a muscle vessel is followed by haematoma formation with progressive fibrosis within the damaged muscle. This complication is more likely to occur when narrow flexible needles are used. With more rigid 25 gauge needles, penetration of the muscle can be more readily perceived and corrected. The immediate treatment of the simple form of trismus is hot saline mouthwashes, and rest by using a soft diet and avoiding forced jaw movements. If pain and tenderness are present at the injection site, suggesting infection as a factor, a course of an antibiotic should be given. If resolution is slow, infra-red radiation may be useful. Drugs with skeletal muscle relaxant properties are of no value in this type of trismus. In the case of delayed onset but persistent complete trismus mentioned above, forcible manipulation under general anaesthesia followed by encouragement of active movement by use of chewing gum is recommended.

(f) Neurological complications

The recorded incidence of damage to nerve trunks by block injections is very low. Theoretically one would expect that the nerves most likely to be traumatized are those which are blocked as they leave bone foraminae, e.g. the mental, infra-orbital and greater palatine. In fact the inferior dental nerve, followed by the lingual nerve, is most often affected.

Prolonged numbness, or more often paraesthesia, of the tissues supplied by the nerve occurs and may persist for a few weeks. The origin is probably haemorrhage in the nerve sheath caused by direct contact with the needle. Evidence of this hypothesis is that in some cases of persistent paraesthesia the patient recalls feeling an 'electric shock' sensation immediately the injection was given. Treatment is by way of an explanation of the cause and reassurance that recovery within a few weeks is likely. It is wise to warn the patient of the bizarre sensation of 'pins and needles' and hyperaesthesia that sometimes accompany recovery of sensation.

A rare complication, that usually only occurs when inexperienced students are giving inferior dental block injections, is unilateral facial palsy. This is usually partial, with the superior branches of the nerve most often affected, causing paralysis of the facial muscles and inability to close the eye. The facial nerve passes through the parotid gland which lies immediately behind the posterior border of the ascending ramus of the mandible. Branches of the nerve are sometimes incompletely encased by the gland. If an injection for the inferior dental nerve is placed too far posteriorly the solution may reach branches of the facial nerve. The treatment consists of reassurance and care that the cornea is not damaged whilst the patient is unable to close the eye. The loss of motor function usually recovers within 2 hours.

(g) Damage to anaesthetized soft tissues

The persistence of soft tissue anaesthesia for longer than necessary is an unfortunate side effect of local anaesthetic injections in the jaws. Self-inflicted trauma by biting the anaesthetized cheek, lips or tongue is not uncommon in children (Fig. 149). An effort should be made to reduce the period of soft tissue anaesthesia by sensible choice of nature and amount of solution used and type of injection given.

(h) Breakage of needles in the tissues

This has become far less common since the introduction of sterile disposable needles that are used once only. Formerly the repeated use of needles, sometimes corroded as a result of inadequate cleansing and storage in antiseptic solutions, led to breakage, particularly if injection techniques involving change of direction of the needle once within the tissues were used. The recovery of needle fragments that are completely beneath the mucosa is a difficult and tedious task.

(i) Disturbance of vision

This is fortunately a rare complication of local anaesthetic injections in the mouth, but is mentioned, for the effects are alarming to both patient and operator. Temporary blurring, double vision and even blindness have been reported.

Inadvertent intra-arterial injection on attempting to block the inferior dental or posterior superior dental nerves is probably responsible for these phenomena. The force of an injection from a cartridge syringe could lead to a retrograde flow of the solution from the inferior or posterior superior dental arteries into the internal maxillary artery, and then *via* its middle meningeal branch to the orbital vessels. It is not uncommon for the middle meningeal artery to contribute to the supply of the orbital contents *via* anastomoses with the lacrimal and ophthalmic arteries. Since the effects wear off as soon as the solution has been absorbed and rarely last more than one hour, the only treatment needed is reassurance and observation of the patient until vision returns to normal. Aspiration prior to nerve block injections would prevent this rare complication. Double vision may also be explained by direct extravascular spread of solution to affect the motor nerves to the extrinsic muscles of the eye. This could occur by passage of solution through the inferior orbital fissure following high posterior superior dental block and maxillary nerve block injections, or *via* the infra-orbital canal following infra-orbital nerve block injections.

REFERENCES MENTIONED IN THE TEXT

ADRIANI, J., ARENS, J., AUTHEMENT, E. & ZEPERNICK, R. (1964) The Comparative Potency and Effectiveness of Topical Anaesthetics in Man. *Clin. Pharmac. Ther.*, **5**, 49.

BJÖRN, H. (1947) The Determination of the Efficiency of Dental Local Anaesthetics. *Svensk Tandläk. Tidskr.*, **40**, 771.

BROWN, G. & LIVINGSTONE WARD, N. (1969) Prilocaine and Lignocaine plus Adrenaline. A Clinical Comparison. *Br. dent. J.*, **126**, 557.

CARDWELL, J. & CAWSON, R. (1969) A Trial of Lignocaine with 1:250,000 Adrenaline. *Br. J. oral Surg.*, **7**, 7.

COWAN, A. (1964) Minimum Dosage Technique in the Clinical Comparison of Representative Modern Local Anaesthetic Agents. *J. dent Res.* **43**, 1228.

COWAN, A. (1965) Comparison of Two Ultrashort Duration Anaesthetic Agents. *J. dent. Res.*, **44**, 13.

GANGEROSA, L. P. & HALIK, F. J. (1967) A Clinical Evaluation of Local Anaesthetic Solutions Containing graded Epinephrine Concentrations. *Archs oral Biol.*, **12**, 611.

RECOMMENDED FOR FURTHER READING

ADATIA, A. K. & GEHRING, E. (1972) Bilateral Inferior Alveolar and Lingual Nerve Block. *Br. dent. J.*, **133**, 377.

ADRIANI, J. (1960) The Clinical Pharmacology of Local Anaesthetics. *Clin. Pharmac. Ther.*, **1**, 645.

AELLIG, W. H., LAURENCE, D. R., O'NEIL, R. & VERRILL, P. J. (1970) Cardiac Effects of Adrenaline and Felypressin as Vasoconstrictors in Local Anaesthesia for Oral Surgery under Diazepam Sedation. *Br. J. Anaesth.*, **42**, 174.

ASTROM, A., EVERS, H. & GOLDMAN, V. (1970) A Study of the Interaction between a Tricyclic Antidepressant and some Local Anaesthetic Solutions Containing Vasoconstrictors. *Proceedings of the 3rd Asian and Australian Congress of Anaesthesiology*. Australia: Butterworth. page 517.

BARKER, B. C. W. & DAVIES, P. L. (1972) The Applied Anatomy of the Pterygomandibular Space. *Br. J. oral Surg.*, **10**, 43.

BERLING, C. (1966) Octapressin as a Vasoconstrictor in Dental Plexus Anaesthesia. *Odont. Revy*, **17**, 369.

HARRIS, S. C. (1957) Aspiration before Injection of Local Anaesthetics. *J. oral Surg.*, **15**, 299.

KAUFMAN, L. (1965) Cardiac Arrhythmias in Dentistry. *Lancet*, ii, 287.

KAY, L. & KILLEY, H. (1967) Trismus following Inferior Dental Nerve Block. *Br. med. J.* iii, 173.

LOCAL ANAESTHETICS (1971) *International Encyclopaedia of Pharmacology and Therapeutics*. 1st Ed. Section 8, Vol. 1. Oxford: Pergamon.

PETERSEN, J. K. (1971) The Mandibular Foramen Block. A Radiographic Study of the Spread of the Analgesic Solution. *Br. J. oral Surg.*, **9**, 126.

CHAPTER SIXTEEN

ANAESTHESIA IN MAXILLO-FACIAL SURGERY

BY

PHILIP MOORE

Patients undergoing operations for maxillo-facial surgery may present considerable problems to the anaesthetist, although the general principles of anaesthesia are the same as in any other branch of surgery. It is the establishment of the airway during induction of anaesthesia and its maintenance during the immediate post-operative period, which provide the major problems.

Operations can be divided into elective and emergency procedures.

Elective Operations

The following procedures are included in this category.

1. Corrective operations on the jaws such as mandibular and maxillary osteotomies, with bone grafts to replace previously resected mandibles, and 'building up' procedures, such as on-lay bone grafts.
2. Removal of tumours of the mandible and maxilla, ranging from the enucleation of simple cysts to the removal of extensive carcinoma of either jaw, the latter often involving the excision of adjacent soft tissues followed by immediate repair. Frequently, block dissection of the glands of the neck is undertaken at the same time, increasing the severity of the surgery and blood loss.
3. Operations on the tongue, the floor of the mouth and submandibular salivary glands.
4. The correction of soft tissue deformities which may be congenital, e.g. pharyngo-plasties and the closure of cleft lips and palates, or which may follow injury, previous surgery or malignant conditions.

Emergency Operations

All cases in this category are the result of trauma to the facial skeleton and/or soft tissues and may be associated with injuries to other parts of the body.

GENERAL CONSIDERATION

Specific criteria for anaesthesia in plastic surgery have been laid down by Apgar *et al.* and these, for the most part, apply to anaesthesia for maxillo-facial surgery. The order and emphasis have been altered, but they are as follows:

1. Recovery should be rapid and smooth. Restlessness and straining can dislodge fixation and dental appliances, soft tissue flaps or pedicles, or may result in haema-toma formation.

2. No technique or agent should be employed which is likely to increase bleeding.
3. Anaesthetic equipment should not encroach, or encroach as little as possible, on the operative field.
4. It is particularly desirable, where repeated anaesthetics are necessary, that the induction of anaesthesia should be as pleasant as possible. The role of the anaesthetist becomes of increasing importance to patients undergoing frequent operations and it is helpful if personal continuity in anaesthetic management can be preserved. The relation between halothane and repeated anaesthetics is discussed on page 107.
5. Finally, there should be no distortion of the operative field. This is important where soft tissues are involved.

The overall management of the anaesthetic and the choice of anaesthetic agents and techniques is, largely, a matter of individual preference. The outstanding problem is that of the establishment and maintenance of an airway before, during and following surgery. The anaesthetic management should aim for a rapid and complete return to consciousness with full recovery of the reflexes at the conclusion of the operation.

In addition to the normal examination and assessment of every patient before anaesthesia, it is necessary in every maxillo-facial case to obtain the full details of their injuries, check local conditions of anatomy (teeth, bridgework, loose crowns, etc.), and discuss with the surgeon the precise nature of the operation contemplated.

ELECTIVE OPERATIONS

In all elective procedures, other than those associated with malignancy, the anaesthetist should remember that there is no urgency in the timing of surgery. It follows, therefore, that general anaesthesia should not be undertaken in the presence of curable or improvable intercurrent disease.

Preoperative Medication

Where no difficulty with intubation is anticipated, preoperative medication presents no specific problems, and is discussed on page 20. A view is held that analgesics are not needed in premedication where there is no pre-existing pain. On the other hand, these drugs often induce a desirable feeling of euphoria and by producing a degree of preoperative analgesia, reduce the need for subsequent analgesia during maintenance also permitting a reduction in the required concentration of non-analgesic anaesthetic agents, such as halothane. In unduly anxious patients, the benzodiazepines, chlordiazepoxide or diazepam may be given for several days preoperatively.

Induction

Most patients prefer an intravenous agent to induce sleep but a few have such a dislike of injections that they prefer an inhalational induction. There is no reason why such patients should be forced to submit to the needle. Children over the age of

2 years should be assessed individually preoperatively and re-assessed at the time of induction of anaesthesia, the anaesthetist being prepared to adjust his induction technique to suit the prevailing circumstances.

The intravenous induction agents most commonly used are thiopentone or methohexitone. The latter has the advantage of leaving less postoperative sedation, but there is an increased incidence of respiratory disturbances and hiccoughs during induction, with a less easy transition to inhalational agents than with thiopentone. If these agents are followed by a short acting muscle relaxant, there is little to choose between them. Regurgitation has been seen in association with hiccoughs before the suxamethonium had taken full effect. Propanidid may be used from individual choice, or where barbiturates are contraindicated, e.g. porphyria (page 26). Intravenous diazepam gives a quiet induction with a smooth transition to inhalational agents with minimal coughing, straining or respiratory depression. It also produces a considerable degree of amnesia. It is eliminated slowly and therefore is not suitable for short procedures where rapid return to consciousness is required. On the other hand, recovery is tranquil and the reflexes return early. Recently, a steroid intravenous induction agent, *Althesin*, initially known by its clinical trial numbers, CT 1341, containing a mixture of pregnanediones, has been introduced. This agent would appear to have a wide safety margin, does not cause thrombophlebitis (c.f. hydroxydione) and, due to its rapid elimination, probably by conjugation in the liver, leads to an early and complete return to consciousness. Its place as an induction agent in anaesthesia has yet to be established (page 192) although it shows promise of replacing both methohexitone and propanidid, particularly in outpatient and day cases.

Choice of Endotracheal Tube

Endotracheal intubation is mandatory in maxillo-facial surgery. The choice between an oral and nasal tube depends upon the site of surgical intervention. In general, greater accessibility for the surgeon in all intra-oral procedures is achieved by nasal intubation, whereas in surgery for the rest of the face an oral tube is more suitable. It is of the utmost importance to prevent blood from reaching the bronchial tree. All oral endotracheal tubes must be cuffed and in addition, a throat pack is inserted. This is not just a 'belt and braces' policy; the pack reduces the amount of blood likely to find its way past the larynx into the trachea above the cuff, or down the oesophagus to the stomach which would predispose to postoperative vomiting. In many intra-oral operations, it is customary to use an uncuffed nasal tube with a pack. If, however, it is anticipated that bleeding is likely to be excessive, then a cuffed nasal tube should be passed even if a tube with a smaller lumen has to be used (page 357).

Pharyngeal Pack (page 268)

The purpose of the pack is to act as a barrier against the passage of blood and foreign material, solid or liquid. Heavy petroleum jelly packs rely on the thick grease to act as an impenetrable barrier. Sponges, gauze rolls dampened with water or petroleum jelly, and even vaginal tampons have been used. These are absorbent and should be changed as soon as they become saturated. The writer prefers a soft gauze roll dipped in hot, white paraffin and wrung out before sterilization. It remains absorbent and is sufficiently greasy to minimize trauma to the mucous membranes. A water soaked pack may dry out and become abrasive. *It should be borne in mind that the responsibility for ensuring that the pack is removed rests firmly with the person who inserted it.* The pack should be in one piece and, if a portion of it cannot be left outside the mouth, a label clearly marked 'throat pack' must be attached to the patient in a conspicuous place. The pack should be placed on either side of the endotracheal tube, starting close to the glottis and filling the pharynx. This will absorb blood from the mouth and also the nasopharynx. If surgery is limited to the lips or front teeth, the tongue may be used to occlude the pharynx and a mouth pack as opposed to a throat pack inserted to hold it in place. Once the pack is positioned, it should not be moved or pushed further back as this will cause severe abrasions of the soft palate and pharynx. It is important to allow the patient to settle before inserting the pack, since swallowing, coughing and tongue movements may displace it. Sufficient packing should be used, but any excess will serve no useful purpose and may get in the way of the operator. It is easier, more reliable and less traumatic to insert the pack under direct vision using a laryngoscope or tongue depressor and Magill forceps, rather than packing blindly with the fingers. At the conclusion of surgery, the pack should be removed with as much care as when it was inserted, since damage can be caused at this stage just as easily as during its insertion.

Maintenance

Maintenance of anaesthesia may be by almost any selected technique, bearing in mind the criteria laid down earlier, namely that no agent or technique should be used which is likely to increase haemorrhage or impair early and smooth recovery. Spontaneous ventilation with nitrous oxide, oxygen and halothane, with or without an analgesic supplement such as intravenous pethidine or pentazocine, is an acceptable technique. The writer frequently uses halothane with intermittent intravenous injections of phenoperidine, starting with an initial dose of 0·4 mg followed by increments of 0·2 mg when indicated by increased depth or rate of respirations, or other response to surgical stimuli. With this dosage, adequate respiratory exchange is maintained and the halothane concentration may be reduced to as little as 0·1% which approximates to the setting at the first mark of the Goldman vaporizer (page 67). Recovery is rapid and smooth with low incidence of postanaesthetic shivering. Alternatively, relaxants, with or without analgesic supplements, may be used with nitrous oxide and oxygen and intermittent positive pressure ventilation (I.P.P.V.). Bleeding is not increased and, again, recovery is smooth and rapid.

Pethidine, chlorpromazine and promethazine given intravenously in varying proportions (the so-called *Lytic Cocktail*), together with nitrous oxide and oxygen gives a quiet anaesthetic but recovery, although smooth, may be prolonged, and reflexes not regained rapidly.

'Neuroleptanalgesia', which employs dissociative anaesthesia and analgesia with the use of droperidol and fentanyl, together with nitrous oxide and oxygen, provides satisfactory conditions. If spontaneous respirations are to be maintained, the dose of fentanyl must not exceed 0·1 to 0·2 mg. Larger doses may only be given in conjunction with I.P.P.V. The cardiovascular system is remarkably stable and there is little, if any, fall in blood-pressure. The dissociation produced by droperidol may continue for 48 hours and patients, particularly those who become ambulant or are allowed to leave hospital on the day following operation, have complained, subsequently, of residual, subjective, dissociative effects.

The Place of Ketamine

Recently, ketamine hydrochloride has been introduced. It is a rapid acting, non-barbiturate general anaesthetic. 2-(o-chlorophenyl)-2-(methylamino) cyclohexanone hydrochloride. It is available in three strengths—10 mg/ml for intravenous use, and 50 mg/ml or 100 mg/ml for intramuscular use. The intravenous dose is 2 mg/kg body weight and the intramuscular dose is 10 mg/kg. Children whose weight is under 25 kg appear to need an increased dose in the order of 12·5 mg/kg intramuscularly. Intravenous doses last for 5 to 10 minutes whereas intramuscular doses last from 12 to 25 minutes. Incremental doses are half the induction dose. This drug produces dissociation and profound analgesia. The anaesthetic state differs fundamentally from conventional anaesthetic conditions in so far as in full dissociation the patient exhibits open eyes, frequently associated with nystagmus. When the eyes close and the patient appears to go to sleep, it is a sign that re-association is occurring and the next incremental dose is due to be given. Purposeful movement in response to surgical stimulation is also an indication for an additional dose. Since the pharyngeal reflexes are not obtunded, it is of limited use in dental surgery. Foreign material is likely to be swallowed rather than inhaled. Although regurgitation and vomiting in patients with full stomachs is less likely to occur under ketamine than under conventional anaesthesia, if it should happen, contamination of the lower respiratory tract may occur. Muscle tone is normal or increased, and operating conditions, in this type of work, far from ideal. Since it is held that the airway is maintained by the retention of muscle tone, it has been recommended for use in patients with airway difficulties. Ketamine has the disadvantage, in adults, of providing a high incidence of emergence reactions, many of which are unpleasant. These may take the form of dreams, some of which are pleasant, but many occur as hallucinatory phenomena which can be terrifying. The horrific factor may be due to the nature of the dreams or because they are recognized as hallucinations. It is the post pubertal or adult patient who is most likely to suffer from these sequelae. Since the drug, particularly when used intravenously, causes an average rise in blood pressure of 30%, it should not be used in severe hypertension or given to patients who are in, or on the brink of, congestive heart failure. Alcoholism, too, is a contraindication to the use of this drug. Although ketamine is not particularly suitable in dental or maxillo-facial surgery, it may well have a place in handling the difficult child. The intramuscular injection frequently causes crying which usually stops as soon as the injection is completed. The main cause of discomfort is probably tissue distension due to the volume of fluid injected. The recent introduction of a solution of 100 mg/ml may help to reduce this disadvantage. There appears, however, to be a high degree of amnesia to the injection in the younger age groups.

Ketamine has become a most useful anaesthetic for pre-pubertal children. Its use in adults in extremely limited because of the high incidence of unpleasant hallucinatory phenomena.

Facial Deformities

There are many congenital and acquired deformities, which may require surgical correction. Over or under development of upper and lower jaws can occur, asymmetrical development of either being possible. Such cases need treatment for both functional and cosmetic reasons. Surgery consists of osteotomies, in which whole sections of mandible or maxilla may be moved forwards or backwards involving bone grafting and fixation of the jaws. The anaesthetic problems associated with these cases are not dissimilar from those encountered in jaw fractures. Other corrective operations include building up processes by 'on-lay' bone grafts, insertion of prosthetic material and soft tissue transposition.

1. Correction of Maxillary and Mandibular Deformities

The Sagittal split intra-oral route (Obwegeser type mandibular osteotomy) may lead to extensive oedema or dissecting haematomata on the deep aspect of the mandible. This may reach the pharyngeal space with no external swelling. Respiratory embarrassment can occur with little warning. This risk can be minimized by delaying jaw fixation or by performing the operation as a two-stage procedure. It is only by very close postoperative observation for the earliest signs of airway obstruction, that the small number of severe complications in these operations can be avoided. Patients should be warned in advance that a tracheostomy may be necessary. However, modification of the operative technique, together with careful postoperative observation, is obviously preferable to routine tracheostomy.

Extensive osteotomies of the maxillae, where the middle third of the face may be moved, lead to considerable blood loss. Such cases justify the use of hypotensive anaesthetic techniques (page 357).

In a number of cases intubation may be difficult, particularly in the patient with an under-developed mandible. It may be impossible to obtain a direct view of the larynx. In such cases, and also in those with trismus or ankylosis of the temperomandibular joints, spontaneous respirations must be preserved until intubation has been achieved. This usually necessitates the use of the blind nasal route.

An extreme degree of the under developed mandible is seen in the Treacher Collins syndrome. It is often associated with a cleft palate, together with other deformities of the maxilla. Abnormalities of ears and eyes are common. A grossly receding chin makes oral intubation difficult or impossible. The case illustrated in Fig. 150 has, so far, been intubated by blind nasal technique only.

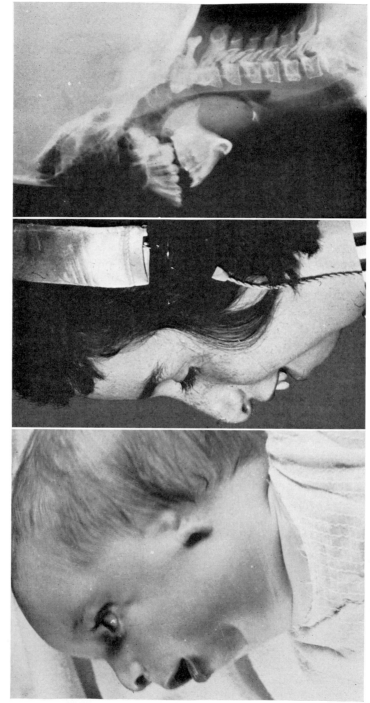

FIG. 150 (a).—Infant with Treacher Collins syndrome showing underdeveloped mandible, flattened malar region, deformity of ear and absence of external aditory meatus. (b) Same child aged 10, wearing hearing aid. (c) Lateral X-ray of skull at the same age showing the skeletal abnormalities described. Note that, when the mouth is opened, the mandible will obstruct the airway and prevent access to the larynx.

The presence of a stomach tube during the postoperative period is often recommended as a safeguard against vomiting, which carries special hazards for the patient whose jaws are wired together. It is doubtful, however, that the stomach can always be emptied by this measure, and indeed the presence of such a tube is not only uncomfortable, but may even promote nausea and vomiting. The final decision must therefore be one of individual assessment of each case.

2. Correction of Cleft Palate and Hare Lip

One of the most common deformities is the cleft palate. It may be partial or complete and is often associated with a cleft lip which may be unilateral or bilateral. The lip (one side only if the defect is bilateral) and the anterior palate are repaired at the same time, either at the age of 3 months or a weight of 5 kg, whichever is reached first. The posterior palate and the second lip cleft, if present, are repaired between the ages of 6 and 12 months since it is desirable to complete the repair before the child learns to speak. Adjustments of lip and nose may need to be carried out when the child is considerably older. There is no urgency to complete the repair and the child should be as fit as possible before the operation. These babies are often underweight due to feeding difficulties, and other congenital defects may be present. The haemoglobin may be low and surgery should not be undertaken until it has reached 10 g/100 ml, nor should the repair be carried out in the presence of pathogenic organisms, in particular, haemolytic streptococci cultured from a throat swab.

The same principles of light anaesthesia and rapid recovery apply to these procedures as in any other operation where the airway may be in jeopardy postoperatively. Premedication is restricted to atropine and the induction is inhalational. Nitrous oxide and oxygen with either halothane or ether are suitable agents both for induction and maintenance. Suxamethonium, intravenously or intramuscularly, may be used to aid intubation. Anaesthesia can be maintained either with spontaneous respiration or with I.P.P.V. associated with a muscle relaxant. Since accidental disconnection of the anaesthetic apparatus can occur beneath the sterile towels with consequent loss of ventilation, spontaneous respiration is often preferred. Following induction with nitrous oxide, oxygen and halothane, 0·25 to 0·5 ml of 1% lignocaine (2·5 to 5 mg) is applied to the glottis by means of a jet from a syringe with a *firmly* attached wide bore needle, previously tested for patency. This ensures that only a small, measured quantity of lignocaine is used. Anaesthesia is continued, to allow time for the lignocaine to take effect, and the endotracheal tube is inserted. The lignocaine allows intubation without coughing or spasm under light anaesthesia and is absorbed sufficiently rapidly to permit full return of the reflexes by the end of the operation. In palatal repairs, it is the surgeon who inserts and removes the throat pack, but where the lip only is involved, this becomes the anaesthetist's responsibility.

Intubation may present difficulties, particularly if the lower jaw is under-developed. The larynx may be difficult to reach and an under-developed epiglottis may add to the problem. It is often easier to use a laryngoscope with a straight blade which lifts the epiglottis directly rather than a curved blade instrument such as the MacIntosh (see Fig. 151). The cross section of the blade is also important; a C shaped cross section of the blade is also important; a C shaped cross section prevents the upper lip from occluding the view and this may be especially helpful where there is a bilateral cleft in which the pre-maxilla is rotated forwards and upwards and may project directly into the field of view (Fig. 152). In addition a broad blade is recom-

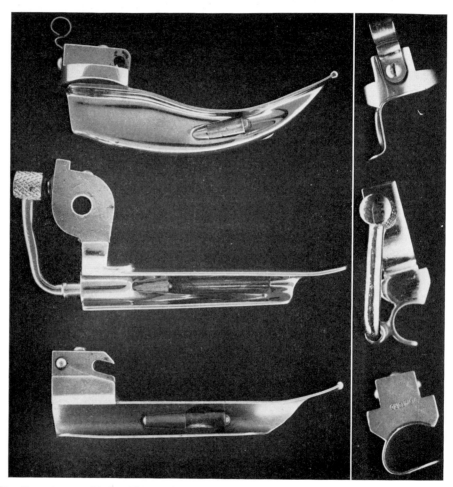

FIG. 151.—Laryngoscope blades. Above. The MacIntosh blade. Middle. The Magill blade. Below. The Oxford Infant blade.

mended, for it is less likely to become lodged in a wide unilateral cleft in the maxilla (Fig. 153). Occasionally, there may be a sub-glottic stenosis so that satisfactory intubation can only be achieved by the use of a smaller tube. It should be stressed again that this is not an urgent operation and if, for any reason at all, intubation is traumatic, or the induction time is unduly prolonged, or the baby undergoes any significant degree of hypoxia, the anaesthetist should swallow his pride, abandon the

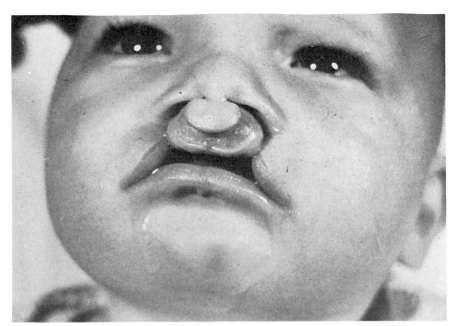

FIG. 152.—Infant with bilateral cleft lip. Note forward and upward rotation of the pre-maxilla

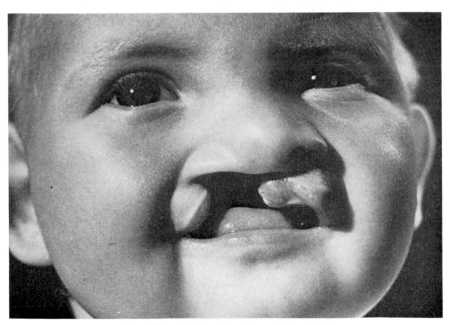

FIG. 153.—Infant with wide unilateral cleft

anaesthetic and postpone the operation until a later date, by which time the normal development and growth of the child may have reduced the problems significantly. Armoured endotracheal tubes of different kinds have been used, e.g. flexo-metallic and nylon or wire reinforced latex tubes. All such tubes tend to be compressed between the mouth gag and the lower alveolus. They also have a tendency to be dislodged during the early manipulation of the mouth gag and later may be pushed

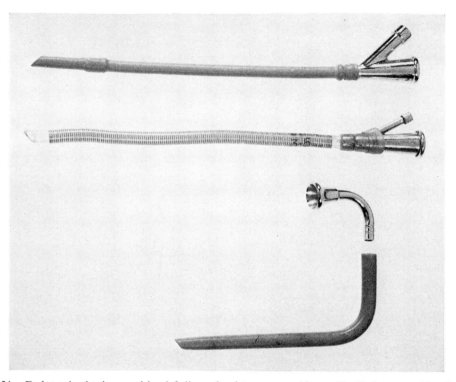

FIG. 154.—Endotracheal tubes used in cleft lip and palate surgery. Above. Magill flexo-metallic tube with wide bore gas inlet. The tip is made of red rubber, the remainder of the tube consisting of a metal spiral covered with thin red rubber or latex. Note the collar at the junction which may press on or pass through the cords causing some degree of trauma. Middle. Woodfield-David metal reinforced latex tube with narrow bore gas inlet. (the size of this inlet is optional with either tube.) The metal spiral is not easily compressed by the mouth gag but, in all such tubes, small areas of the inner layer of latex can separate from the metal, form bubbles and occlude the lumen. Nylon reinforced tubes (not illustrated), although "kink proof" are compressed too easily to be of value in these cases. Below. An Oxford right-angled tube with a Magill oral connection which, when inserted in the tube, supports it where it is most likely to be compressed.

further down the trachea to enter one or other bronchus, usually the right. The Oxford right angled tube (Fig. 154) would seem to be the most satisfactory. It is uncuffed for the small child, sits nicely under the gag and, in the writer's experience, does not lead to endobronchial anaesthesia. A right angled Magill connection prevents compression between the gag and either the lower alveolar margin, or the teeth in the older child. There are two periods when loss of airway is most likely to occur.

The first is during the insertion and opening of the mouth gag by the surgeon and is due to compression or dislodgement of the tube, and the second follows the insertion of the throat pack in palatal repairs. The anaesthetist must check very carefully at both these times that there is no diminution of respiratory exchange and he must listen with a stethoscope to ensure that air entry is present in both left and right upper lobes. The occurrence of these complications has been minimized since the introduction of the Oxford tube.

Different types of mouth gag are used, but all have a slit or groove in the tongue

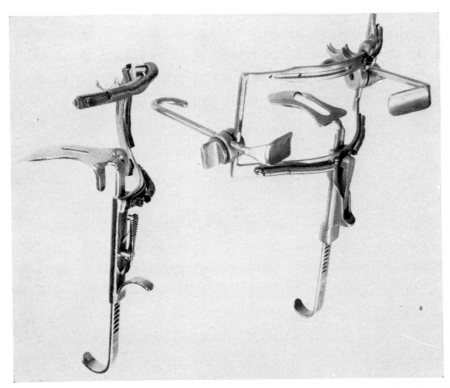

Fig. 155.—Cleft palate mouth gags. Left. Kilner-Dott mouth gag. Right. Dingman gag with adjustable cheek retractors.

depressor which maintains the position of the oral tube (Fig. 155). Unlike the tonsil gag, the cleft palate gag does not need to expose the posterior pharynx, the blade thus being wider and shorter than the Boyle-Davis gag. Although a sandbag is placed under the baby's shoulders, extreme extension of the neck is not necessary. Maintenance of anaesthesia with spontaneous respirations is by means of nitrous oxide and oxygen, supplemented by halothane or other suitable inhalational agent. The rapid recovery associated with halothane is an advantage. An Ayre's T-piece principle or Mapleson type E circuit (Fig. 124) is used with a gas flow of at least twice the child's minute volume. Frequently, the operator uses a small amount of local anaesthetic and adrenaline to reduce bleeding, and this permits anaesthesia to be maintained at a very light plane. At the conclusion of surgery, the throat pack is removed, pharyngeal toilet is carried out, and since neither an oral airway nor a pharyngeal tube may be used, for fear of disrupting the repair, a tongue stitch is inserted to enable it to be pulled forward in an emergency, and the child is turned on his side. It is imperative to obtain a rapid return to consciousness and, as a rule, very little postoperative sedation is needed.

The most likely anaesthetic complications following this operation are respiratory. Some degree of stridor occurs in a small number of cases and usually responds to nursing in warm moist air in a steam tent. Very rarely, laryngeal oedema may develop, in which case stridor is pronounced and signs of respiratory obstruction are evident. The baby should be nursed in a humidified oxygen tent, hydrocortisone (50 mg i.m.) given promptly, and if the laryngeal obstruction is not relieved the child should be re-intubated. It should always be possible to avoid a tracheostomy in these cases, since the oedema usually subsides rapidly and the airway is maintained by the endotracheal tube. Laryngeal oedema occurred more frequently in the past when trauma associated with endotracheal intubation was not uncommon, and little attention was paid to the presence of pathogenic organisms in the throat.

In spite of all preventative measures, some contamination of the lower respiratory tract may occur, usually in the immediate postoperative period. This may lead to pulmonary infections and atelectasis. Treatment consists of antibiotics and oxygen therapy where necessary.

Malignant Disease

Surgery for the removal of malignant tumours of the jaws is extensive and leads to considerable loss of blood. Maxillary tumours may involve the removal of the complete maxilla on the affected side together with the zygoma and orbital floor. Central tumours require the excision of the middle third including the nasal bones. Malignant disease below the maxilla occurs in the mandible, tongue and floor of the mouth. Treatment consists of surgical removal of part of the mandible, partial glossectomy, which may mean the lateral half of the tongue or the anterior two-thirds, and extensive excision of the floor of the mouth and underlying muscles. Block dissection of the glands of the neck is usually carried out at the same time. This will be either unilateral or, in the case of a centrally placed growth, submental. Following partial removal of the mandible, the remaining fragment may be immobilized by being splinted to the maxilla with inter-dental wires or locking bars. Postoperative airway difficulties depend upon the extent of destruction of the muscles controlling the tongue and the removal of their mandibular support. Mandibulectomy, which stops short of the midline interferes little with airway control, but should it extend across the midline, or involve both horizontal rami, tracheostomy is essential. Soft tissue loss in these operations can be extensive. The mucous lining of the mouth may be difficult to close, and skin loss may necessitate rotation, transposition flaps, or free split skin grafts to repair the defect. Occasionally, the mandibular defect may be repaired at the same operation by means of a bone graft or prosthesis.

Essential anaesthetic requirements are:

(1) Complete control of the airway with a cuffed endotracheal tube, which may be sited orally where the maxillae only are involved, but should be nasal for all others. Even in hemi-maxillectomy a cuffed nasal tube down the contra-lateral nostril is more convenient for the surgeon and easier to stabilise than an oral tube.

(2) A throat pack.

(3) A stomach tube passed before the operation since this may be a difficult procedure at the conclusion.

(4) An intravenous infusion. Blood should be cross matched and available immediately. Apart from the risk of blood loss during surgery, these patients may be anaemic so their preoperative haemoglobin must be estimated. Difficulties in intubation can result from the size of the tumour, trismus, ankylosis of the tempero-mandibular joints, induration of the soft tissues with malignant infiltration, radiotherapy or scarring from previous surgery. The oral cavity and nasopharynx may be contaminated with pus, necrotic material and blood. It is most important to avoid extending such contamination to the lower respiratory tract. Dental cap splints may have been applied preoperatively; they can further restrict access to the mouth and care must be taken to avoid damaging or dislodging them. If no difficulty in intubation is anticipated, induction of anaesthesia may be by means of an intravenous anaesthetic followed by suxamethonium, but where difficulty is expected, induction of anaesthesia should follow the lines described in *Difficulties of Intubation* (page 368).

If a tracheostomy is considered necessary, it should be carried out initially. With a tracheostomy, postoperative airway problems are minimized whereas, without one, the problems are similar to those following acute trauma (page 363). An additional hazard is created by pressure dressings around the neck and the lower part of the face where plastic repair has been carried out.

The malignant case, in which there is considerable blood loss, and where accurate dissection is important, fully justifies the use of induced hypotension.

Induced Hypotension

Controlled hypotension leads to greatly reduced blood loss during surgery, which lessens or abolishes the need for blood transfusion. The surgeon is presented with relatively bloodless operating conditions, thus enabling him to perform a cleaner dissection more rapidly.

In order to produce a significant reduction in bleeding, the systolic blood-pressure should be lowered to 70 mm/Hg or less. More moderate falls do not give a dry field and merely rob the patient of the ability to compensate for any blood loss sustained.

The basic mechanism involved in hypotensive techniques is that of lowering the peripheral resistance. In addition, posture contributes to the reduction in bleeding at the operative site by (a) increasing the overall fall in blood-pressure and (b) elevating the part of the body undergoing surgery, thus decreasing its local vascularity.

While a normal cardiovascular system can withstand considerable falls of blood-pressure without obvious harm, diseased and narrowed arteries which are unable to dilate may, where the pressure is low, lead to inadequate tissue perfusion and, since the rate of flow is reduced, thrombosis within the vessels and tissue ischaemia. Cerebral ischaemia or thrombosis may lead to temporary or permanent brain damage. Cardiac ischaemia, myocardial infarction, retinal artery thrombosis, liver necrosis, and renal damage have been reported.

The healthy, young patient probably runs very little risk from prolonged hypotension, but the older patient who may suffer from known or unrecognized arterial disease must, inevitably, run a greater risk than he would if his blood-pressure were maintained within normal limits.

Sometimes other methods of reducing blood loss are preferable to hypotension. Where the operative field is limited, the use of local vaso-constrictors can be helpful. Following induction of general anaesthesia infiltration with a local analgesic and adrenaline (1 in 320,000 to 1 in 400,000) has been used for block dissections of the glands of the neck, where the patient's cardiovascular system has been sufficiently diseased to preclude the use of hypotension. A satisfactorily dry field is produced for the first 90 minutes, but bleeding becomes troublesome in the later stages of the operation. It does, however, allow the surgeon time to carry out the difficult parts of the dissection.

Methods of Producing Induced Hypotension

The induction of anaesthesia, prior to the use of induced hypotension, must be as smooth as possible, avoiding straining and coughing which would raise venous pressure. Care must be taken to ensure that the airway is faultless, since any degree of obstruction with concomitant hypoxia, coupled with a low blood-pressure, may be disastrous. There is often a significant fall in blood-pressure after premedication and, almost certainly, after the induction of anaesthesia. This fall may be accentuated by posture where the patient is placed in the 'head up' position. However, under light anaesthesia where autonomic control is not lost, surgical stimulation, together with the redistribution of the induction agents, rapidly leads to some return of vasomotor tone and an increase in blood-pressure. The following methods of producing controlled hypotension are in current use.

1. **Deep Anaesthesia.**—Deep anaesthesia with halothane causes a fall in blood-pressure. This fall is due to a variety of mechanisms which may result in a reduction in both cardiac output and peripheral resistance (page 105). The use of deep anaesthesia with halothane, necessitating high concentrations of the inspired vapour, is not without the risk of overdosage and respiratory depression leading to carbon dioxide retention. This combination encourages the development of cardiac arrhythmias, e.g. bradycardia, ventricular ectopics, ventricular tachycardia and even

ventricular fibrillation. Furthermore, after prolonged deep anaesthesia with halothane, recovery may be slow and there may be an increased incidence of postoperative shivering.

2. **Light Anaesthesia, Paralysis and I.P.P.V.**—Lighter anaesthesia with halothane combined with curare and I.P.P.V. produces a similar effect with a more rapid recovery of both blood-pressure and consciousness. The fall in blood-pressure is increased by the ganglion blocking effect of curare. As a rule, a fairly small dose of curare (15 to 30 mg) is all that is needed, and the patient is ventilated with oxygen and halothane, or nitrous oxide, oxygen and halothane, the halothane concentration being in the order of 0·5 to 2%. The blood pressure can be titrated against the concentration of halothane with this combination of drugs, and normal pressure can be restored rapidly by stopping the halothane and reversing the curare.

3. **Ganglionic Blockade.**—The use of specific ganglion blocking agents is one of the more usual ways of artificially lowering the blood-pressure. The two ganglion blocking agents currently available are pentolinium tartrate (Ansolysen) and trimetaphan camphorsulphonate (Arfonad).

Pentolinium tartrate ($C_{23}H_{42}O_{12}N_2$) is pentamethylene 1:5-Bis (1-methylpyrrolidinium) hydrogen tartrate. Its properties are similar to those of the hexamethonium salts, inhibiting transmission in autonomic ganglia by the competitive inhibition of acetylcholine. It is approximately five times as potent and has a longer action than hexamethonium and does not antagonize the neuromuscular blocking action of decamethonium. The dose is 10 to 20 mg of a 0·5% solution intravenously. The drug is excreted in the urine.

Trimetaphan ($C_{32}H_{40}O_5N_2S_2$) is 4:6-Dibenzyl-5-oxo-l-thia-4:6-diazatricyclo $(6:3:0:0^{3:7})$ undecanium $(+)$-β-camphor-sulphonate. This is a ganglion blocking agent of rapid onset and short duration (5 to 20 minutes). In addition to its ganglion blocking effect, it has a histamine liberating action and a direct vasodilator effect on small blood vessels. Tachyphylaxis may be produced with repeated doses. Compensatory tachycardia may develop in the younger patient, and is associated with failure to achieve adequate levels of hypotension. The drug is partly destroyed by cholinesterase, the remainder being excreted by the kidneys.

Trimetaphan may be used as a continuous 0·1% intravenous infusion, the drip rate being titrated against the systolic blood-pressure level. It may also be used as an intermittent intravenous injection, the effect lasting from 5 to 20 minutes. The dose varies according to the cardiovascular state of the patient, and with the anaesthetic agents and techniques employed. A healthy young adult may need as much as 50 mg as an initial dose, followed by 10 to 30 mg at 10 to 15 minute intervals, whereas an elderly, atherosclerotic patient having halothane may need as little as 5 to 15 mg and less in subsequent doses. In many cases, an initial fall of blood-pressure to the required level is produced rapidly by trimetaphan and the level maintained by halothane, no further trimetaphan being required even after its initial effects have completely worn off.

With both ganglion blocking agents, tachycardia may occur with consequent failure to lower the blood-pressure and increased capillary oozing. Halothane, in combination with a ganglion blocking agent, has already been discussed. Tachycardia may also be prevented by the use of a specific β adrenergic blocking agent such as practolol or propranolol (page 23).

4. **Sodium Nitroprusside.**—Recently, sodium nitroprusside has been used to produce hypotension. It does not block the autonomic system but produces vasodilatation by direct action on the blood vessels. The degree of fall in blood-pressure does not appear to be easy to control, although normal pressure is restored rapidly when the drug is discontinued. It is given as a 0·01% infusion. At the present time the use of this drug must be considered to be in an experimental stage.

There are two alternatives in the whole approach to hypotensive techniques. The first is the production of hypotension for a short period of time allowing the blood-pressure to return to normal before the end of the operation. This allows the surgeon to complete his dissection with a relatively dry operative field and to ligate or diathermy all bleeding points as the blood-pressure rises before closure of the wound. This approach can be achieved by any of the methods described, but if a ganglion blocking agent is used, it should be short-acting, and may be given as the sole hypotensive agent, or, in minimal dosage, in conjunction with halothane and posture. Restoration of the blood-pressure is rapid, but it must be remembered that it is likely to be labile for some hours afterwards and sudden changes in posture should be avoided.

In the second method, a long-acting ganglion blocker is used and the whole operation completed with a low systolic pressure. Postoperatively, the blood-pressure is allowed to rise slowly to its normal level. If the blood-pressure is to remain low for a prolonged period, haemostasis during surgery must be meticulous.

Whichever method of reducing the blood-pressure is used, it must be borne in mind that the patient has been robbed of his normal mechanisms of compensating for haemorrhage. It is, therefore, not only imperative that any blood loss must be replaced immediately by blood transfusion, but it is also of the greatest importance that no degree of hypoxia or hypercarbia is allowed. The airway must be faultless and the inspired oxygen concentration high. Following the use of any hypotensive technique, the patient should be observed very closely for some hours postoperatively. Blood-pressure should be checked every 15 minutes and care should be taken to avoid unnecessary changes of posture. The patient should be nursed flat and supplementary oxygen added to the inspired air. Elevation of the head should be allowed only when the blood-pressure approximates to normal levels and is maintained in the new posture. The blood-pressure must be checked after any such change in position. Ideally, the patient should spend some hours in a well staffed and fully equipped recovery ward, but where this is not available, individual intensive care must be instituted and with every requirement for resuscitation at hand. Blood loss must be carefully observed and, should haemorrhage occur, replacement must be immediate. When induced hypotension is used, co-operation within the whole surgical team is of the utmost importance. The writer feels that hypotensive techniques should be used only where they benefit the patient and not purely for the convenience of the surgeon or at the whim of the anaesthetist. The risk of the complications of hypotension should be no greater than the risk of the condition necessitating surgery, or the risk of the surgical procedure itself. This restricts its use to cases of malignant disease, to cases of non-malignant disease where blood loss may be considerable, and in other cases where reduced bleeding will enable a surgeon to perform an operation which would otherwise be difficult or hazardous. There is also a case for the use of induced hypotension in patients who have a rare blood group, and perhaps in people undergoing surgery whose religious beliefs preclude the use of blood transfusions.

EMERGENCY OPERATIONS

This category includes all injuries of the facial skeleton, sometimes associated with soft tissue damage and injuries to other parts of the body. In cases of multiple injury, the treatment of severe thoracic, intracranial or intra-abdominal damage must take priority over maxillo-facial problems, unless the latter are associated with serious bleeding or loss of airway. It must be stressed that resuscitation with adequate fluid replacement should be carried out, or at least instituted, before surgery is undertaken.

Contrary to what might be expected, it is unusual for a patient with maxillo-facial injuries to present in a shocked condition unless any of the concomitant injuries, mentioned above, are present.

Fractures of the Facial Skeleton

1. Fractures of the zygoma present little problem from the anaesthetic point of view. The repair can be a simple elevation of the zygomatic arch or may involve wiring or pinning of the fragments. If the maxillary sinuses are involved, blood may reach the pharynx during surgery.
2. Nasal fractures must be assumed to have bled copiously at the time of injury and there is the strong possibility that the stomach will contain blood. As with any such problem, precautions must be taken during induction of anaesthesia to deal with vomiting or regurgitation, and prevent contamination of the trachea and bronchial tree. It is equally certain that correction of such fractures will lead to further copious haemorrhage. It is advisable to reduce bleeding to the minimum, a useful technique, following induction of anaesthesia and intubation, being to shrink the nasal mucous membranes by the application of 10% cocaine on cotton-wool applicators, three in each nostril. The first is inserted as far as possible in an upward direction, the second under the middle turbinates, and the third along the floor of the nose. They should be left in position for at least 15 minutes. Although approximately 3 ml of 10% cocaine are required to soak the six cotton-wool applica-

tors, minimal absorption ensures that toxic effects are rarely encountered. It is unnecessary to add adrenaline to the cocaine, since vasoconstriction is not increased and, with adrenaline, there is a greater likelihood of a reactive hyperaemia when the effect of the drug has worn off.

3. Fractures of the mandible may be simple, multiple, or compound into the mouth. In simple fractures of the mandible, with minimal displacement, it is important to cause as little disturbance to the fracture as possible. The wide opening of the mouth associated with the passage of a laryngoscope may convert a simple fracture

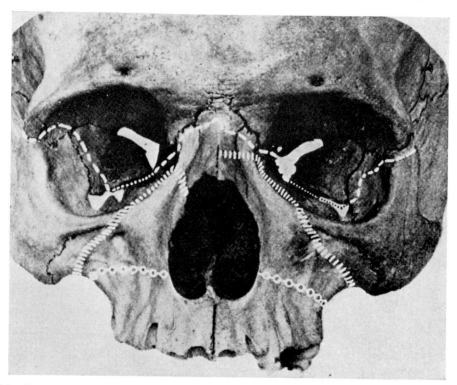

Fig. 156.—Common sites of maxillary fractures as classified by Le Fort. Le Fort I. -o-o-o-o- Le Fort II. IIIIIIII Le Fort III. — — — — — — — —

into a compound one, or may cause greater displacement of the bone fragments than already exists. Blind nasal intubation is helpful in such cases and the throat pack should be inserted with a tongue depressor, rather than a laryngoscope, with minimal movement of the mandible. It is unlikely that there will be any foreign material in the mouth or nasopharynx in these cases.

4. Maxillary fractures have been classified by Le Fort (Fig. 156). Le Fort I is a transverse maxillary fracture above the palate; a Le Fort II is a pyramidal fracture involving the nasal bones and infra-orbital margins, whilst a Le Fort III consists of a transverse fracture across the zygoma, orbital floor, ethmoids and sphenoids. The

whole middle third of the maxillae may be 'floating'. Le Fort fractures II and III are often associated with cerebro-spinal fluid rhinorrhoea.

Severe fractures of the face present the two major problems of loss of airway and haemorrhage. Proper first aid measures, before the patient reaches hospital, can be life saving. Unless major vessels are involved, bleeding is not usually severe, and it is the airway that is of paramount importance. The patient should be transported either face down or in the lateral position, depending upon the effect on his airway, so that blood will gravitate outwards and not enter the lower respiratory tract. On arrival

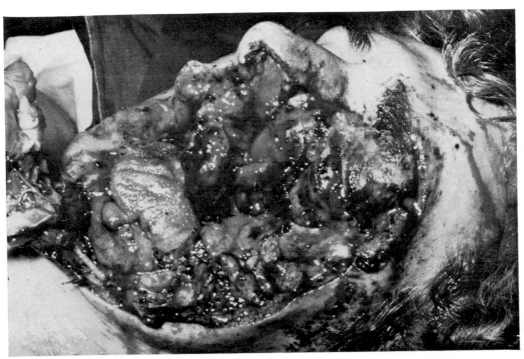

Fig. 157.—Severe facial injury following a road traffic accident.

in hospital, respiratory and circulatory problems must be dealt with immediately, even if that entails giving a general anaesthetic to an unstarved patient. When the patient reaches the anaesthetist, his first consideration is the establishment and maintenance of the airway. The stomach may be full of blood and, if the accident occurred shortly after a meal, will also contain food. It is useless to wait for natural emptying of the stomach, and not practical to empty it by passing a stomach tube or by induced emesis. Anaesthesia should be undertaken without delay, with full pre-parations for dealing with massive vomiting or regurgitation. The stomach may be emptied by means of a naso-gastric tube after the establishment of a secure airway.

Where disruption of the facial skeleton and soft tissues is extensive, further dis-placement by the anaesthetist is of little consequence (Fig. 157). The airway must be secured, followed by nasopharyngeal and tracheobronchial toilet. If it is known or suspected that foreign bodies such as loose teeth, bone fragments, or pieces of denture have entered the trachea, it is at this stage that bronchoscopy must be undertaken, the only exception being where haemorrhage is so extensive that this must be dealt with first.

Prior to induction it is essential to have available a selection of cuffed and uncuffed oral and nasal tubes, laryngoscopes and bronchoscopes checked to be in working order, Magill forceps, and powerful suction, already working, with a wide bore suction nozzle and a selection of suction catheters. A tracheostomy set should be readily available. Anaesthesia should be induced with the patient in whatever position is needed to maintain a satisfactory airway. It must be possible to tilt the patient head down if regurgitation occurs; induction, therefore, must be undertaken either on a tilting trolley or an operating table.

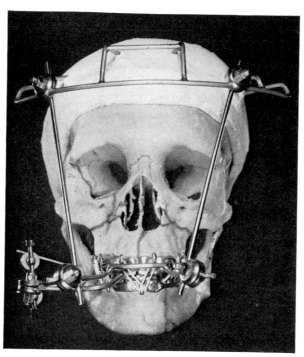

FIG. 158—Skull marked with multiple maxillary and mandibular fractures showing a variety of methods of fixation. These include a plaster head-cap with external locking bars to dental cap splints, pin fixation of the right ascending mandibular ramus and inter-dental locking bars together with rubber bands

Anaesthesia should be induced with an intravenous agent in suitable dosage for the patient's general condition, followed by a short acting muscle relaxant and the passage of an endotracheal tube, cricoid pressure being used to prevent regurgitation. The greater the disruption of tissues, the less relaxation is required and in some cases, none at all. If no active bleeding is taking place and a reasonable airway exists, anaesthesia may be deepened with inhalational agents, spontaneous respirations being maintained and the use of a muscle relaxant with its resultant apnoea thus being avoided. This is particularly important if there is any doubt over the ability to obtain access to the larynx.

In the majority of mandibular fractures, fixation is obtained by splinting the mandible and maxilla together by means of interdental or circumferential wiring, locking cap splints and/or interosseous pinning with external locking bars. Maxillary fractures, after reduction, are secured by means of wires and dental cap splints locked externally to the cranium, usually to a plaster head cap or halo frame (Fig.

158). Recently, a 'box' fixation has been devised consisting of a cranio-mandibular fixation with external locking bars between the mandible and the supra-orbital region, the maxilla being sandwiched between and wired or splinted to the mandible (Fig. 159). In all cases of mandibular fractures, in cases where both mandibular and maxillary fractures co-exist, and in maxillary fractures where the 'box' method is used, nasotracheal intubation is essential. Very rarely, with extensive maxillary damage and excessive bleeding, it may be necessary to pass an orotracheal tube while the bleeding is controlled and the fractures reduced, and then a change made to a nasal tube before final fixation and locking of the fragments.

Where a nasal tube is used in maxillary fractures, there is no place for blind intubation since blood and debris may be carried into the trachea unobserved. A well lubricated Magill tube, preferably cuffed, is passed gently through the nostril and into the nasopharynx. The tube should contain a suction catheter to prevent blockage by foreign material during its passage through the nose. Once in the pharynx, the tip of the tube should be under direct vision, the suction catheter removed, and direct suction with a throat sucker used to clear the pharynx while the tube is passed through the glottis. The cuff is inflated and time may now be spent in further pharyngeal toilet and the passage of a stomach tube if this is deemed necessary. The throat pack is inserted at this stage.

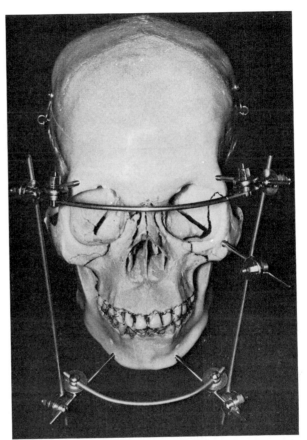

Fig. 159.—Skull with "box" fixation showing inter-dental wiring and an additional pin holding the left, fractured zygoma in place

Further tracheobronchial toilet may be carried out with a suction catheter. It should be remembered that the cuff should always be inflated during suction through the endotracheal tube once through the glottis, both at this stage and at the conclusion of the operation, since a negative pressure in the trachea will suck blood and debris through the glottis, causing further contamination of the lower respiratory tract.

A view is held that orotracheal tubes should be used always in this type of case and mandibulo-maxillary fixation completed after recovery of consciousness.

Reasons for this opinion include the provision of a better airway with a tube of larger bore than can be passed through the nose, avoidance of tracheobronchial contamination, ease of re-establishing the airway if there is difficulty during recovery and a reduction of the likelihood of meningitis if cerebro-spinal fluid rhinorrhoea, from fractures of the cribriform plate, is present. On the other hand, fixation is more efficient if carried out under general anaesthesia; the airway is adequate through a nasotracheal tube; with reasonable care, tracheobronchial contamination is avoidable; lastly, meningitis is rare, the few cases which have occurred being difficult to connect with nasotracheal intubation or the use of nasopharyngeal airways. Moreover, even where nasal fractures are present, it is quite possible for the surgeon to manipulate both septum and nasal bones adequately with the nasotracheal tube in position.

Maintenance of anaesthesia throughout these operations may be by any of the previously mentioned techniques, the importance of a rapid and full recovery again being stressed. In all but the most minor fractures, intravenous fluids will be needed

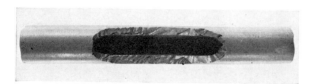

FIG. 160.—Buccal airway. This, placed anterior to the teeth with the open ends inside the cheeks, holds the lips apart and provides an oral airway when the jaws are wired together

and blood loss should be replaced. If during the course of the operation the pack becomes severely contaminated, it is wise to replace it with a fresh one. Careful oral toilet should be carried out by the operator and checked by the anaesthetist before the jaws are fastened together. The throat pack may have to be removed at this stage but, quite often, there is a gap in the patient's dentition through which it may be removed at the conclusion of surgery. Every care must be taken to clear the nasopharynx before, during and after the removal of the endotracheal tube. This is far easier to state than to accomplish. It is inevitable that there will be some residual bleeding, thus demanding that laryngeal and pharyngeal reflexes are present, and that the patient is able to maintain his airway. If this appears difficult, a tongue stitch may be used, the thread emerging from a gap, if present. However, more often reliance is placed on nasopharyngeal airways in one or both nostrils. These may be flanged tubes (page 142) or shortened endotracheal tubes secured with large safety pins. In addition to its function as an airway, such a tube may serve to prevent the development of secondary intracranial aerocoeles. These result from air being forced through the fracture line by raised nasopharyngeal pressure and may give rise to meningitis. The use of nasopharyngeal airways, so far from increasing this likelihood should help to prevent it by relieving any pressure which may build up in the nasopharynx due to coughing or straining in the post-operative period.

In a few cases a buccal airway consisting of a piece of rubber tubing with a section removed, as illustrated (Fig. 160), may be used for a short period.

Patients recovering from these operations should, ideally, be nursed in an intensive care unit. Failing this, they should be kept for some time in a recovery area. On return to the ward they still need intensive nursing care. Reliable suction and oxygen must be instantly available, as must also wire cutters, screwdrivers and spanners in order to be able to remove dental fixation should an emergency arise. A laryngoscope, endotracheal tubes, and tracheostomy set must be part of the bedside equipment, all of which must be checked frequently and maintained in perfect working order. In the immediate recovery period it would be ideal to nurse the

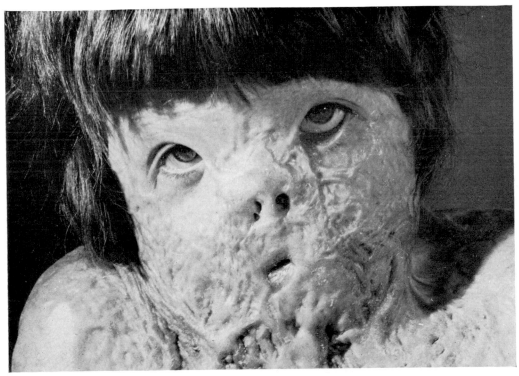

FIG. 161.—Severe contractures following facial burns. This case never required a tracheostomy, blind nasal intubation being used with each anaesthetic

patient in a lateral position but this, quite often, is not possible due to the external dental fixation.

A few cases present so much disruption of tissues in the submandibular region that they will be unable to maintain their airway on full recovery; such cases require tracheostomy, which may be performed either before or at the conclusion of the operation. Indications for tracheostomy are given on page 374.

Post-operative sedation should be kept to a minimum, pain being the only indication for giving opiates. Even in the presence of pain, it may be wiser to use pentazocine which is said to give rise to minimum respiratory depression. Anti-emetics can be given with caution, although the writer does not use them routinely.

Difficulties of Intubation

Cases where difficulties in intubation are associated with acute injury have already been discussed. A further group consists of cases where it is difficult or impossible to obtain an adequate view of the glottis. The most problematical in this group are the congenital malformations of the mandible, e.g. Treacher Collins and Pierre Robin syndromes, which are extreme examples of the under-developed mandible. In addition to the other deformities, infants with the Pierre Robin syndrome are often

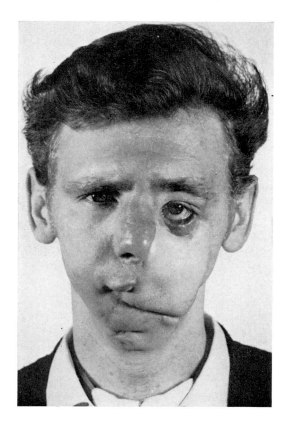

FIG. 162.—An intermediate stage in the repair of the case illustrated in Fig. 157. The facial flap occludes the left nostril and most of the mouth. This patient was given a tracheostomy at his first operation because of the injuries to the floor of the mouth. Subsequently, this was allowed to close and blind intubation through the right nostril was the only way to establish an airway

both blind and mentally retarded. The mandible is so under-developed that the patient has little or no control over the tongue and so presents as an intensive nursing care problem, needing to be nursed face down to maintain an airway. Surgery is rarely required at this stage, and it is only if they survive the neonatal period that they will need anaesthesia for surgical correction of their deformities. The mildest example, frequently met with in all branches of surgery, is the patient with a receding chin and prominent upper teeth. Laryngoscopy is always difficult and may become impossible at some stage between these two extremes.

Other conditions which make laryngoscopy impossible include microstoma, which may be congenital (Fig. 161); or follow scarring from any cause such as facial burns surgical repair with facial flaps and pedicles (Fig. 162); the Abbé flap where a wedge from the lower lip is rotated into the upper lip for a period of 2 weeks, leaving two small openings neither of which is adequate for intubation (Fig. 163). It may be impossible to open the mouth because of severe trismus or from ankylosis of one or both tempero-mandibular joints. Dental appliances or mandibulo-maxillary fixation, though they may be removed in an emergency, form a relative indication for not opening the mouth. Finally, large tumours can prevent laryngoscopy, and radio-therapy and previous surgery may add to the problems.

In all cases where laryngoscopy may be impossible, and where difficulty in the maintenance of the airway is anticipated after loss of consciousness, great care must be taken not to lose the existing airway during induction of anaesthesia. Intravenous drugs causing respiratory depression may be administered only in minimal 'sleep'

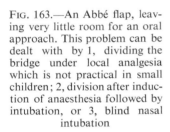

Fig. 163.—An Abbé flap, leaving very little room for an oral approach. This problem can be dealt with by 1, dividing the bridge under local analgesia which is not practical in small children; 2, division after induction of anaesthesia followed by intubation, or 3, blind nasal intubation

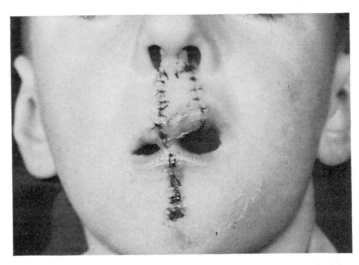

doses followed by inhalational agents to deepen anaesthesia. Sometimes an oral airway will prove adequate but quite often it is necessary to pass a nasopharyngeal tube behind the tongue to establish a satisfactory airway. Coughing, straining and breath holding should be avoided and care taken to avoid haemorrhage from the nose which can lead to laryngeal spasm. Intravenous diazepam is useful, as it rarely causes significant respiratory depression, and transition to inhalational agents is smoother than with other induction agents. In some cases it may be deemed safer to rely on an inhalational induction.

In the majority of these cases the difficulty may be overcome by the passage of a nasotracheal tube by a 'blind' intubation technique. Passing a blind nasal endo-tracheal tube, like most practical manoeuvres, is a skill which can only be acquired by practice.

The disadvantages of nasal intubation (e.g. smaller tube, compression of tube by septal spur, nasal bleeding, adenoid tissue) depend mainly upon the tube being passed through the nose, rather than its blind introduction into the larynx, although the risk of introducing foreign material into the trachea is greater than when under direct visual control. In fact, passing the tube blind avoids the additional risk of damage which is possible with the use of a laryngoscope (e.g. damage to teeth or pharynx and tearing of the anterior tonsillar pillar due to stretching). The writer feels that it is quite justified, when the nasal route is indicated by the surgery, both to learn and practise blind nasal techniques in cases on whom laryngoscopy can be easily performed, should the 'blind' technique fail. The anaesthetist will thus be confident in his ability, when he meets the patient where laryngoscopy is impossible.

Techniques (see also Chapter 13)

Basically, the problem of passing a blind nasotracheal tube consists of matching the curve between the external nares and the glottis with the curve of the tube. Tubes with greater or lesser degrees of curvature are a matter of individual preference. The patient may then be positioned to allow easy passage of the tube. Any one of the following anaesthetic techniques may be used.

1. **Relaxed and Apnoeic.**—This state is produced by an intravenous induction agent and muscle relaxant (usually suxamethonium). All the muscles are relaxed, the tissues are slack and the glottis is open. It is relatively easy to manipulate the tube into the trachea. However, it cannot be too strongly emphasized that the use of a muscle relaxant with the loss of spontaneous respiration is extremely dangerous where the possible loss of the airway and the inability to carry out laryngoscopy exists. If any doubt is present, spontaneous respirations with maintenance of airway must be retained, and the use of muscle relaxants is absolutely contraindicated.

2. **Deep Anaesthesia.**—Deep inhalational anaesthesia with maintenance of spontaneous respiration gives satisfactory conditions.

3. **Light Anaesthesia.**—Light anaesthesia with the inhalation of carbon dioxide to increase the depth of respirations also provides satisfactory conditions. When using carbon dioxide it is wiser to employ a high concentration for a short time than a low concentration for a long time. The effect required is achieved rapidly and the excess carbon dioxide is eliminated equally rapidly.

Immediately after induction, a nasal decongestant containing ephedrine, or 10% cocaine which is the only local analgesic with a vasoconstrictive action, may be instilled or sprayed into one or both nostrils. This should reduce the likelihood of nasal haemorrhage.

Opinions differ regarding the best position for blind nasal intubation, since it depends so much on individual technique, the curvature of the tube and the patient's anatomy. In the average case, the head and shoulders should lie on one firm pillow and the 'sniffing the morning air' position adopted. Magill tubes are made with the bevel pointing medially and designed to be passed through the right nostril. There is less risk of turbinates being impacted in the lumen of the tube, its oblique tip approaching the glottis at the correct angle.

With the patient breathing deeply, the anaesthetist occludes the left nostril with his left thumb, keeps the patient's lips closed with his index and middle fingers, supports the chin with his ring finger leaving his little finger free to push the larynx backwards or to one side if necessary (Fig. 164). The tube, well lubricated, is passed along the floor of the right nostril, through the nasopharynx and into the pharynx behind the tongue, coming to rest in front of the glottic opening. The tube should be twisted gently from side to side during its passage through the nose to minimize trauma. Major obstructions consist of septal spurs and the prominent body of the

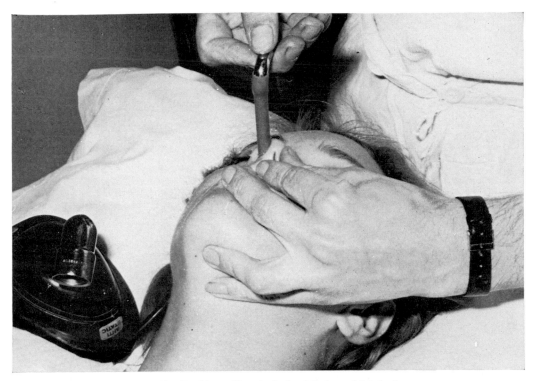

FIG. 164.—Position of hands during blind nasal intubation

sixth cervical vertebra. With the tube in this position there should be a clear airway through its lumen which can be both heard and also felt in the palm of the hand. The cords are more widely abducted during inspiration than during expiration, so that it is important to time the passage of the tube during the inspiratory phase. This is more easily carried out by watching for the expiratory phase and following it rapidly by the passage of the tube. The final passage of the tube through the glottic opening should be a rapid movement and it is important to recognize success or failure quickly so that no time is lost in withdrawing the point of the tube and making another attempt.

If the tube does not pass easily, repeated attempts should be made with minor alterations in the position of the head. The likely incorrect positions of the tube are behind the larynx and down the oesophagus, in one or other of the piriform fossae (this can be seen or felt externally), or the tip may impact on the anterior commissure. In the last position, acute flexion of the head on the neck will often allow it to pass easily. In the other positions, rotation of the head to either side, increased extension of the head and rotation of the tube may be of help.

Should anaesthesia become light, there is a risk of laryngeal spasm and the anaesthetic should be deepened *via* the tube still in the pharynx before making another

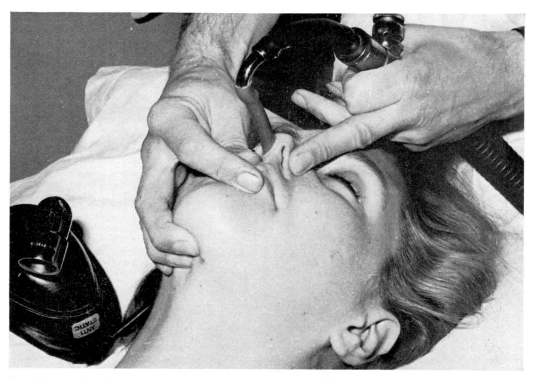

FIG. 165.—Position for deepening anaesthesia with the tube in the naso-pharynx, either between attempts at intubation or during induction where no other airway can be maintained. Note the occlusion of the left nostril and the mouth

attempt (Fig. 165). Preliminary spraying of the cords, blind through the mouth or nose during inspiration, when it is safe to do so, will avoid laryngospasm and facilitate the passage of the tube.

Use has been made of the hyperventilation occurring after induction of anaesthesia with propanidid. Speed is essential and if the tube does not enter the glottis, spasm is likely to occur and the anaesthetic has either to be deepened rapidly or suxamethonium given. It might be argued that propanidid plus a tube thrust into the larynx under very light anaesthesia, possibly with failure of intubation followed rapidly by intravenous suxamethonium, could lead to undesirable cardiac reflexes.

Many surgical procedures, where laryngoscopy is impossible, can be carried out with a nasotracheal tube. Some, however, require an oral endotracheal tube (e.g. repair of cleft palate in Treacher Collins syndrome), and this gives rise to considerable anaesthetic difficulty. The problem may be tackled in one of the following ways. Firstly, anaesthesia must be deep enough to relax the jaw as much as possible while maintaining spontaneous respiration. Then the patient is placed in the optimum position for laryngoscopy. The neck should be flexed and the head extended at the atlanto-occipital joint and supported on two pillows, or by an assistant. By this means, as near an approach to the larynx as possible can be made with the laryngoscope. It is wise to have an assortment of laryngoscope blades at hand, since different designs

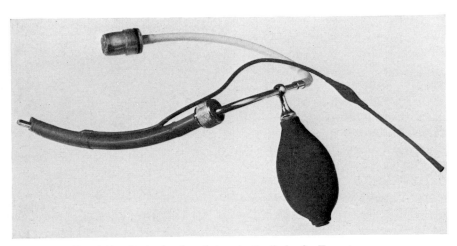

FIG. 166.—Oral tube threaded on to the limb of a Forrester spray

may suit different cases. After spraying the larynx with local analgesic by means of a curved spray, blind oral intubation may be attempted with an orotracheal tube stiffened with a blunt ended stilette. This may be of soft malleable metal or consist of a plastic or gum-elastic bougie. The stilette supplied for 'Oxford' tubes can be useful and, in adults, the tube may be threaded on to the limb of the 'Forrester' spray (Fig. 166).

When there is no room in the mouth for these manoeuvres and, as sometimes happens, the opening of the mouth makes the approach to the larynx even more difficult, it may be possible to pass a small nasal tube blind—pass it well down and extract it through the mouth. If its lumen is too small to allow an adequate airway, it can be used as a stilette and guide for a larger diameter tube to be passed over it.

A method has been described by which a crico-thyroid puncture is performed using a Tuohy epidural needle, an epidural catheter being passed through its lumen upwards into the pharynx, from which its end is extracted through the mouth, and the catheter again used as a guide for the endotracheal tube. This method might carry the risk of severe laryngeal spasm and bleeding. The introduction of flexible fibre-optic systems has given the anaesthetist an additional aid in this type of case.

The 'Bronchofiberscope', lubricated and inserted in the required size of endotracheal tube, can be passed, nasally or orally, under direct vision. The writer, so far, has had no experience in its use but this instrument may well be the answer to intubation, where direct vision of the glottis with a laryngoscope is impossible. It is obtainable in diameters of 5, 4 and 3 mm and has an internal channel which can be used for spraying with local analgesic solutions or for suction.

Failing all else a tracheostomy may have to be the ultimate resort.

Each case must be dealt with on its own merits and the anaesthetist should have all the equipment he may need ready to hand, since he may have to change his technique to meet the varied circumstances. He must have assistance and a tracheostomy set with someone, other than himself, available to perform the operation in an emergency. In this type of case, where there is any doubt regarding certainty of intubation, the cardinal rule is to make sure that neither spontaneous respiration nor the patency of the airway is lost after induction of anaesthesia.

Indications for Tracheostomy

1. **Maxillo-Facial Injury associated with loss of Consciousness.**—The reduction in airway dead space following a tracheostomy frequently leads to marked improvement in the patient's condition. If a short period of I.P.P.V. is required because of central respiratory depression, it can usually be managed satisfactorily *via* a cuffed endotracheal tube.

2. **Thoracic Cage Injuries.**—Major injuries of the thoracic cage, often with a 'flail' segment and damage to lung tissue, require I.P.P.V. for several weeks. Tracheostomy may also be essential when there is pre-existing severe respiratory disease.

3. **Loss of Tongue Control.**—This may be due to trauma or resection of the floor of the mouth.

4. **Supra-Laryngeal Obstruction.**—Loss, or potential loss, of the airway above the larynx, may result from oedema or dissecting haematoma of the pharynx and glottic region. This includes fractures of the hyoid bone or swelling in the hyoid region and direct injuries to the larynx itself.

A relative indication for tracheostomy is inexperience on the part of the anaesthetist in the management of severe maxillo-facial injuries in the lack of adequate nursing care. Tracheostomy may also be considered when the anaesthetist does not feel confident that he can obtain control of the airway in such cases as severe trismus, ankylosis of the tempero-mandibular joints, or in Ludwig's Angina.

Tracheostomy is by no means free from complications, and requires skilled observation and constant supervision, and should therefore not be undertaken lightly. Where, however, there is serious doubt regarding the patency of the airway, it should not be withheld. It is safe to say that when both medical and nursing staff are skilled in the management of cases of this kind, fewer tracheostomies are likely to be performed.

The post-operative management of a tracheostomy aims at keeping the tube patent and removing secretions from the lower respiratory tract. Suction through the tube should be carried out at hourly intervals, or more frequently if secretions are collecting rapidly. A sterile catheter should be used, preferably with an angled tip which may be directed into either right or left main bronchi. Cold, dry inspired air rapidly causes crust formation in the trachea and bronchi, so that it is essential to provide warm humidified air. This is achieved by using a blower humidifier unit which delivers air saturated with water vapour at a temperature of approximately 36° C.

Tracheostomy tubes may be made of (a) metal, consisting of an inner and outer tube, the inner tube being removed for cleaning at four-hourly intervals, or (b) rubber or plastic which may be cuffed or uncuffed. The cuffed variety is essential if the patient is on I.P.P.V. Under these conditions, the respired gases will be delivered, warmed and humidified, by the ventilator. The cuff should be deflated and re-inflated at regular intervals (every 4 to 6 hours). This should be supervised very carefully since more damage can result from over re-inflation than from leaving the cuff continuously inflated for a much longer period. Except during the administration of anaesthesia, it is quite unnecessary for a patient, breathing spontaneously, to have a tracheostomy tube with an inflated cuff.

CONCLUSION

As stated at the beginning of the chapter, preservation of a patent airway, sometimes under very difficult conditions, is the outstanding problem in anaesthesia for maxillo-facial surgery. To sum up in a single sentence, the anaesthetist in outlook and technique should be adaptable and, whatever the circumstances, should possess the ability to keep both his own head and the patient's airway.

INDEX

(Page numbers in bold type indicate main reference)

A.A.D.—13

Breath holding, 263
Breathlessness, *see dyspnoea*
Breathsounds, 132
Brevital, *see Methohexitone*
Brietal, *see Methohexitone*
Bronchiectasis, 281
Bronchitis, 4, 148, 281
Bronchodilators, 150
Bronchofiberscope, 374
Bronchospasm, 4, 25, 132, **148**
Bruising, prevention of, 206
Butanilicaine, **304**, 309
Buthalitone sodium, 193
Butobarbitone, **28**, 271
Butterfly needles, 212, 242
Butyrophenones, 34

C

Calcium in cardiac arrest, 177
Carbon dioxide, 89
    cardiac dysrhythmia and, 259
    carriage in body, 93
    cerebral blood-flow and, 94
    excess of, *see Hypercarbia*
    low gas flows and, 59
    physical properties of, 93
Carbamino haemoglobin, 93
Carbocaine, *see Mepivacaine*
Carbonic anhydrase, 93
Cardiac arrest, 172
    disease, *see Cardiovascular disease*
    dysrythmia, 106, 166, 171, 257
    massage, 173, 177
    monitors, 87
    output, 164
        effect on drug dose, 182
        halothane and, 105
    resuscitation team, 176
Cardiomyopathy
    anaesthesia in, 279
    epilepsy and, 5, 166, 219
Cardiovascular disease
    adrenaline in, 3
    anaesthesia and, 2, 274
    coronary infarction and, 3, 170
    premedication and, 275
Cardiovascular system
    atropine, effect on, 20
    barbiturates, effect on, 24, 185
    halothane, effect on, 105
    local anaesthetics, effect on, 298
    methoxyflurane, effect on, 108
    nitrous oxide, effect on, 100
    supervision of, 133, 163
    trichlorethylene, effect on, 109
Carotid pulse, *see Pulse*
Carpopedal spasm, *see Spasm*
Cartridges, local anaesthetic, 317

Catarrh, 281
Catecholamines, 306
Catechol-o-methyl transferase, 8
    monoamine oxidase inhibitors and, 8
Cawthorne's laryngotomy knife, 148
Cephaloridine, 218, 274
Cerebral
    aneurysm, 168
    arteriosclerosis, 168
        effect on intravenous drug dosage, 183
        blood-flow, 94, 105, 164
    haemorrhage, 169
    hypoxia in children, 231
    ischaemia, 357
    thrombosis, 3, 357
Cetrimide antiseptic solution, 240
Cetylpyridium chloride, 314
Chair, dental, 71
    conventional (Ritter), 71, 73
    contoured, 74
Chest movement, 132
Children's anaesthesia, 215
    induction techniques, 222
    medical considerations in, 217
    nasal intubation and, 219
    premedication in, *see Premedication*
    psychological approach to, 215
    recovery from, 230
    role of parent in, 217
    unco-operative child and, 217, 228
    upper respiratory obstruction and, 219
Chloral hydrate, 29
Chlordiazepoxide, 38
Chloride shift, 93
Chlorhexidine, 322
Chloroform, 97, **111**
Chlorothiazide, 11
Chlorpheniramine, 26, 41, 151, 338
Chlorpromazine, 32
Chlorthalidone, 11, 293
Cholinesterase, 84
Choline theophyllinate, 150
Chorea, 16
Cilliary activity, 100, 107, 110, 144
Circulation, 133
    cerebral, 105
    coronary, 106
Circuit
    Magill (semi-open)—Mapleson A, 59, 60
    Mapleson I (closed circuit), 59
    Mapleson E, Jackson-Rees, 264, 272, 355
Citanest, *see Prilocaine*
Cleft palate, 350
Closed circuit, *see Circuit*
Clothing, 18
Clubbing of fingers, 16
Cobefrin, *see Nordifrin*
Cocaine, 23, 266, 301, 360
    nasal spray, 369